Ken Gaagaard

MANAGED CARE AND CHRONIC ILLNESS

Challenges and Opportunities

Edited by

Peter D. Fox, PhD
PDF Incorporated
Chevy Chase, Maryland

Teresa Fama, MS
Group Health Foundation
Washington, DC

AN ASPEN PUBLICATION®
Aspen Publishers, Inc.
Gaithersburg, Maryland
1996

Library of Congress Cataloging-in-Publication Data

Managed care and chronic illness: Challenges and opportunities / edited by Peter D. Fox,
Teresa Fama.
p. cm.
Includes bibliographical references and index.
ISBN 0-8342-0844-X
1. Chronic diseases—Treatment. 2. Managed care plans (Medical
care) I. Fox, Peter D. II. Fama, Teresa.
RA644.5.M345 1996
362.1—dc20
96-20321
CIP

Orders: (800) 638-8437
Customer Service: (800) 234-1660

About Aspen Publishers • For more than 35 years, Aspen has been a leading professional publisher in a variety of disciplines. Aspen's vast information resources are
available in both print and electronic formats. We are committed to providing the
highest quality information available in the most appropriate format for our customers. Visit Aspen's Internet site for more information resources, directories, articles,
and a searchable version of Aspen's full catalog, including the most recent publications: **http://www.aspenpub.com**
Aspen Publishers, Inc. • The hallmark of quality in publishing
Member of the worldwide Wolters Kluwer group

Editorial Resources: Lenda Hill
Library of Congress Catalog Card Number: 96-20321
ISBN: 0-8342-0844-X

Printed in the United States of America

1 2 3 4 5

Table of Contents

Contributors vii

Foreword xi

Preface xiii

Part I—Overview 1

1—Managed Care and Chronic Illness: An Overview 3
    Peter D. Fox and Teresa Fama

2—Managed Care and Chronic Care: Challenges and
    Opportunities 8
    Lewis G. Sandy and Rosemary Gibson

3—Choosing Chronic Disease Measures for HEDIS:
    Conceptual Framework and Review of Seven
    Clinical Areas 18
    Elizabeth A. McGlynn

Part II—Care Management 59

4—Components of a Successful Case
    Management Program 61
    Sherry L. Aliotta

5—Case Management: Meeting the Needs of Chronically Ill
    Patients in an HMO 73
    Ronnie Grower, Bonnie Hillegass, and Fran Nelson

6—The Role of Health Organizations in Integrating Care
    for Persons with Special Health Care Needs 93
    David Siegel and Nancy Combs Habel

Part III—Reorganizing Primary Care 101

7—Improving Outcomes in Chronic Illness 103
    Edward H. Wagner, Brian T. Austin, and Michael Von Korff

8—Kaiser Colorado's Cooperative Health Care Clinic:
    A Group Approach to Patient Care 125
    John C. Scott and Barbara J. Robertson

Part IV—Disease Management 133

9—The Community Medical Alliance: An Integrated System
    of Care in Greater Boston for People with Severe
    Disability and AIDS 135
    Robert J. Master, Tony Dreyfus, Sharon Connors, Carol Tobias,
    Zhiyuan Zhou, and Richard Kronick

10—A Systems Approach to Asthma Care 154
    Thomas F. Plaut, Tom Howell, Susan M. Walsh, Mary Pastor, and Teresa Jones

11—The Treatment of Chronic Benign Pain Syndrome in
    Capitated Health Care 173
    Jaylene Kent

12—Physician Attitudes Toward Computerized Practice
    Guidelines 183
    Ellen Aliberti and Timmothy J. Holt

Part V—Children with Special Needs 195

13—Enhancing Preventive and Primary Care for Children
    with Chronic or Disabling Conditions Served in
    Health Maintenance Organizations 197
    Margaret A. McManus and Harriette B. Fox

14—Caring for Children with Special Need in HMOs:
    The Consumer's Perspective 213
    Betsy Anderson

Part VI—Mental Health 221

**15—Evolution of Services for the Chronically Mentally Ill in a
      Managed Care Setting: A Case Study** 223
Steve Stelovich

**16—A Medicaid Mental Health Carve-Out Program:
      The Massachusetts Experience** 233
Christopher W. Counihan, Deborah Nelson, and Elizabeth Pattullo

**17—Commentary: Managing Care for Mental Illness:
      Paradox and Pitfalls** 245
Leslie J. Scallett

Part VII—Using Data to Design Programs 257

**18—USQA Health Profile Database as a Tool for Health
      Plan Quality Improvement** 259
*Nicholas A. Hanchak, James F. Murray, Alex Hirsch, Patricia D. McDermott,
and Neil Schlackman*

**19—Using Clinical Data in Program Design:
      A Family Support Program for Families with
      Preterm Infants** 276
Maryjoan Ladden

**20—Using Data to Design Systems of Care for Adults
      with Chronic Illness** 286
Gerri S. Lamb, Vicky Mahn, and Rebecca Dahl

Index 299

Contributors

Ellen Aliberti, RN, MS
Health Services Program Manager for
  Long-Term Care
PacifiCare of California
Cypress, CA

Sherry L. Aliotta, RN, BSN, CCM
Regional Director
Prudential Health Care
Utilization Management/Case
  Management Department
Woodland Hills, CA

Betsy Anderson
Director of the CAPP Project
Federation for Children with Special
  Needs
Boston, MA

Brian T. Austin
Manager
W.A. (Sandy) MacColl Institute for
  Healthcare Innovation
Seattle, WA

Sharon Connors
Health Care Consultant
Medimetrix Group
Boston, MA

Christopher W. Counihan, MSW
Regional Manager
First Mental Health/MHMA
Boston, MA

Rebecca Dahl, PhD, RN
Research Specialist
Carondelet Health Network
Tucson, AZ

Tony Dreyfus, MCP
Consultant
Medicaid Working Group
Boston, MA

Teresa Fama, MS
Deputy Director
Chronic Care Initiatives in HMOs (a
  Robert Wood Johnson Foundation
  National Program Office)
Washington, DC

Harriette B. Fox, MSS
President
Fox Health Policy Consultants
Washington, DC

Peter D. Fox, PhD
President
PDF Incorporated
Chevy Chase, MD

Rosemary Gibson
Program Officer
Robert Wood Johnson Foundation
Princeton, NJ

Ronnie Grower, MA
Director of Quality Improvement and
  Research
Sierra Health Services, Inc.
Las Vegas, NV

Nancy Combs Habel, MA
Director of Communications
Center for Health Promotion and
   Disease Prevention
Henry Ford Health System
Detroit, MI

Nicholas A. Hanchak, MD
President
U.S. Quality Algorithms, Inc.
U.S. Healthcare, Inc.
Blue Bell, PA

Bonnie Hillegass
Assistant Vice President of Health
   Care Operations
Sierra Health Services, Inc.
Las Vegas, NV

Alex Hirsch
Director, Clinical Studies and
   Analysis
U.S. Quality Algorithms, Inc.
U.S. Healthcare, Inc.
Blue Bell, PA

Timmothy J. Holt, MD, MPH
Director of Older Adult Services
St. Mary's Medical Center
Long Beach, CA

Tom Howell, MSN, FNP, RN-C, CCM
Manager
Health Services Department
Principal Health Care of Louisiana
New Orleans, LA

Teresa Jones, BA
Research Associate
Asthma Consultants
Amherst, MA

Jaylene Kent, PhD
Chief of Behavioral Medicine
Department of Family Practice
Kaiser Permanente Medical Center at
   Santa Teresa
San Jose, CA

Richard Kronick, PhD
Assistant Professor
Department of Family and
   Community Medicine
University of California at San Diego
La Jolla, CA

Maryjoan Ladden, PhD, RN, CS
Nurse Researcher
Pediatric Nurse Practitioner
Department of Ambulatory Care and
   Prevention
Harvard Medical School and Harvard
   Pilgrim Health Care
Boston, MA

Gerri S. Lamb, PhD, RN, FAAN
Director
Carondelet Community Nursing
   Organization
Tucson, AZ

Vicky Mahn, MS, RN
Systems Associate for Quality
Carondelet Health Network
Tucson, AZ

Robert J. Master, MD
Principal Investigator
Medicaid Working Group
Boston, MA

Patricia D. McDermott, RN
Member, Research and Development
   Team
U.S. Quality Algorithms, Inc.
U.S. Healthcare, Inc.
Blue Bell, PA

Elizabeth A. McGlynn, PhD
Health Policy Analyst
RAND
Santa Monica, CA

Margaret A. McManus, MHS
President
McManus Health Policy, Inc.
Washington, DC

James F. Murray, PhD
Director, Health Services Research
U.S. Quality Algorithms, Inc.
U.S. Healthcare, Inc.
Blue Bell, PA

Deborah Nelson, PhD
Director of Quality Management
First Mental Health/MHMA
Boston, MA

Fran Nelson
Project Manager of Quality
  Improvement and Research
Sierra Health Services, Inc.
Las Vegas, NV

Mary Pastor, RN
Assistant Director of Health
  Operations
Principal Health Care, Inc.
Rockville, MD

Elizabeth Pattullo, MEd
Executive Director of First Mental
  Health/MHMA
Boston, MA

Thomas F. Plaut, MD
Director
Asthma Consultants
Amherst, MA

Barbara J. Robertson, RN, PhD
Senior Program Manager
Kaiser Permanente
Denver, CO

Lewis G. Sandy, MD
Vice President for Program
Robert Wood Johnson Foundation
Princeton, NJ

Leslie J. Scallet, JD
Founder and Executive Director
Mental Health Policy Resource
  Center
Washington, DC

Neil Schlackman, MD, FAAP
Chairman of Corporate Quality
  Improvement
U.S. Quality Algorithms, Inc.
U.S. Healthcare, Inc.
Blue Bell, PA

John C. Scott, MD
Internist and Geriatrician
Colorado Permanente Medical Group
Denver, CO

David Siegel, MD, MPH
Vice President and Medical Director
Health Alliance Plan
Chief Health Officer
Center for Health Promotion and
  Disease Prevention
Henry Ford Health System
Detroit, MI

Steve Stelovich, MD
Associate Medical Director
Harvard Pilgrim Health Care
Medical Groups Division
Brookline, MA

Carol Tobias, MMHS
Project Director
Medicaid Working Group
Boston, MA

Michael Von Korff, ScD
Associate Director
Research Group Health Cooperative's
  Center for Health Studies
Seattle, WA

Edward H. Wagner, MD, MPH
Physician/Epidemiologist
Director of Group Health
  Cooperative's Center for Health
  Studies
W.A. (Sandy) MacColl Institute for
  Healthcare Innovation
Seattle, WA

Susan M. Walsh, RN, CCM
Consultant
Principal Health Care of Louisiana
New Orleans, LA

Zhiyuan Zhou, PhD
Senior Research Associate
Upjohn Pharmaceuticals
Kalamazoo, MI

Foreword

One of the most far-reaching economic and clinical challenges facing the health care industry is the growing demand for chronic care services. As the current demographic bulge passes from middle age into old age retirement, managed care delivery systems will be overwhelmed by the prevalence of chronic illness and the accompanying cost burden. Reengineering the current approach to care is an economic necessity for health care delivery systems and society.

Managed care providers and payers must learn how to manage chronic care as well as acute care in order to meet the financial and social needs of customers. The future of managed care and chronic care services are inextricably joined, yet few delivery systems, hospitals, or medical groups have adequate knowledge and resources to manage chronically ill patients and individuals who are at-risk for chronic illness.

The ability to manage all dimensions of chronic care is a litmus test for HMOs, PPOs, and health care vendors. It is a critical performance indicator and a barometer of an organization's vision and commitment to quality. It is also a core competency that will affect profitability and customer satisfaction, thus determining market share. The ability to effectively manage chronic care and enhance the lives of chronically ill patients is a strong predictor of a delivery system's success.

Source: Adapted from two forthcoming books with permission from P. Boland, *The Capitation Sourcebook: A Practical Guide to Managing At-Risk Arrangements,* and *Redesigning Healthcare Delivery: A Practical Guide to Reengineering, Restructuring, and Renewal,* © 1996, BOLAND HEALTHCARE, INC.

Managed care delivery systems are deeply rooted in the acute care model of curative medicine. This model is not geared to an aging population whose chronic illnesses cannot be cured but who need relief of symptoms and prevention of further dysfunction. It calls for a bio-psychosocial model (i.e., medical, social, and community orientation) that encompasses far more than physiological factors commonly associated with acute care treatment. The goal of chronic care management is not curative; the emphasis is on quality of life and level of function.

A multidisciplinary team is required to integrate primary and specialty care with home-based and community-based services. Both patient and family perspectives must be integrated into the care process for treatment to be effective and valued. This approach means redesigning and reorienting current medical management practices—including capitation—that are often based more on the needs of health care organizations and providers than on patients or health plan members. This critical success factor must be acknowledged by the managed care industry as their top priority for the decade ahead.

Organized delivery systems have the potential to improve care for members with chronic conditions because they can intervene at a system level as well as the individual patient or provider level. *Managed Care and Chronic Illness* illustrates that delivery systems can effectively manage chronic care in a variety of settings. It offers concrete examples of how providers can successfully combine acute and chronic care management to improve patient functioning and quality of life. It is a valuable resource for health care industry leaders and policymakers to use in designing better ways of delivering chronic care services within the context of managed care.

Peter Boland, PhD
President and Publisher
BOLAND HEALTHCARE, INC.
Berkeley, California

Preface

Health maintenance organizations (HMOs) and other managed care organizations are enrolling increasing numbers of people with chronic conditions. This is particularly the case for health plans that enroll individuals who are eligible for Medicare or Medicaid.

Persons with chronic conditions require care that is fundamentally different from acute care medicine, which has traditionally been the focus of the American health care system. Chronic conditions such as diabetes and congestive heart failure often result in an ongoing functional impairment. These conditions are diverse, however, and differ on such dimensions as the severity of the condition; whether the condition is physical, mental, or some combination; whether or not it is amenable for improvement; and the nature of the family and other support systems that are available. Although chronic conditions cannot be cured, they can be effectively managed to allow maximum functioning. The fragmentation that characterizes the traditional fee-for-service system has in many respects militated against the kinds of care that the chronically ill need and that are the subject of this book.

Prepaid financing, which underlies much of managed care, introduces greater flexibility in services delivery upon which most health plans are only beginning to capitalize. Elements of this flexibility include the use of a broad range of professional providers, better coordination with community-based social services, greater attention to the psychological and social needs of patients, selective provision of a broader array of services (e.g., paying attention to physical safety in the home), and a more holistic approach generally. For the full potential of managed care to be realized, however, health plans and providers will have to adopt new approaches and unlearn certain practices—notably those associated with episodic acute care—practices that are deeply rooted in medical training.

This book illustrates the range of activities that are being undertaken within HMOs to improve the management of chronic conditions. Among the topics discussed are (1) the conceptual basis for chronic care and suggestions on how best to intervene; (2) reorganization of the primary care system; (3) the needs of special populations such as children, the chronically mentally ill, and others with specific conditions; (4) approaches to implementing case management; and (5) data as a tool for health plan quality improvement and program design.

This book does not purport to be comprehensive. Nonetheless, the chapters taken as a whole convey the richness of the initiatives that are being undertaken. Tempering this excitement, however, is the sense that many of the interventions have been implemented only sporadically—not unusual for those that are at an early stage of evolution—as well as the lack of empirical research in many instances to support their adoption.

Finally, we are indebted to the many people who have made this book possible. Above all, we appreciate the support from The Robert Wood Johnson Foundation, which funds the "Chronic Care Initiatives in HMOs" program that we direct. At the Foundation, we would particularly mention Rosemary Gibson, Program Officer, who is responsible for overseeing that program; Lewis G. Sandy, MD, Vice President, who took a strong interest in our efforts from the beginning; and Nancy L. Barrand, Senior Program Officer, who played a significant role in starting and shaping the program.

We would also like to thank the American Association of Health Plans and its nonprofit and educational arm, the Group Health Foundation, which has served as our administrative home and has been supportive of our efforts while allowing us total intellectual and substantive freedom. We would also like to thank Peter Boland, former Editor of *Managed Care Quarterly*, who originated the idea of this book and Lisa Lopez, who helped with the editing of earlier drafts.

Peter D. Fox
Teresa Fama

I

Overview

1
Overview

Managed Care and Chronic Illness: An Overview

Peter D. Fox and Teresa Fama

HMOs and other managed care organizations are searching for new ways of caring for people with chronic illness, reflecting at least two phenomena. The first is the prevalence of chronic illness and the concomitant cost burden. Internists, for example, spend a majority of their time treating people with chronic illness, and by one estimate, chronic illness accounts for some 80 percent of all medical expenses.[1] The second phenomenon is the recent explosive growth in Medicare risk contracting, resulting in health care plans having to manage the care of significant numbers of seniors. During the twelve-month period ending April 1995, the number of plans with Medicare risk contracts increased 38 percent, from 118 to 163, and the number of enrollees increased 31 percent, from 1,938,000 to 2,540,000.[2]

The growth in managed care raises a number of issues with respect to people with chronic illness. One issue is whether HMOs enroll their fair share of people with chronic illness, or, stated more negatively, whether HMOs market or organize their delivery systems to discourage enrollment among the chronically ill. For those under the age of 65, evidence from two recent studies shows that people with chronic illness enroll in HMOs in roughly the same proportion as in indemnity plans.[3,4] Among the elderly, the best available evidence indicates that HMOs do benefit from favorable selection.[5] However, that study is based on 1990 data, and one can hypothesize that the findings would remain valid today for *new*

Source: Reprinted from P.D. Fox and T. Fama, Managed Care and Chronic Illness, *Managed Care Quarterly*, Vol. 4, No. 2, pp. 1–4, © 1996, Aspen Publishers, Inc.

Medicare contractors, but not for Medicare contractors with mature programs in mature markets.

Another issue is how to address the fears among people with chronic illness or disabilities who are faced with requirements to join managed care plans. They may be concerned with losing access to physicians with whom they have had long-term attachments; they may have doubts about whether the health care plan will regard them as valued customers or, instead, as expensive nuisances; and they may fear that the plan will discourage access to appropriate services by methods such as by not offering adequate specialty care.

Quality of care, however measured, is also an issue under any system of care. Quality of care under different financing and delivery arrangements should be a matter of empirical study, not value judgments or a priori reasoning. The incentives embodied in capitation have the potential to improve care by:

- Incorporating flexibility in decision making because plans are not bound by the rigid rules that characterize fee-for-service Medicare, Medicaid, and much commercial indemnity insurance. For example, formal coverage guidelines become floors, not ceilings, and HMOs have the incentive to provide nonmedical services, for example, services in the home beyond stated policy, when these substitute for more expensive medical services.
- Generating incentives to promote patient empowerment and engage in prevention, particularly to reduce hospitalization.
- Providing a mechanism to shift compensation to reward cognitive services and services by nonphysician providers such as social workers and nurse practitioners.
- Allowing for local decision making by patients, providers, and plans rather than through edicts from remote third parties in Baltimore (the Medicare capital), Hartford (the insurance capital), or elsewhere.

However, whether and how these incentives are operationalized, and what impact they have on the patient, has not been adequately studied. In addition, such care improvements may occur more frequently for the more common chronic conditions such as asthma and diabetes that are prevalent and highly visible through various "report card" efforts than they do for rarer conditions such as multiple sclerosis and cystic fibrosis. Many advocates for children with special needs, in particular, believe such to be the case.

Yet another issue is the boundaries between HMOs and community-based social service programs. What should be expected of the HMO in terms of (1) offering services that are beyond the contractual obligation of the HMO, and (2) coordinating or making referrals to community-based social services that the plan does not provide? As with indemnity plans, HMOs are contracted to provide medical care, not social services. However, HMOs often provide services that are not traditionally considered medical as a means of preventing future service use, especially inpatient. Examples observed include eliminating hazards in the home for people who are frail or disabled, creating support groups for people with chronic illness as well as for people who have recently lost a spouse, and offering limited respite care for caregivers of people with frailty or disability. Many HMOs make referrals, such as to community-based housing, nutritional, or financial counseling programs.

Although the concerns and issues discussed above are real, examples abound of innovations in HMOs. These include:

- Screening of Medicare enrollees to identify those who have chronic illness to promote early intervention, including case management.
- Providing more extensive primary care than typically exists in traditional insurance. For example, to reduce emergency room and hospital inpatient use, many HMOs make primary care service available to long-term nursing home patients considerably in excess of the Medicare fee-for-service guidelines. In addition, some HMOs are experimenting with providing primary care in the ambulatory setting in nontraditional ways (e.g., group primary care visits for patients with similar chronic conditions).
- Offering transportation, other than the ambulance, for people with mobility problems who are seeking care, particularly as the ambulance's destination is typically the hospital emergency room rather than the physician's office.
- Offering targeted educational and self-care efforts, such as for patients with hypertension, diabetes, and arthritis.
- Making the home safer for those at risk of falls by such measures as removing slippery throw rugs and cords strung across the room, improving the lighting, and fixing steps.
- Creating "friendly visiting" or "friendly telephone" programs whereby either volunteers or staff stay in regular contact with homebound patients to identify changes in medical condition as well as reduce social isolation, which can create demands on the medical system.

The amount of innovation in HMOs appears to be sporadic, however. A common allegation is that HMOs may prefer not to have the reputation of excellence in caring for high-cost patients in order to attract as few as possible. However, whatever their motivations, HMOs do attract significant numbers of people with chronic conditions.[6] More to the point, many health care plans largely retain a fee-for-service mindset, and their providers may be only vaguely aware of the service delivery opportunities embodied in prepaid capitated financing. One contributing factor is that HMO physicians and other providers are trained in medical schools, hospitals, and (more rarely) in ambulatory care centers—organizations that have been slow to adapt to managed care health plans in which their graduates will practice and are oriented more to acute than chronic care.

Traditional cost management measures, that is, some combination of financial incentives, corporate culture, and administrative controls such as prior authorization and concurrent review, are insufficient in caring for people with chronic illness. For example, telephone calls to 911, the portal of entry to the emergency room and all that follows, cannot be precertified. Also, primary care physicians, regardless of the financial incentives they face, cannot reach their full potential without an adequate knowledge base, information systems to enhance clinical decision making, and professional support by well-trained nurses and other health professionals.

Managed care organizations and their providers need to adopt philosophies, and the operational programs to implement them, of outreach, early identification of problems, and both secondary prevention (i.e., identifying and treating the disease at an early stage) and tertiary prevention (i.e., reducing impairment, disability, and suffering associated with having an illness). The interrelationships between medical and social problems do not disappear by being ignored. For example, a grieving widow or a disabled person living alone in a physically hazardous setting is in grave danger of accessing the medical care system via the ambulance and the emergency room—sooner rather than later.

Chronic care requires a different perspective than acute care, and a different paradigm for providers and health care plans. Some of the differences are presented in Table 1–1. They include:

- a focus on relief of symptoms rather than cure;
- the imperative of patient participation in the care process ("patient empowerment");
- active roles for significant others, mostly immediate family;
- unclear boundaries among providers and between traditional medical services and the social services delivery system; and
- technical quality and patient (as well as family) satisfaction being more interdependent than for acute care.

Finally, there is a paucity of research to support desirable changes. As one illustration, HMOs differ widely in their reliance on case management, ranging from only performing case management in the inpatient setting to extensive programs for community-dwelling chronically ill.[7] Not having ambulatory case management programs may indeed result in

Table 1-1 Differences in Caring for People with Acute Versus Chronic Illness[8]

	Acute Care	*Chronic care*
Underlying objective	Cure	Relief of symptoms, ability to adapt to illness
Focus of patient descriptor	Diagnosis	Diagnosis and functional status
Outcomes	Often objectively defined	Subjectively defined
Elements of care	May be purely physical	Almost always includes a psychological component
Need for patient empowerment	Moderate	Essential
Nature of treatment	Brief and intensive	Long-term and, commonly, low-level
Relation with social service system	Minimal	Significant
Caregivers	Medical professionals	Important roles for family members and nonmedical caregivers

higher cost and missed opportunities to improve service delivery. However, the empirical basis for selecting one approach over another is lacking. Thus, implementing a process for evaluation and feedback should be a component of any strategy to improve how care is delivered to people with chronic conditions.

REFERENCES

1. Lohr, K.N. et al. "Chronic Disease in a General Adult Population: Findings from the Rand Health Insurance Experiment." *The Western Journal of Medicine* 145(4) (1986): 537–545.
2. Office of Managed Care, Health Care Financing Administration. *Medicare Managed Care Contract Report.* June 1, 1995.
3. Fama, T., Fox, P.D., and White, L.A. "Do HMOs Care for the Chronically Ill?" *Health Affairs* 14(1) (1995): 234–243.
4. Taylor, A.K., Beauregard, K.M., and Vistnes, J.P. "Who Belongs to HMOs: A Comparison of Fee-for-Service Versus HMO Enrollees." *Medical Care Research and Review* 52(3) (1995): 389–408.
5. Brown, R.S., et al. "Do Health Maintenance Organizations Work for Medicare?" *Health Care Financing Review* 15(1) (1993): 7–23.
6. See, for example, Fama, Fox, and White, "Do HMOs Care for the Chronically Ill?"
7. Pacala, J.T., et al. "Case Management of Older Adults in Health Maintenance Organizations." *Journal of the American Geriatric Society* 43 (1995): 538–542.
8. Adapted from Vladeck, B. Presentation to meeting of the American Association of Retired Persons and the National Academy for State Health Policy, November 15–16, 1993, Washington, DC.

2

Managed Care and Chronic Care: Challenges and Opportunities

Lewis G. Sandy and Rosemary Gibson

Managed care, for decades an interesting experiment grafted onto a "usual and customary" fee-for-service (FFS) health care system, is poised to dominate the nation's medical care delivery system. More than 90 percent of the employed population now obtain their care from some form of "managed" health care system. State Medicaid programs already have embraced managed care for mothers and their children, and some states are beginning to enroll persons with serious disabling conditions. The last bastion of fee-for-service medicine, Medicare, appears to be following suit. The number of Medicare risk contract enrollees grew by nearly 30 percent between 1994 and 1995,[1] and 164 health plans now have Medicare risk contract products.[2] As managed care enrolls an ever-increasing proportion of the population, increased attention will need to be paid to the care of persons with serious chronic conditions. These trends offer challenges and opportunities for managed care organizations.

Although a recent analysis suggests that among the employed insured population, HMOs have the same proportion of persons with chronic illness as the FFS sector,[3] HMOs have not fully capitalized on the opportunity to improve care to this population. The high cost of chronic illness, which is in part due to suboptimal management of chronic conditions, makes it imperative that managed care organizations examine ways to provide improved care. For example, the cost of diabetes and attendant

Source: Reprinted from L.G. Sandy and R. Gibson, Managed Care and Chronic Care: Challenges and Opportunities, *Managed Care Quarterly*, Vol. 4, No. 2, pp. 5–11, © 1996, Aspen Publishers, Inc.

comorbidities can range as high as 15 percent of total health plan costs.[4] Chronic conditions, therefore, are "big ticket" items, and delivery system innovations that improve the effectiveness and efficiency of care merit close scrutiny. Whereas the fee-for-service system has limited financial incentives to improve health care for this population, competition in the marketplace necessitates improvement. Managed care plans that can deliver on price and quality will prevail in the long run.

CHRONIC CONDITIONS: WHAT IS THE SCOPE?

What are chronic conditions? They are long-term conditions that encompass diseases, injuries with long sequelae, and prolonged structural, sensory, and communication abnormalities. They manifest themselves in physical or mental impairments, and they emerge both at birth and throughout the lifespan.[5]

Based on more than two decades of grantmaking supporting research, demonstrations, and evaluations in this area for populations as diverse as the physically disabled, children with special health care needs, and persons with AIDS, chronic mental illness, and chronic medical conditions such as diabetes, the Robert Wood Johnson Foundation made "improving services for people with chronic conditions" one of its major priorities for the 1990s. For this purpose, persons with chronic illness are defined as those who have ongoing functional impairment, from whatever cause. Based on this definition, nearly 40 million Americans have chronic illness.[6] Although the elderly have a higher proportion of persons with chronic illness, overall only one third of persons with chronic illness are elderly, while one third are children and one third are working age adults.

CHRONIC ILLNESS AND THE CHANGING NATURE OF MEDICINE

Earlier this century it was uncertain whether an encounter with the health care system increased or decreased the odds of survival. Today, modern medicine creates a spectacular success on a daily basis. The emerging scientific understanding of normal and abnormal physiology, the development of antibiotics, insulin, and other therapeutics, and the high-technology diagnostic and therapeutic armamentarium that exist today, offer new opportunities to prevent, manage, and cure disease. One of the byproducts of this capability, however, is the transformation of many acute diseases into chronic illnesses. Insulin, for example, transformed juvenile onset diabetes from a rapidly fatal condition to a chronic one. Many other, less dramatic examples have combined to alter the epidemiology of late twentieth-century illness. Patients who may have died of acute myocardial infarction in an earlier era now survive their acute event and live with chronic congestive heart failure. Advances in caring for premature neonates has created "NICU alumni" with chronic respiratory conditions. Children with cystic fibrosis, once rarely surviving to adolescence, now regularly reach adulthood. HIV infection is best understood and managed as a chronic condition. As medical science advances, these transformations will continue and accelerate.

The success of biomedical science and clinical medicine has helped to increase life expectancy. Since 1960—within the lifetime of the baby boomer population—the life expectancy of women at age 65 has increased 17.7 percent.[7] Not only is the population aging, the fastest growth rate is in the over-85 population, a segment with a high prevalence of chronic illness.

CHRONIC CARE: THE IDEAL AND THE REALITY

This shift from acute to chronic illness would not signify a major problem if the health care delivery system were prepared to handle it. The curative model of medical practice is not well suited to a population whose illnesses cannot be cured. Instead, the dictum in medicine to "cure sometimes, comfort always" takes on renewed salience in the management of chronic illness. Different models of care and new delivery systems, therefore, are needed.

What are some major differences in chronic care as compared to acute care? First, chronic illness typically has a fluctuating and unpredictable course with exacerbations and improvement. Second, the patients and their families or other caregivers need to be active participants in the process of care if treatments are to be successful. Third, chronic illness is best understood with a biopsychosocial model of illness, one that takes into account the patients' psychology, preferences, social situation, and other factors far beyond physiologic factors.

Quality of life for persons with chronic conditions is determined only in part by medical care. Today's medical science may not yet be able to increase function in a spinal cord injured patient, but adaptive technology can help the patient function at a much higher level. Since maximizing function involves nonmedical interventions, the boundaries between the traditional medical care system and other systems overlap. Moreover, the prevention of further dysfunction, rather than cure, becomes the desired outcome. As noted by the Institute of Medicine:

> To accommodate the changing needs of an increasingly older society we must broaden the traditional goals of health—curing disease and

preventing its occurrence—to include preventing the ill from becoming disabled and helping the disabled cope with and prevent further disability.[8]

Patients with chronic illness typically find themselves trying to traverse a dysfunctional health care financing and delivery system built on an acute care model. Care is fragmented and episodic. It is common for patients to see multiple specialty physicians at the tertiary care medical center, but it is rare for one physician to oversee the patient's entire care requirements, or assume responsibility for helping patients and their families coordinate care. Patient education and active participation in care are limited. Overuse of expensive diagnostic and therapeutic technologies occurs at the expense of low-tech supportive services, often home- and community-based. Medicare will pay $10,000 for a hip fracture hospitalization, but not $500 for installing rails at home to prevent a fall. Medicaid will pay handsomely for acute hospitalizations for children with serious chronic conditions, while very low reimbursement for primary care in the physician's office discourages physicians from seeing these patients. Although variable by state, low Medicaid reimbursement may also encourage excessively brief visits that do not permit sufficient exploration of chronic care issues. Better service delivery systems can be adopted that rationalize care for the chronically ill.

AN OPTIMAL CHRONIC CARE DELIVERY SYSTEM

Effective models of chronic care developed for special populations of persons with chronic illness are characterized by several main features:

1. Integration of primary and specialty care.

Most persons with chronic illness require both in-depth specialized expertise in the expert management of their condition(s) coupled with breadth of perspective and a generalist orientation to effectively manage the complex interplay of medical and social factors that affect patients and families. As a result, most of the most effective care models provide integration of primary care and specialty care.

2. Integration of medical care with home- and community-based services.

Similarly, effective management of chronic illness not only requires good medical care, but also the use of home- and community-based services such as visiting nurse services, meals on wheels, transportation, "friendly visiting," respite care services, housekeeping services, and minor home repair. It does little use to educate diabetes patients about appropriate diet if they are unable to prepare meals.

3. Integrating patient and family perspectives into the care process.

Since chronic care by definition is ongoing, patients and caregivers must be active participants in care, not passive recipients of services. Provider training in patient-centered communication, use of detailed satisfaction information, and a consumer-oriented focus are key. A few models go even further and provide patients with vouchers that enable them to purchase directly the services they need.

4. Emphasis on functional status and quality of life.

Chronic illness usually cannot be cured, and has a natural progression toward increasing functional limitation. The goal of care is not solely medical in nature, but must take into account patients' quality of life and level of function. Effective chronic care systems measure and track function, and trained providers elicit patient preferences and intervene appropriately to improve quality of life. Special attention is paid to advance directives, delivering care in the least intrusive setting, and involving families in the process of care.

5. Delivering care in multidisciplinary care teams.

No one provider can deliver all the care required by patients with serious chronic conditions. Nurses, case managers, social workers, and even van drivers each have unique competencies to bring to bear on the care of a patient. Effective systems use multidisciplinary teams to provide integrated care. These teams may be physically co-located in a staff or group HMO or group practice, or may be "virtual teams" in smaller practices or IPAs. Nevertheless, they function as a team. The Program for All-Inclusive Care for the Elderly (PACE) provides an optimal model of an interdisciplinary approach to caregiving for a very frail elderly population.[9]

OPPORTUNITIES FOR MANAGED CARE

Managed care offers a number of features that have potential to improve care for persons with chronic illness. First, managed care systems have the potential to intervene at a system level, as opposed to the individual patient or provider level. That simple and obvious fact has enormous capacity to overcome the fragmentation of a poorly organized fee-for-service sector. Second, capitated financing allows reallocation of resources to better meet the needs of persons with chronic conditions. Unconstrained by narrow, contractually defined benefits, health plans have flexibility to devote resources to home- and community-based services, outreach, case management, patient education, and prevention. Third, the capitated prepaid financing environment of managed care creates a financial incentive to provide cost-effective care in the most appropriate setting. Fourth, the primary care orientation of managed care delivery systems, emphasizing generalist physicians, nurse practitioners, and other health providers, can be more appropriate for caring for many persons with chronic illness than specialty-oriented hospitals and other practice settings.

On the other hand, managed care organizations may not fully embrace the required level of system development. On average, persons with chronic illness may be a small proportion of a health plan's overall membership. They are, however, disproportionately high utilizers of medical services. For example, 9.8 percent of all Medicare beneficiaries (most of whom have chronic conditions) account for 68.4 percent of all Medicare expenditures.[10] Second, chronic conditions encompass many relatively uncommon conditions (e.g., ALS, cardiomyopathy, muscular dystrophy) along with more highly prevalent chronic illnesses (e.g., congestive heart failure, emphysema, diabetes). Although most systems development has occurred in these more common conditions, HMOs should be sensitive to rare conditions among their members, which may require highly specialized expertise. Third, the highest proportion of persons with chronic illness have been in publicly financed systems such as Medicaid and Medicare; this, however, is changing rapidly. Fourth, current quality measures and external accrediting bodies, such as the HEDIS indicators and the NCQA accrediting process, emphasize acute and preventive services in their indicators and reporting requirements.

CHALLENGES TO THE FIELD

The managed care industry will need to rise to the challenge of providing high-quality, cost-effective care to persons with chronic illness. Where should an HMO begin? We suggest three initial steps to begin the process of improvement. First, analyze the enrolled population. Persons with chronic conditions can be grouped into three major categories: children with special needs, working aged disabled, and the elderly. HMOs can begin by systematically analyzing their enrollment database to identify persons with chronic conditions within these age strata. Only by identifying persons with chronic conditions within the HMO can targeted efforts begin. Screening systems at enrollment are another method often employed to identify new members with complex chronic conditions.

Second, managed care plans can begin disease-specific improvement programs for chronic conditions such as asthma, congestive heart failure, diabetes, and Alzheimer's disease. There are innumerable opportunities to narrow the gap between current practice and "best practices," resulting in both lower costs and higher quality. For example, optimal diabetes care requires intensive patient education, active monitoring, and a multidisciplinary care team, as shown in the Diabetes Care and Complications (DCCT) trial.[11] Care of congestive heart failure can be improved by provision of home scales to monitor weight, aggressive use of ACE inhibitors, and telephone management systems.[12] Other well-documented performance gaps exist in the areas of pain management,[13] behavioral health (especially somatization disorders, depression, and anxiety),[14] and substance abuse detection and treatment.[15]

Third, plans can adopt a systems orientation to improving key areas in the HMO delivery system. Although HMOs generally have well-functioning acute care delivery systems, optimal chronic care requires redesign in certain key support areas. For example, information systems need to be redesigned to compile and analyze information longitudinally and to assess, track, and monitor functional status. Case management, home and community care, and informal care systems are also features of effective chronic care that need to be developed or adapted by HMOs. Existing HMO, medical group, or hospital utilization management, case management, home health, quality assurance, and utilization review entities should increase their focus on chronic care.

Another key challenge for managed care organizations is enhancing the capacity of primary care providers to manage the care of persons with physical disabilities. In fee-for-service medicine, such patients often have poor access to primary care. When patients do have access, the limited prevalence of certain conditions makes it unlikely that primary care physicians have the knowledge base necessary to competently manage such patient care. For example, paraplegic patients may be treated by a urologist for a urinary tract infection or by a plastic surgeon for a decubitus ulcer, but may not have the requisite primary care to prevent such conditions in the first place. Managed care organizations have incentive to ensure such patients have primary care to obviate exacerbations of preventable complications. Overlapping special competencies within primary care practices or networks for patients with serious chronic conditions may be a promising approach.

Enrollment and network development are another key challenge for managed care organizations in adapting their delivery systems in a timely fashion to an accelerated pace of enrollment of persons with serious chronic conditions. Is managed care ready? What unique enrollment strategies are needed, for example, for a managed care plan to enroll persons with developmental disabilities? What referral networks will be established for children with serious chronic medical conditions? The design of medical and social support models that make the best use of managed care's potential for the disabled and others with serious chronic conditions is still in its infancy. As plans engage in marketing and enrollment of these populations—and develop appropriate referral systems—managed care plans will probably find it helpful to consult with prospective users (and their families) to yield information about services that are more clinically appropriate and satisfactory to the patient.[16]

The growth in Medicare managed care is a harbinger for yet another complex issue for managed care: caring for patients at the end of life. A significant portion of expenditures in health care are spent in the last year of life. HMO managers (perhaps more so than clinicians) may have concerns about developing palliative care interventions for the terminally ill, even though major advances in palliative care offer great promise in relieving suffering at the end of life. The financial incentives inherent in managed care heighten sensitivities to caring for patients at the end stage of illness. Nonetheless, managed care, in its most optimal configuration, offers significant opportunity to care for the dying in a compassionate and humane way.

ISSUES CONFRONTING HMOs

Although managed care has unrealized potential to develop better chronic care systems, a number of thorny issues need to be addressed if this potential is to be fully realized. One current controversy is the "carve-out." Some health plans have "carved out" mental health, substance abuse, cancer care, HIV care, and other chronic conditions into special networks that are either subcapitated or on a unique fee schedule. No rigorous studies of these carve-outs exist, but such carve-outs can fragment care, especially for patients with multiple chronic conditions.

Second, managed care plans will increasingly encounter the "boundary problem." Effective chronic care requires going beyond a medical model, and even beyond a medically oriented biopsychosocial model, to one that encompasses medical, social, and community perspectives. Managed care plans might, for example, contract with community-based agencies to provide support services and health promotion to a population of elders concentrated in an urban high-rise building or other defined geographic area. Such services can help the elderly maintain their independence and improve their perception of health and well-being. These activities, although beyond the scope of the traditional medical care system, can help obviate the need for acute services. For children with serious chronic medical conditions, the school setting is frequently the locus for dispensing medication and overall health maintenance. Will HMOs promote effective communication between the plan's primary or specialty physician and school nurses and teachers? Is this the HMOs' responsibility? Is it the managed care plans' responsibility to pay for the wheelchair for the disabled child, or is it the purview of special education funds? These and other boundary questions are in abundance, and no consensus is likely to emerge in the foreseeable future.

Finally, good chronic care is critically dependent on both the formal and informal systems of care among families, friends, and neighbors. Most elderly live at home, and many rely on family members for transportation, personal care, and household chores. HMOs need to recognize the importance of informal caregiving; and some are even going beyond recognition toward action. For example, the Robert Wood Johnson Foundation is supporting the development of volunteer service credit programs in managed care organizations.[17] Service credit programs match older people in need of supportive services with a volunteer—usually another older person— able to provide the service. Volunteers receive a "credit" for each service hour they provide, which can be redeemed for services they need. These programs have the aim of helping enrollees remain independent and active in the community.

Medical care in the United States is deeply rooted in the acute model of illness, and systems of care have been established accordingly. The distinctive character of chronic conditions necessitates a reorientation of clinical practice, medical education, and the way in which medical and nonmedical services are organized.

As managed care continues to grow, particularly in the Medicare and Medicaid programs, it is being held to a higher standard than fee-for-service medicine. Many health care experts believe that HMOs can provide good basic health care and preventive services to relatively healthy employed populations. Some are skeptical, however, of managed care's capacity to deliver high-quality care to sick or vulnerable populations. Managed care has the potential to deliver on its potential to improve health care delivery, and the current market trends now make it imperative that HMOs deliver on that promise. How the managed care industry responds to this challenge is critical to the industry's long-term success.

If the nation learned anything from recent national health care reform debates, it is that health care is both profoundly important to people and intensely personal. Analytical debates over health care financing and delivery issues do not resonate with the general public. They want to know, "What does it all mean for me?" and, "Can I get the care that I need when I need it?"

Policy makers and the public are counting on managed care to improve quality, control costs, and add value to the health care equation. If plans cannot deliver that to persons with chronic conditions, the nation may eventually reconsider whether marketed-oriented managed care should be the organizing framework for health care in the United States.

REFERENCES

1. Health Care Financing Administration (HCFA). *Medicare Managed Care Contract Report.* Baltimore: Office of Managed Care. April 1, 1994 and April 1, 1995.
2. HCFA. *Medicare Managed Care Contract Report.* Baltimore: Office of Managed Care. June 1, 1995.
3. Fama, T.F., Fox, P.F., and White, L.A. "Do HMOs Care for the Chronically Ill?" *Health Affairs* 14 (Spring 1995): 234.
4. Personal Communication with Jonathan Brown, Investigator, Center for Health Research, Kaiser Permanente Northwest Region, Portland, Oregon, July 21, 1995.
5. Verbrugge, L.M., and Patrick, D. "Seven Chronic Conditions: Their Impact on US Adults' Activity Levels and Use of Medical Services." *American Journal of Public Health* 85(2) (February 1995): 173.
6. Institute of Medicine. *Disability in America: Toward a National Agenda for Prevention.* Eds. A.M. Pope and A.R. Tarlov. Washington, D.C.: National Academy Press, 1991.
7. Cassel, C., Rudberg, M., and Olshansky, S. "The Price of Success: Health Care in An Aging Society." *Health Affairs* (Summer 1992): 88.
8. Institute of Medicine. *The Second Fifty Years: Promoting Health and Preventing Disability.* Washington, D.C.: National Academy Press, 1991, p. vii.
9. Kane, R., Illston, L., and Miller, N. "Qualitative Analysis of the Program of All-inclusive Care for the Elderly (PACE)." *The Gerontologist* 32(6): 771–780.
10. Health Care Financing Administration. *Health Care Financing Review: Statistical Supplement.* Baltimore: Department of Health and Human Services (DHHS), HCFA, Office of Research and Demonstrations, February 1995.
11. The Diabetes Control and Complications Trial Research. "The Effect of Intensive Treatment of Diabetes on the Development and Progression of Long-Term Complication in Insulin-dependent Diabetes Mellitus." *New England Journal of Medicine* 329(14) (September 30, 1993): 977–986.
12. Baker, D.W., et al. "Management of Heart Failure. I. Pharmacologic Treatment." *Journal of the American Medical Association* 272(17) (November 2, 1994): 1361–1366.
13. Cleeland, C.S., et al. "Pain and its Treatment in Outpatients with Metastatic Cancer." *New England Journal of Medicine* 330(9):(March 3, 1994): 592–596.
14. Tulkin, S.R. "Behavioral Medicine Programs That Work." *HMO Practice* 9(2) (June 1995): 57.
15. Research Triangle Institute. *The Impact of Health Care Reforms and Managed Care on the Availability, Financing, and Cost of Substance Abuse Treatment.* Final Report. Washington, D.C., June 1995.
16. Roper, W. Presentation at Annual Meeting, Chronic Care Initiative in HMOs. Washington, D.C., April 27–28, 1995.
17. "Service Credit Banking in Managed Care," a national program of The Robert Wood Johnson Foundation, Princeton, New Jersey.

3

Choosing Chronic Disease Measures for HEDIS: Conceptual Framework and Review of Seven Clinical Areas

Elizabeth A. McGlynn

Expenditures on care for chronic diseases are consuming an ever-growing portion of the U.S. health care budget. In the RAND Health Insurance Experiment, about 30 percent of adults ages 18–61 had one chronic condition; 16 percent had two or more.[1] About 80% of health care resources are spent on care for chronic diseases.[2] As policy makers struggle with mechanisms for making the delivery of this care more cost-effective, methods for monitoring the quality of services for chronic disease must also be developed. Few quality measures are available today that assess care for chronic conditions. The Health Plan Employer Data and Information System (HEDIS) version 2.0 contains nine measures of quality; four pertain to preventive services, two pertain to prenatal care, and three relate to care for chronic conditions (i.e., hospitalization rates for childhood asthma, annual eye examinations for diabetics, and follow-up visits following hospitalization for major affective disorders).

Concern has been expressed by the developers of HEDIS that the current chronic disease measures may not adequately capture the most critical dimensions of quality for chronic diseases. The National Committee for Quality Assurance (NCQA) appointed a steering committee in September 1994 to address this concern and to identify chronic conditions for new performance measurement development. This article formed the basis of the NCQA steering committee's discussion for selecting chronic conditions for

Source: Reprinted from E.A. McGlynn, Choosing Chronic Disease Measures for HEDIS: Conceptual Framework and Review of Seven Clinical Areas, *Managed Care Quarterly*, Vol. 4, No. 3, pp. 54–77, © 1996, Aspen Publishers, Inc.

HEDIS. In particular, the article outlines a conceptual framework for selecting chronic diseases and aspects of care for quality assessment, reviews what is known about the efficacy of providing care in seven disease categories that meet those criteria, and makes recommendations regarding promising areas for the development of quality measures. Although this article was originally written to support the NCQA steering committee's work, the information that is reviewed might also be used to structure and focus disease management programs.

CRITERIA FOR SELECTING DISEASES FOR QUALITY ASSESSMENT

Building on previous RAND work,[3] five criteria for selecting chronic conditions for which quality assessment measures should be developed are recommended:

- The condition is highly prevalent or has a significant effect on mortality and morbidity in the population.
- There is reasonable scientific evidence that efficacious or effective interventions exist to prevent the chronic disease from developing (i.e., primary prevention), to identify and treat the disease at an early stage (i.e., secondary prevention), or to reduce impairment, disability, and suffering associated with having an illness (i.e., tertiary prevention).
- Improving the quality of service delivery will enhance the health of the population.
- The recommended interventions do not impose unreasonable costs on the organization.
- The recommended interventions are under the control of health plans.

The first criterion is important for both conceptual and logistical reasons. Conceptually, attention is focused on how well health care is being delivered for the most common health problems faced by the population. From a logistical viewpoint, choosing highly prevalent conditions will facilitate identifying a sufficient number of cases for review so that statistically valid conclusions can be drawn.

The second criterion underscores that health plans and providers should be held accountable only for those interventions that meet rigorous standards of scientific proof or professional consensus. The health care system should not be encouraged to deliver care of uncertain benefit and systems that have not embraced unproven practices should not be penalized. Many health services provided in this country do not meet these standards; some services may never be subjected to rigorous evaluation because of concerns about the ethics of withholding treatment (i.e., as would be necessary for a no treatment control group) or providing a treatment that is believed to be less desirable (i.e., as would be necessary to test competing treatments). For these areas, studies with less rigorous designs or consensus opinion will form the basis for review criteria.

The third criterion suggests that evaluation should focus on interventions that have a significant positive impact on the health of the population. Because one of the potential effects of quality monitoring may be to shift health plan resources to areas that are being evaluated over areas that are not subject to assessment, this should occur only for services where improved quality is likely to make a real contribution to the overall health of the population. The health impact of improved quality is a function of both the efficacy or effectiveness of an intervention and the extent to which current practice is failing to adhere to the recommended strategy.

The fourth criterion acknowledges the limited resources available for health care today. Information on the cost effectiveness of many interventions is limited, but it remains important as a framework for evaluating potential assessment areas. Cost effectiveness should be considered in a general sense (i.e., over the course of the individual lifetime) rather than at the level of the health plan; many health plans may not realize the differential in cost effectiveness between interventions within the time an individual is enrolled in the health plan. Nonetheless, in thinking about the potential for quality assessment measures to affect resource allocation decisions, it is important to evaluate whether shifting resources to the measured areas will have a deleterious effect on health plan finances.

The final criterion recognizes that not all interventions are under the control of health plans. Many primary prevention campaigns have been most effective in a public health rather than private health context. For example, initial survival after a myocardial infarction may be more a function of the adequacy of the trauma system in an area than the quality of medical care; after admission, the focal point of responsibility shifts more clearly to the health plan. Some interventions may be highly dependent on patient compliance and this may vary depending on the characteristics of the enrolled population. For example, return to work after a back injury may be more dependent on workers compensation benefits than the quality of care provided.

REVIEW OF POTENTIAL CONDITIONS FOR INCLUSION

Based on previous work, some current reviews of the literature, and discussions with NCQA staff and the chair of the steering committee for this project, seven conditions were selected for evaluation:

1. coronary artery disease
2. breast cancer
3. colorectal cancer
4. low back pain
5. major depression
6. diabetes mellitus
7. childhood asthma

For each of these conditions, this article will review what is known about that condition on each of the five evaluation criteria:

1. importance of the condition
2. availability of efficacious or effective interventions
3. the potential for improving quality
4. the cost effectiveness of the intervention
5. the extent to which the intervention is under the control of the health plan.

The final section of the article offers recommendations for the development of measures of quality for chronic disease care based on the findings from this review.

Coronary Artery Disease

Importance

Mortality from coronary artery disease (CAD) has been declining in the United States over the past two decades, but CAD and related diagnoses are a major cause of morbidity and mortality among adults.[4] In 1990, almost 500,000 deaths were attributable to CAD. From 1973 through 1987, cardiovascular mortality decreased 42 percent in the age group under 54 years and decreased 33 percent in the age group 55–84 years.[5] Annually, about 1.5 million people are newly diagnosed with CAD and the direct and indirect health care costs are estimated to be $47 billion.[6]

Efficacy or Effectiveness of Interventions

There are a number of risk factors that, if modified, can prevent development of CAD, including elevated serum cholesterol, low levels of high-density lipoprotein cholesterol, uncontrolled hypertension, cigarette smoking, obesity, and physical inactivity.

An analysis of 19 randomized trials that evaluated the effect of *cholesterol reduction* on total mortality and the incidence of CAD found that reducing cholesterol was effective in lowering the incidence of CAD but reductions had to be at least 8–9 percent to effectively reduce total mortality.[7] For every one percent reduction in cholesterol, an estimated 2.5 percent reduction in disease incidence was found. The trials showed greater effect from cholesterol-lowering drugs than from dietary modifications. The U.S. Preventive Services Task Force (USPSTF) has recommended that all adults have their blood cholesterol and serum cholesterol checked every five years.[8]

Hypertension is a risk factor for CAD as well as for stroke and cerebrovascular disease. If the average diastolic blood pressure for the entire population was reduced by 6–8 mm Hg, the incidence of CAD would be reduced by 25 percent.[9] Although there is general agreement that high blood pressure control should contribute to reductions in the incidence of and mortality from CAD, the hypertension intervention trials involving diuretics and beta blockers have not demonstrated significant reductions in CAD.[10] This may be because multiple risk factors for heart disease (e.g., serum cholesterol and smoking) tend to cluster together and multifactorial treatment may be required. The Public Health Service (PHS) recommends that blood pressure be measured regularly to screen for hypertension in all individuals who are three years of age or older and that the measurements be made every two years if the last blood pressure readings were in the normal range (140 mm Hg systolic and 85 mm Hg diastolic) and annually if the last diastolic blood pressure was 85–89 mm Hg. Once hypertension is confirmed, the patient should receive counseling about exercise, weight reduction, dietary sodium intake, and alcohol consumption. The *Healthy People 2000* objectives for the nation call for 50 percent of persons with hypertension to have their blood pressure under control and for 90 percent to be taking actions to bring their blood pressure under control.[11]

Smoking is responsible for over 115,000 deaths annually from CAD.[12] About 27 percent of American adults smoke.[13] Smoking cessation can contribute to reductions in deaths from CAD; the benefits become evident as soon as two years after quitting.[14] Clinical trials of smoking cessation techniques have concluded that effectiveness depends on several factors, including: use of multiple modes, frequent contact with the patient, longer length intervention, the use of face-to-face techniques, and both physician and nonphysician staff.[15,16] Nicotine gum can increase long-term smoking cessation rates by about one third.[17] Patient factors are also important (e.g., level of dependence, motivation to quit). A meta-analysis of 38 clinical trials found differences in cessation rates of unselected patients to be 8 percent after six months and 6 percent after one year.[18]

Obesity is a risk factor for CAD[19]; about 10 percent of women and 20 percent of men in the Framingham study were obese.[20] It is difficult to assess the independent effect of weight reduction on cardiovascular risk because of the close association between obesity and other risk factors (e.g., hypercholesterolemia). Many weight reduction interventions that have been studied demonstrate short-term efficacy but the results are not maintained in the long term.[21,22] The best results have been achieved in conservative programs that involve behavior therapy, nutrition education, and exercise programs and that are typically targeted at persons with mild to moderate obesity.[23] The USPSTF recommends that persons who are 20 percent or more above their desired weight (as determined by standard life insurance tables) be referred to appropriate nutritional and exercise counseling.[24]

The relationship between cardiovascular fitness and *exercise* is strongly positive, but the clinical and public health implications of this finding are less clear.[25] Efficacy studies limited to secondary prevention trials report a 66 percent compliance rate and a 15 percent reduction in total mortality. Two recent studies have found that regular exercise provides a protective effect against triggering sudden onset of a myocardial infarction during strenuous exercise.[26,27] The risk of heart attack among sedentary people during vigorous exercise was seven times greater in one study[28] and 100 times greater in the other study[29] than during lighter activity or no activity. In both studies, among people who exercise regularly, there was no increase in the risk of heart attack. There is some suggestion that regular, heavy exertion exercise may prevent the development and progression of heart disease.[30,31]

The other preventive strategy that has been recommended (by the USPSTF) for men is *low doses of aspirin* on alternate days to prevent a first myocardial infarction.[32] A review of three female cohort studies did not support a general recommendation that asymptomatic women take aspirin as a preventive measure; there was some evidence of benefit among high-risk women.[33]

Thus, a number of primary prevention strategies have been suggested as important for reducing the likelihood of developing CAD. The risk profile of the population enrolled in a health plan may provide some measure of the potential for preventing the development of heart disease. In the short run, the success of programs designed to modify these risk factors might be examined.

There are a number of secondary and tertiary prevention interventions available for the treatment of heart disease. Lowering plasma cholesterol can slow the progression of established coronary artery disease.[34] Effective medications are available for the treatment of chronic angina[35] and unstable angina.[36] Improved prehospital care for acute myocardial infarction has been shown to reduce mortality.[37] Major advances have been made in the acute[38–44] and postacute[45] treatment of myocardial infarction. Some deaths among patients hospitalized for acute myocardial infarction may be preventable.[46] Thrombolytic therapy after acute myocardial infarction may reduce mortality among those hospitalized by an average of 24 percent[47] with the largest benefit accruing to those receiving therapy within six hours of the onset of symptoms. The benefits of thrombolytic therapy are even greater among the elderly; 2.1 nonelderly lives versus 4.2 elderly lives per 100 admissions for heart attack would be saved with this therapy.[48] Similarly, the use of beta blockers after myocardial infarction proportionally reduces the risk of death by about 22 percent.[49]

Three leading cardiac procedures are used in the diagnosis and treatment of persons with heart disease: coronary angiography, coronary artery bypass graft surgery (CABG), and percutaneous transluminal coronary angioplasty (PTCA). Previous studies of angiography and CABG have found significant numbers of these interventions performed for inappropriate clinical indications.[50,51] Although more recent studies have reported considerably lower rates of inappropriate procedure use,[52–54] these studies were done in New York State, which has an active program to monitor outcomes of cardiac procedures. It is likely that other regions of the country would not produce the impressive results found in New York State.

Potential for Improving Quality

Considerable potential exists for improving the quality of care for persons at risk for developing or who have already developed CAD, including primary, secondary, and tertiary interventions.

About 10 percent of adults have serum cholesterol levels that are associated with a fourfold increase in the risk of coronary death.[54] The recent HEDIS pilot study found that among persons continuously enrolled for five years in any one of the 21 participating health plans, 67 percent had a cholesterol screen in the previous five years; the range by individual health plan was from 34 to 87 percent.[55] Reducing cholesterol levels by 10 percent among half of the high-risk population has been estimated to result in a 3.5 percent reduction in coronary mortality.[56] Thus, continued efforts to identify persons with high cholesterol and to reduce cholesterol levels will contribute to reduced incidence of heart disease and coronary deaths.

The second National Health and Nutrition Examination Survey (NHANES II) found that 54 percent of adults with hypertension were aware they had high blood pressure, but only 11 percent had their blood pressure under control. Another study found that 66 percent of hypertensives knew they had high blood pressure but only 24 percent had their blood pressure under control.[57] A recent study of unionized New York City health care workers found that 71 percent of hypertensives were aware of their condition but only 12 percent had their blood pressure controlled.[58] The findings of this study are particularly important for quality improvement because the study subjects had fairly high levels of physician visits (9.6 annually in the uncontrolled group versus 19.4 in the controlled group).[59]

The USPSTF has estimated that if every primary care provider offered the brief smoking cessation counseling intervention that has been shown to be effective[60] to all of their patients who currently smoke, an additional 1 million Americans would quit smoking annually; currently 1.3 million quit annually.[61] One study found that more than one third of smokers seen in university internal medicine practices reported that a physician had never suggested that they stop smoking.[62]

Increasing the use of thrombolytic therapy for persons with a recent myocardial infarction from 40 to about 75 percent of eligible patients has been estimated to reduce mortality by 9.3 percent.[63] On average, only about 18 percent of all patients with a heart attack currently receive thrombolytic therapy.[64] Similarly, increasing the use of beta blockade after myocardial infarction from 40 to 75 percent of eligibles could reduce coronary mortality by 8.4 percent.[65]

Because coronary angiography is the most common cardiac procedure and provides a pathway to both CABG surgery and PTCA, examining the appropriateness of use of this procedure may be an excellent quality indicator. In addition to examining appropriateness, examining the volume of procedures performed by hospitals providing care for managed care enrollees might provide additional indirect evidence of quality.

Cost Effectiveness of Interventions

An Australian study investigated the cost effectiveness of three alternative strategies for reducing blood cholesterol levels: a high-risk strategy (identifying and treating men with cholesterol levels greater than 6.5 mmol/L with diet and drug), a moderate/high-risk strategy (diet counseling for those with 5.5 to 6.5 mmol/L cholesterol levels plus the same strategy for high-risk persons), and a population strategy (dietary change for the entire population regardless of cholesterol levels). The cost effectiveness ratios (costs per heart disease events saved) in Australian dollars were $482,224 (high-risk), $369,098 (moderate/high-risk), and $46,667 (population-based). The authors suggest further research on strategies to alter the eating habits of the entire population.[66] A U.S. study comparing targeted versus population-wide interventions for lowering serum cholesterol also concluded that population-wide strategies were indicated.[67]

Another study compared the cost effectiveness of treatment alternatives for elevated serum cholesterol, hypertension, and symptomatic CAD in reducing the risk of CAD.[68] The author concluded that the recommendations from the National Cholesterol Education program went beyond the scientific evidence and did not adequately account for problems with adherence to diet and drug regimens as well as the costs of widespread implementation. The cost effectiveness of drug treatment for both high cholesterol and hypertension depends on the target population.

Evaluations of thrombolytic therapy[69] and beta blockage[70] have demonstrated the cost effectiveness of these therapeutic interventions.

An analysis of the cost effectiveness of CABG surgery as compared to medical therapy found that surgery was an excellent value for persons with three vessel or left main disease and a reasonable value for persons with two vessel disease who had severe angina that was uncontrollable by medication.[71] The results of cost effectiveness comparisons of CABG and PTCA are dependent on the time frame evaluated because of the high rate of PTCA failure; five-year costs are $39,656 for CABG and $32,838 for PTCA.[72]

Health Plan Role in Providing Intervention

The role of health plans in providing secondary and tertiary interventions for the treatment of CAD is noncontroversial. The considerable expense and potential for negative outcomes associated with mismanaging these patients suggests careful attention to best practices is warranted. More controversial may be the role of the health plan in risk factor modification. For many of these activities, the health plan itself may not reap the benefits of the intervention (i.e., if the person does not remain with the health plan for life). The surveillance and intervention programs are not inexpensive and health plans may argue that public health interventions for certain aspects of risk factor modification (e.g., smoking cessation, dietary changes) may be more appropriate. The presence of quality indicators in these areas, however, would send a strong signal that health plans should be responsible for offering these interventions.

Breast Cancer

Importance

The prevalence of breast cancer is estimated to be 1,332 per 100,000 women; it is the most common site of cancer among women. The prevalence of cancer increases with age; 949 per 100,000 women age 35–54 have a diagnosis of breast cancer, compared with 3,881 per 100,000 among women age 75 or older. Among those with breast cancer, about one third were diagnosed between the ages of 45 and 54.[73]

Because of high survival rates relative to other cancers, breast cancer is the second leading cause of cancer deaths for women (lung cancer being the first) with nearly 40,000 deaths annually.[74] The incidence of the disease is quite high. Based on current trends, one in eight women will develop breast cancer in her lifetime and one in 33 will die from breast cancer.[75,76]

Efficacy or Effectiveness of Interventions

Although risk factors associated with the development of breast cancer have been identified, most are not modifiable (e.g., previous breast cancer, family history, nulliparity, late first pregnancy). The efficacy of modifying other risk factors (e.g., estrogen therapy, high-fat diet, alcohol consumption) has not been proven.[77]

Secondary prevention, that is, early identification of breast cancer, is an important intervention for this disease. Over 90 percent of women diagnosed with localized breast cancer survive for five years compared with only 18 percent of women diagnosed with metastatic breast cancer.[78] Screening breast examination and mammography have been promoted as mechanisms for early identification; evidence suggests that mammography can detect breast cancer at earlier stages than physical examination alone.[79] Screening mammography has been shown in randomized trials to reduce mortality by up to 40 percent among women age 50 and older.[80,81] Although mammography may be effective among women under age 50, the benefits are smaller and the decision to screen is likely to be more individualized.[82]

The primary treatment of early breast cancer is surgical.[83,84] Chemotherapy is routinely used for premenopausal patients with involved lymph nodes; tamoxifen is used if patients are postmenopausal, especially if their tumors contain estrogen receptor.[85] A meta-analysis of randomized trials of adjuvant therapy in early stage breast cancer concluded that the use of tamoxifen improves relapse-free time and overall survival rates for postmenopausal women, including those older than age 70.[86]

Potential for Improving Quality

Early detection remains the most effective way of improving the outcomes of breast cancer. Based on information from the National Health Interview Survey, the proportion of women age 40 and older who had ever received a screening mammogram increased from 17 percent in 1987 to 33 percent in 1990.[87] The National Cancer Institute reports that about 25 percent of women age 50 and older had a mammography in the previous two years. Although there is clear room for improvement among all women, African American and Hispanic women are at higher risk for late stage detection. Managed care plans may do better than the national average; the HEDIS pilot project reported that among women aged 52 to 64 who had been continuously enrolled in one of the 21 participating health plans for at least two years, 71 percent had received a screening mammography in the previous two years; the range for individual health plans was from 43 to 83 percent.

One way of improving the rate of screening mammography is to increase the number of primary care physicians who recommend this procedure to women. A 1985 survey found that fewer than 50 percent of primary care physicians ever recommended screening mammography to their female patients.[88] Failure to receive a recommendation for mammography is one of the most common reasons women give for not obtaining the procedure[89]; when mammography is recommended, two out of three women comply.[90]

Estimates about the effectiveness of screening mammography in improving the stage at detection and subsequent decrease in mortality rely on assumptions about the quality of the mammography and the adequacy of follow-up, diagnostic workup, and therapeutic procedures. These aspects of breast cancer treatment have been studied less frequently and may warrant further attention. For example, the new AHCPR clinical guideline on quality mammography recommends that diagnostic workup of an abnormal mammogram be conducted within a month of the abnormal finding.[91]

Cost Effectiveness of Interventions

An analysis of the cost effectiveness of mammography among women aged 50–70 in The Netherlands found that the cost effectiveness ratio was about $3,000 to $5,000 per year of life gained.[92] The authors reported limited effect on quality of life; estimates of the cost per quality adjusted life year gained was $4,050. The cost effectiveness ratio for women 40–70 was $5,400, but the incremental cost per additional life year gained was $35,000.[93]

A study on the cost effectiveness of mammograms conducted for the National Cancer Institute found that the cost was $7,000 to $8,000 per year of life gained.[94] The study was designed to reconcile the conflicting estimates that have emerged from other studies; the range from other studies has been $3,000 to $130,000 per year of life saved.

Health Plan Role in Providing Intervention

Screening for and treatment of breast cancer are clearly within the mandate of the health plan. Further, there is evidence that programs to remind women to obtain mammography successfully increase the rates of use of this procedure (42 percent of reminder group versus 28 percent of the control group).[95]

The additional steps in the treatment of breast cancer—notifying patients of the results of tests, follow-up of abnormal tests, diagnostic workup, and therapeutic interventions—may also be important in the overall quality of care for breast cancer. There is much less information available, however, on how well those steps are being accomplished in the treatment process.

Colorectal Cancer

Importance

Colorectal cancer is the second leading cause of death from cancer, accounting for 14 percent of cancer deaths in men and 15 percent of cancer deaths among women.[96] Annually, about 150,000 new cases of colorectal cancer are found and 60,900 individuals die from the disease. On average, about 6 percent of adults will develop this condition during their lifetime. The probability of developing colorectal cancer increases if certain risk factors are present, including: inflammatory bowel disease, familial polyposis syndromes, family cancer syndromes, history of colorectal cancer in a first degree relative, and a personal history of neoplasms.[97] The other major risk factor is age; the incidence of disease increases for men from about 12 per 100,000 in the age 40–44 population to 244 in the age 65–69 population.[98] The rates for women are comparable to men up to about age 49, but then increase at a slower rate.

Efficacy or Effectiveness of Interventions

Although associations between diet and the risk of developing colorectal cancer have been shown,[99] there is no evidence that dietary modification interventions are efficacious or effective in reducing the risk of developing the condition.

Secondary prevention interventions have been the focus of most research in this area because detection at an early stage substantially improves five-year survival rates; 85 percent of those whose cancer is detected at Duke's stage A or B survive five years, compared to 38 percent whose cancer is detected at Duke's stage C or D.[100] Currently, only about 34 percent of colorectal cancers are detected at the early stage. Five screening interventions are currently used to identify colorectal cancer: digital rectal examination, sigmoidoscopy, fecal occult blood testing, air contrast barium enemas, and colonoscopy. Because of differences in the cost and risks associated with these different screening procedures, the first three have been suggested for use in screening the general asymptomatic population and the last two have been recommended for use only among those at increased risk for developing the disease either due to the presence of symptoms or certain risk factors.[101]

Digital Rectal Examination. This screening procedure is a physical examination in which the physician inserts a finger into the rectum and searches for possible polyps. It is the simplest and least expensive to conduct. No studies have demonstrated reductions in mortality due to this screening procedure.[102] The potential effectiveness of this intervention is limited because only about 10 percent of adenomas and cancers can be detected by this exam.[103] The American Cancer Society recommends annual digital rectal examinations for men and women over age 40. Recommendations for routine digital rectal examinations are not included in the guidelines from the National Cancer Institute, the American College of Physicians, the American Society of Colon and Rectal Surgeons, the American Gastroenterological Association, and the American Society for Gastrointestinal Endoscopy, the U.S. Preventive Services Task Force, or the Canadian Task Force on the Periodic Health Examination. Many of these groups do recommend routine screening, however, digital rectal examination is not the preferred method.[104]

Sigmoidoscopy. This screening procedure consists of inserting a scope in the rectum so that the distal colon and rectum can be visually inspected for signs of adenomatous polyps. About 25–30 percent of cancers are detectable with a rigid sigmoidoscope and 50–60 percent are detectable with a 60–65 centimeter flexible sigmoidoscope. No randomized trials of the efficacy of this procedure have been conducted.[105]

There have been two large uncontrolled studies of screening sigmoidoscopy. The Strang Cancer Prevention Clinic (New York) examined the results of 47,091 screening sigmoidoscopy examinations performed on 26,196 patients, 89 percent of whom were asymptomatic.[106] The detection rate for colorectal cancer was 2.2 per 1,000 examinations; 76.5 percent were discovered through sigmoidoscopy; 81 percent of cases were localized and the five-year survival rate was 88 percent. A study at the University of Minnesota conducted initial screening sigmoidoscopy on about 21,150 patients and then followed up with annual repeat examinations. Considerably lower rates of colorectal cancer were found during the follow-up period than was expected.[107] These studies contain several biases that limit interpretability of the results.[108,109]

Sigmoidoscopy was studied as part of a randomized controlled trial of multiphasic health screening conducted by Kaiser Permanente of Northern California. Significantly fewer deaths from colorectal cancer were found in the study group than in the control group (12 versus 29 deaths) over the 16-year study. A re-examination of these results found that most of the cancers were detected after the occurrence of symptoms, although detection was earlier for study patients than control patients.[110] The authors speculate that encouraging annual health examinations may have made the study group more health conscious and more likely to seek care for symptoms at an earlier point. A case-control study conducted at Kaiser

Permanente of Northern California found that a significantly smaller proportion of case subjects (those dying from colon or rectal cancer from 1971 to 1988) had undergone screening sigmoidoscopy compared to control subjects (8.8 percent versus 24.2 percent); the adjusted odds ratio was 0.41.[111] The authors conclude that screening is effective and that conducting routine screening of asymptomatic populations at 10-year intervals may be as effective as more frequent screening.

The American Cancer Society recommends sigmoidoscopy every three to five years beginning at age 50. The USPSTF did not make a definitive recommendation in favor of or against sigmoidoscopy because they neither wanted to discourage current uses of sigmoidoscopy nor encourage additional use.[112]

Fecal Occult Blood Testing. This procedure involves testing stool samples collected over three consecutive days for the presence of occult blood; the test is designed to detect cancers or adenomas that are bleeding consistently. The sensitivity of the test has been shown to be quite low (50 percent for known cancers and about 25 percent for adenomas). The true efficacy of the test has been estimated to be about 10–30 percent.[113]

Five randomized controlled trials of fecal occult blood screening are currently under way and interim results have been reported from one trial. The randomized trial assigned 46,551 participants ranging in age from 50 to 80 to one of three conditions: annual screening, biannual screening, and a control group. The follow-up period was 13 years. The trial found that annual fecal occult blood testing, with rehydration of the samples, decreased the 13-year cumulative mortality rate from colorectal cancer by 33 percent as compared with the control group.[114] The annual screening group had colon cancer detected at an earlier stage than control group members.

A re-analysis of the results from this trial using a mathematical model suggested that chance selection for colonoscopy explained about one third to one half of the mortality reduction observed in the trial. The high false positive rate for fecal occult blood testing increases rates of rule-out colonoscopy; over the length of the trial, everyone would eventually get a rule-out colonoscopy, suggesting that this is the screening method that should be evaluated.

Air contrast barium enema has the capacity to identify about 92 percent of lesions in the large bowel and has a sensitivity of about 85 percent.[115] The false positive rate for barium enemas is about three to four percent. The major drawbacks to this method are discomfort for the patient and the expense of the procedure. This examination method is generally used in combination with other tests, such as fecal occult blood testing, and has not been recommended for screening asymptomatic populations.

Colonoscopy is a screening procedure that allows for visualization of the entire bowel area. About 95 percent of cancers within the region viewed by the colonoscope can be detected; it has a sensitivity rate of 95 percent. Because biopsies can be taken during a colonoscopic examination, the false positive rate is effectively zero. The major drawbacks to the use of colonoscopy in asymptomatic populations are the discomfort to the patient and the cost. No trials have been conducted to examine the efficacy of colonoscopy in screening persons with average risk.

The principal treatment for colorectal cancer is surgery, although in recent years multimodal approaches have become more common.[116] There is a relationship between therapeutic approach and stage of presentation; surgery alone is used for 91 percent of stage 0, 93 percent of stage I, and 83 percent of stage II colon cancer. For stage III colon cancer, 63 percent receive surgery alone, 3 percent have surgery and radiation, 28 percent have surgery and chemotherapy, 3 percent have surgery, radiation, and chemotherapy, 1 percent have chemotherapy alone, and 2 percent have some other treatment or no treatment. For stage IV, 42 percent have surgery only, 2 percent have surgery and radiation, 31 percent have surgery and chemotherapy, 3 percent have surgery, radiation, and chemotherapy, 7 percent have chemotherapy only, and 16 percent have another treatment or no treatment.[117]

Potential for Improving Quality

There is a clear link between stage of cancer at diagnosis and five-year survival rates; little evidence exists to suggest that different therapeutic strategies contribute substantially to improved survival. Identifying individuals at early stages requires screening, but there is little consensus about the frequency or method of screening that should be used for asymptomatic populations. There is greater agreement about the frequency and methods for persons who are at increased risk of developing colorectal cancer. At a minimum, those persons who are at increased risk should be identified and closely monitored.

Cost Effectiveness of Interventions

The various screening tests for colorectal cancer have quite different costs and levels of effectiveness. For example, Eddy[118] reports the costs of these screening tests based on an informal survey as: fecal occult blood test ($5); rigid sigmoidoscopy ($70); 35 centimeter flexible sigmoidoscopy ($100); 60 centimeter flexible sigmoidoscopy ($135); air contrast barium enema ($200); and colonoscopy ($500). Eddy[119] examined the cost effectiveness of 11 combinations of tests and interval frequency and recommended that, for persons over age 50, an annual fecal occult blood test be done in combination with a 70 centimeter flexible sigmoidoscopy every three to five years. For high-risk persons, an air contrast barium enema or colonoscopy was recommended every three to five years instead of the sigmoidoscopy.

Health Plan Role in Providing Intervention

Both screening and treatment fall under the traditional role of health plan activities; thus, if a standard can be agreed upon, health plans can be held accountable for compliance with that standard. Two considerations for health plans should be mentioned. First, although there is no firm agreement on the intervals between screening, much of the evidence for asymptomatic populations suggests that as little as three and as many as 10 years may elapse between screening tests. Given the turnover in health plan enrollment, this suggests the need for health plans to maintain good information on an individual's screening history in order to maximize the probability that the individual obtains screening at appropriate intervals. For new enrollees, this may require obtaining a history that includes receiving results from the most recent test as a baseline for subsequent testing. Second, greater consensus exists on the recommendations regarding screening for high-risk persons and these recommendations involve more intensive strategies (both increased frequency of screening and use of more expensive procedures). This implies that the health plan must have information that will facilitate the identification of persons at high risk for colorectal cancer. The risk factors could be obtained in a comprehensive history. Similar to the first point, information on risk is critical if the health plan is to play a proactive role in early identification of colorectal cancer.

Low Back Pain

Importance

There are a number of methodological challenges in estimating the prevalence of low back pain,[120] but it is the second leading cause of work absenteeism in the United States.[121] The lifetime prevalence of low back pain has been estimated to be 60–80 percent and the one-year prevalence is 15–20 percent.[122] Among the working age population, about half report symptoms of back pain during a one-year period.[123,124] About 5–10 percent of patients experience chronic problems,[125] but these individuals account for nearly 60 percent of expenditures for this problem.

Estimates of the direct medical costs of low back pain treatment range from $20–$50 billion[126] and the cost to the nation when work loss days are included increases substantially. It has been estimated that the work loss time plus disability payments can cost three times the expenditures on medical treatment.[127]

Efficacy or Effectiveness of Interventions

There is no strong evidence to suggest that preventive strategies for low back pain are efficacious or effective. The literature evaluating the effectiveness of four prevention strategies was recently reviewed.[128] The strategies included back and aerobic exercises, education, mechanical supports, and risk factor modification. The authors did not examine worksite-specific preventive measures, although all of the prevention studies included in the review were conducted in work settings. The review concluded that exercise is mildly protective, there is no support for the use of educational strategies, there is insufficient evidence to recommend the use of orthotic devices for prevention, and there is no proof that risk factor modification will reduce the incidence of low back pain.[129]

The Agency for Health Care Policy and Research has recently published a clinical practice guideline on the assessment and treatment of acute low back problems in adults.[130] The medical history is important in assessing whether the patient is suffering from a serious underlying condition such as cancer or spinal infection. The guideline recommends that the history include questions about: age, history of cancer, unexplained weight loss, immunosuppression, duration of symptoms responsiveness to previous therapy, pain that is worse at rest, history of intravenous drug use, and urinary or other infection. Symptoms of leg pain or problems walking due to leg pain may suggest neurological problems (e.g., herniated disc, spinal stenosis). The elements of the suggested medical history along with estimates of the sensitivity and specificity of those elements of the history are provided in the guideline document; an algorithm is provided for the use of responses to the initial assessment. The panel points out that a number of factors (e.g., work status, educational level, workers compensation issues, depression) may affect patients' responses regarding symptoms and may also influence treatment outcomes.

Elements of the physical examination (inspection, palpation, observation, specialized neuromuscular evaluation) are also reviewed along with estimates of their sensitivity and specificity. The guideline concludes that for 95 percent of patients with acute low back problems, no special interventions or diagnostic tests are required within the first month of symptoms. A brief summary of the clinical care methods for which the panel had strong recommendations are given here.[131]

Symptom education. The panel recommends educating patients about: expectations for recovery and recurrence, safe and effective methods of symptom control, reasonable activity modifications, methods for limiting recurrence of symptoms, why special investigations are not warranted, and the effectiveness and risks of diagnostic and treatment measures if symptoms persist. The panel indicated that symptom education may reduce utilization of medical care, decrease patient apprehension, and increase the speed of recovery.

Medications. The panel concluded that both acetaminophen and nonsteroidal anti-inflammatory drugs (NSAIDs) were adequate for achieving pain relief; acetaminophen may have fewer side effects. Muscle relaxants were found to be no better than NSAIDs in relieving low back symptoms and they have greater side effects, especially drowsiness. Opioids were found to be no more effective than NSAIDs or acetaminophen in providing pain relief; side effects include decreased reaction time, clouded judgment, drowsiness, and risk of physical dependence. A number of other medications (e.g., oral steroids, colchicine, antidepressants) were not recommended for the treatment of low back pain.

Physical treatments. Spinal manipulation for patients without radiculopathy is effective in reducing pain and may speed recovery within the first month. The evidence after one month is inconclusive. Transcutaneous electrical nerve stimulation (TENS), lumbar corsets and support belts, shoe lifts and supports, spinal traction, biofeedback, trigger point injections, ligamentous and sclerosant injections, facet joint injections, epidural injections, and acupuncture were not recommended for the treatment of acute back pain. For patients with radiculopathy, epidural steroid injections were considered an option after failure of conservative treatment and as a means of avoiding surgery.

Activity modifications. The panel recommended that patients with acute low back problems temporarily limit heavy lifting, prolonged sitting, and bending or twisting the spine. The activity limitations should take into account the age and clinical status of the patient as well as the demands of the patient's job. These modifications should be considered time-limited and the clinician may want to lay out goals for a return to normal activity.

Bed rest. Prolonged bed rest (i.e., more than four days) was not recommended because it may increase rather than decrease debilitation. The panel recommended a gradual return to normal activities and bed rest of short duration only for patients with severe initial symptoms of primary leg pain.

Exercise. The panel recommended that the initial goal of exercise programs be to prevent debilitation due to inactivity and then to improve activity tolerance with the goal of returning patients to their highest level of functioning. Exercise programs designed to improve general endurance (aerobic fitness) and muscular strength of the back and abdomen were considered particularly beneficial.

Special diagnostic tests. For patients whose symptoms with the recommended treatments listed above persist longer than one month, additional diagnostic and treatment procedures may be considered. The tests are of two types: tests for evidence of physiologic dysfunction and tests for evidence of anatomic causes of dysfunction. Tests in the former category include electromyography, sensory evoked potentials, thermography, general laboratory screening tests, and bone scan. The appropriate indications for and timing of these tests are provided in the guideline document. Tests in the latter category include plain myelography, magnetic resonance imaging, computerized axial tomography (CT) scan, CT-myelography, discography, and CT-discography. These tests must be combined with information from the medical history, physical examination, and/or physiologic tests because these imaging studies can be difficult to interpret and many patients may not show defects.

Surgery. Lumbar discectomy may provide faster pain relief in patients with severe and disabling leg symptoms who have failed to improve after one to two months of adequate nonsurgical treatment. However, there is little difference in outcomes for patients at four to ten years as compared with conservative care, and the procedure is quite expensive. Among methods of discectomy, direct methods of nerve root decompression were recommended over indirect methods. The role of patient preferences was emphasized but only if adequate information about efficacy, risks, and expectations is presented.

Surgery for spinal stenosis was not recommended within the first three months of symptoms. Decisions about this surgery should take into account the patient's lifestyle, preference, other medical problems, and the risk of surgery. Elderly patients in general should be managed with conservative therapy.

Spinal fusion was not recommended during the first three months of symptoms in the absence of fracture, dislocation, or complications of tumor or infection. Spinal fusion was recommended for consideration following decompression in patients with combined degenerative spondylolisthesis, stenosis, and radiculopathy. Patients under age 30 with significant spondylolisthesis and severe leg pain may also be considered candidates for spinal fusion.

Potential for Improving Quality

Many patients with low back pain who are unable to perform their usual activities may be receiving care that is either inappropriate or suboptimal.[132] The evidence includes substantial variations in the rates of hospitalization and surgery for low back problems[133,134] and variations in the use of diagnostic tests.[135] For example, in a study conducted in Washington state, the rate of surgery for low back pain varied 15-fold among the 39 counties in the state.[136] The likely explanation for this variation is difference in physician practice style. A study of the effect of practice style in managing back pain on patient outcomes found that a low-intensity intervention style characterized by self-care, fewer prescription medications, and less bed rest produced long-term pain and functional outcomes that were similar to more intensive styles and were less costly and associated with higher levels of patient satisfaction.[137] There are also patients that appear to have more disability after treatment than before, particularly those who have undergone surgery, those treated with extended bed rest, and those treated with extended use of high-dose opioids.[138]

The lack of consensus on appropriate treatments for low back pain suggests that there is likely to be considerable variation in practice across the country. The recent promulgation of a clinical practice guideline by the AHCPR offers an opportunity for developing tools for monitoring the use of both recommended and nonrecommended practices. This may provide a substantial incentive for decreasing the variation in care and reducing poor quality care.

Cost Effectiveness of Interventions

The costs of different treatment alternatives for low back pain vary considerably. The AHCPR panel characterized costs in three categories: low cost (less than $200), moderate cost ($200–1,000), and high cost (more than $1,000). The effectiveness of different intervention strategies is summarized above. No formal cost effectiveness analyses have been conducted, but the AHCPR panel took cost into account in making some of its recommendations and the bulk of evidence would appear to favor less resource intensive over more intensive interventions.

One study that examined the costs and outcomes of three different management styles for back pain found that the one-year costs of treatment ranged from $428 on average for patients seen by "low intensity" physicians to $768 on average for patients seen by "high intensity" physicians.[139] The differences were reduced somewhat when case mix variables were taken into account. Because the lower intensity practice style produced similar outcomes, that style would certainly be judged to be more cost-effective.

Health Plan Role in Providing Intervention

Both the initial assessment and treatment of low back pain fall under the traditional role of the health plan. Population-based preventive strategies have not been shown to be effective, but work-site specific interventions may be effective; this suggests a role for employers rather than the health care system.

In examining the guidelines, health plans may develop protocols that bring practice into line with what the panel has recommended. This may have the benefit of reducing costs without a decline in patient function. The availability of certain interventions (e.g., spinal manipulation) may vary by health plan and an assessment of their benefit as compared to more expensive alternatives that may be available should be assessed by plans in determining the range of treatment options for low back pain.

Major Depression

Importance

Major depression and recurrent depression (dysthymia) are among the most highly prevalent mental disorders in adults; about 17 percent of adults are diagnosed with major depression sometime during their life and the annual prevalence is about 10 percent among adults.[140] Major depression is more commonly found in women and in nonelderly populations.[141] The lifetime prevalence of depression is lower among African Americans than among non-Hispanic whites.[142] Among general medical outpatients, the prevalence of major depression is 5–9 percent and the prevalence of dysthymia is 6 percent.[143]

Depression has a substantial impact on functioning.[144] This impact on functioning translates into significant economic costs for society.[145] Direct treatment costs are estimated to be $12.4 billion. Mortality costs due to suicide (i.e., lost years of work) are estimated at $7.5 billion; morbidity costs due to reduction in productivity have been estimated at $23.7 billion.[146]

Efficacy or Effectiveness of Interventions

The treatment for depression includes several phases:

1. detection and assessment
2. treatment of the acute phase
3. continuation therapy to prevent early relapse
4. ongoing maintenance therapy to prevent recurrence.[147]

Clinical trials have demonstrated the efficacy of specific treatments at different phases. The USPHS estimates that properly implemented psychologic and pharmacologic treatments are effective more than 8 times out of 10.[148] AHCPR has published a clinical practice guideline on detection, diagnosis, and treatment of major depression in primary care.[149]

About 65–70 percent of patients with acute major depression respond to antidepressant medication.[150] The effectiveness of antidepressant medication was similar between patients in specialty mental health care and patients in primary care settings. Brief psychotherapies have been demonstrated to be efficacious as the sole treatment for persons with mild to moderate acute depression; about 47–55 percent respond positively. Little difference has been found in efficacy between group and individual psychotherapy in the acute phase; controversy exists around the use of psychotherapy in the continuation phase of treatment.[151,152]

Based on evidence from a few randomized trials, continuation treatment with the same dose and type of medication used in the acute phase is recommended for four to nine months after the patient has returned to a clinically well state.[153] Early discontinuation of treatment is associated with a 25 percent relapse rate within two months.[154] Several months of follow-up will facilitate early identification of a recurrence. For patients experiencing a recurrence, the new episode should be treated like a new acute phase. The benefit of continuation psychotherapy alone has neither been proven nor disproven in two ongoing continuation studies[155,156] and one randomized controlled trial.[157]

The World Health Organization recommends maintenance therapy for patients who have experienced two episodes within a five-year period.[158] The Depression Guideline Panel[159] very strongly recommended maintenance medication for persons with three or more episodes of depressive disorder; maintenance medication was strongly recommended for persons with two episodes and a family history of bipolar disorder, a history of recurrence within one year after previously effective medication was discontinued, a family history of recurrent major depression, a first episode of depression before age 20, and if both episodes were severe, sudden or life-threatening in the past three years. The panel recommended that maintenance medication be given at the same dosage that was used successfully during the acute phase. Maintenance psychotherapy (minimum once per month) does not appear to prevent a recurrence although it may delay the onset of a subsequent episode.[160] More frequent maintenance psychotherapy has not been evaluated.

Potential for Improving Quality

Many individuals with major depression may not receive appropriate or high-quality care. About half of persons with depression receive no therapeutic care.[161] Among those who are being treated for major depression, about half receive care only in the general medical sector rather than from specialty providers.[162] General medical clinicians fail to detect current depressive disorder in about half of patients with the problem and this increases to about 60 percent failure to detect in prepaid practices.[163,164]

Only 20–30 percent of general medical patients with depression are prescribed antidepressant medications and 30 percent of those with prescriptions are receiving a subtherapeutic dosage.[165,166] Minor tranquilizers are often used to treat depression[167,168] despite the lack of evidence for efficacy.[169]

The appropriateness of medication use among ethnic minority patients is even lower than that found for white patients.[170] General medical clinicians use brief counseling for half of their depressed patients.[171] Primary care is often the sole source of care for minorities and for the elderly.[172,173]

Thus, there is considerable evidence of quality problems in the detection and treatment of depression. Given its high prevalence and substantial impact on functioning, improved quality of care for this disorder is likely to have substantial positive impact on the health of the population.

Cost Effectiveness of Interventions

Studies of cost effectiveness of care for depression are rare.[174] A recent study using a decision-analysis simulation approach suggested that the greatest opportunity for improving the cost effectiveness of care is in the general medical sector; the mechanism for improvement is to increase the percentage of patients who use an effective dosage of antidepressant medication or who receive counseling for depression.[175]

Health Plan Role in Providing Intervention

The interventions for detection and treatment of depression are clearly under the control of health plans. Perhaps the biggest challenge for health plans is improving care delivered by primary care physicians. Studies investigating effective methods of changing provider behavior have shown some positive effects of feedback on detection[176-178]; others have found no effect[179] or a negative effect.[180] Clinical psychosocial skills of primary care physicians have been improved by approaches relying on videotaping, role-playing, case vignettes, or case management seminars.[181,182]

Diabetes Mellitus

Importance

Approximately seven million Americans have been diagnosed with diabetes mellitus and an additional five million may have the disease and be unaware of it.[183] Diabetes is an underlying cause of death for 37,000 persons and a contributing factor in another 100,000 deaths.[184] Complications related to diabetes are quite high, with an estimated 5,800 cases of blindness, 40,000 amputations, and 4,000 cases of renal failure annually.[185]

There are two types of diabetes mellitus. Type I (insulin dependent or IDDM) and Type II (non–insulin dependent or NIDDM) are quite different in their epidemiology and risk of complications. Type I most often afflicts children and young adults whereas Type II (accounting for 92 percent of all diabetes cases) tends to afflict older adults. Type II diabetes is more likely to be mild and asymptomatic and may frequently be undetected and untreated. Type I is more serious and generally requires ongoing insulin therapy.

IDDM is one of the more common chronic conditions among children. The prevalence is estimated to be 1.2 to 1.9 cases per 1,000 children[186] and the peak age at onset is between 10 and 14 years of age[187]; the peak age of onset for girls is earlier (10–12 years old) than for boys, probably due to earlier onset of puberty. There is both seasonal and geographic variation in the incidence of cases with more cases being diagnosed in cooler months and more cases being identified in cooler climates. There is no significant difference in the prevalence of IDDM between males and females. There are racial differences in the incidence of IDDM with whites being considerably more likely to develop IDDM than nonwhites.[188]

Efficacy or Effectiveness of Interventions

Primary prevention of either Type I or Type II diabetes is currently considered infeasible. Secondary and tertiary prevention of acute and long-term complications of the disease are the principal focus of treatment strategies.

Annually, more than 67,000 cases of acute metabolic complications (ketoacidosis or nonketotic hyperosmolar coma) occur.[189] Although there is evidence that some acute complications of diabetes can be reduced or prevented through improved management,[190] many may not be preventable and some management strategies may actually increase the likelihood of complications.[191,192] However, both ketoacidosis and hyperosmolar coma can be effectively treated in the hospital, implying that death from these conditions is preventable and high rates of deaths due to acute complications may signal possible problems of quality.[193]

The longer-term management of IDDM presents a challenge for the health professional, child, and family. The major goals of treatment are: (1) normal physical and emotional development; (2) reduction in symptoms associated with excessive glycemic excursion; and (3) lessening of the long-term complications. Children who are undertreated are likely to experience growth retardation and delays in sexual maturation. Children with IDDM are at risk for hypoglycemia, which can cause an altered level of consciousness, seizures, and brain damage. Long-term problems include significant retinal, renal, and nerve damage. Management of the disease is important and requires education of the family and the child so that they can participate in independent decision making around daily decisions related to diet, activities, and insulin dose adjustment to reduce hyperglycemia and hypoglycemia. Avoiding metabolic abnormalities requires monitoring blood glucose multiple times daily as well as intermittent urinary ketone checks. Frequent health care visits are recommended to monitor HbA_{1C} levels, blood lipids, and blood pressure, although no specific guidelines exist that specify the exact number of recommended visits.[194]

The Diabetes Control and Complications Trial established that intensive insulin therapy was superior to conventional therapy in delaying the onset and slowing the progression of retinopathy, nephropathy, and neuropathy in patients with IDDM.[195] In the primary prevention cohort, the adjusted mean risk of developing retinopathy was reduced by 76 percent in the intensive insulin therapy group as compared to the conventional therapy group. In the secondary prevention group, the progression of retinopathy was slowed by 54 percent in the intensive as compared to the conventional therapy group. Intensive therapy also resulted in significant reductions in the occurrence of microalbuminuria, albuminuria, and clinical neuropathy. The major adverse event was a two- to threefold increase in severe hypoglycemia.

Prevention of long-term complications may be feasible using strategies other than tight glycemic control. For example, patient education programs may improve outcomes among persons with diabetes.[196] Annual eye examinations have been recommended to identify and treat proliferative retinopathy and diabetic macular edema, cataracts, and glaucoma at an early stage.[197] The incidence of foot infections may be reduced by patient education about foot care and encouraging smoking cessation[198]; among those who develop foot infections, medical and surgical management may reduce morbidity.[199,200] Persons with diabetes are at increased risk of developing hypertension and hypercholesterolemia.[201] Attention to the prevention and treatment of these risk factors may reduce the incidence of cardiovascular complications. Decline in renal function may be mitigated for patients with diabetic nephropathy through aggressive treatment of hypertension[202] or microalbuminuria.[203]

Potential for Improving Quality

The evidence suggests that substantial shortcomings exist in the care of diabetics. One study found that only one third of diabetics seen by university internists were under adequate control[204]; among diabetics with hypertension, 40 percent were found to have poorly controlled blood pressures.[205] Foot examinations are infrequently done in physician visits.[206] The recent HEDIS Pilot Project found that overall annual funduscopic examinations were performed for 47 percent of persons in the 21 participating health plans, with a range from 12 to 58 percent.[207] These exams may need to be done by ophthalmologists because primary care physicians may not be able to perform an adequate funduscopic examination.[208]

Because the DCCT results are only recently available, there may be considerable variation in the use of intensive insulin therapy versus conventional therapeutic approaches. This may represent one area of potential improvement in the quality of care for persons with IDDM.

Cost Effectiveness of Interventions

Probably because there are not many alternatives in diabetes treatment, few studies examining cost effectiveness have been conducted. One study examining classroom versus individual education found that classroom education was more cost-effective, and more conducive to learning than individual instruction.[209] Failure to adequately treat individuals who have diabetes is likely to result in complications, hospitalization, and death; these are likely to be extremely expensive relative to the cost of high-quality care.

Health Plan Role in Providing Intervention

The health plan role in providing treatment of diabetes, both Type I and Type II, is consistent with a traditional role. Perhaps the greatest challenge is the provision of educational interventions designed to facilitate self-management of the disease. This may be best accomplished by special clinics. For example, the DCCT treatment team included diabetologists, nurses, dietitians, and behavioral specialists. During the first month of the trial, the treatment team was in daily phone contact with study participants. Such team management may be beyond the coverage of many insurance policies, but may be more feasible to accomplish in the managed care setting than in a solo practice.

Childhood Asthma

Importance

Asthma is the most common childhood chronic condition with an estimated prevalence rate between 5 and 10 percent. Asthma accounts for 23 percent of school absence days and remains one of the primary reasons for hospitalizing children.[210] Children with severe asthma miss more than twice as many school days as healthy children.[211] Data from the National Health Interview Survey suggest that the prevalence of asthma in the pediatric population increased by 29 percent between 1980 and 1987. Moreover, the hospitalization rates for children less than 15 years of age with asthma have increased substantially over the past 20 years.[212] Of even greater concern is the 46 percent increase in death rates from asthma that were reported between 1980 and 1989 despite therapeutic advances in diagnosis and treatment.[213–215]

Efficacy or Effectiveness of Interventions

Research and clinical data indicate that effective treatment exists for children with asthma.[216–218] The goals of asthma management are to: (1) maximize functional status of children as indicated by their ability to participate in normal activities; (2) maximize symptom relief (i.e., minimize frequency of attacks, maximize pulmonary function); (3) facilitate child and family empowerment by maximizing self-efficacy in symptom control and treatment regimens; and (4) limit side effects of treatments and interventions.[219]

NHLBI issued guidelines for the diagnosis and management of asthma, including childhood asthma, in 1991.[220] Guidelines were established for different clinical presentations of asthma (mild, moderate, and severe) and for different health care settings (home, emergency room, hospital). Subsequently, an American Academy of Pediatrics (AAP) quality committee developed a practice parameter for the office-based management of acute exacerbations of childhood asthma.[221] Critics of the guidelines have emphasized the lack of scientific rigor in their development and challenges in complying with the required structural elements; nonetheless, these guidelines have become the national standard for asthma care.

The NHLBI classification of asthma by severity of disease uses several characteristics to distinguish among patients at different levels, including: frequency of exacerbations, frequency of symptoms, degree of exercise tolerance, frequency of nocturnal asthma, school attendance, and pulmonary function. The initial classification is based on categorizing the patient on these dimensions prior to treatment. After optimal treatment is established, the guidelines classify severity by also taking into account response to and duration of therapy.

For children with asthma, the therapeutic recommendations include both medication and patient education.[222] The dose, method of administration, and type of medication vary with the severity of disease. All children and families should receive education about self-management of the disease (e.g., early identification of acute exacerbations and plans for action to resolve such episodes, identification and elimination of environmental triggers in the home).

The AAP practice parameter was developed based on information obtained from the scientific literature and a nominal group process consensus for areas without scientific evidence. The committee developed a clinical algorithm that identified key decisions related to the medication strategy for patients with an acute exacerbation. The committee also made statements regarding the resources, knowledge, and skills required to treat acute exacerbations.

The *basic office resources* for the assessment and treatment of an acute exacerbation that were recommended include[223]:

- capability to treat hypoxia through delivery of oxygen by nasal cannula or mask
- peak expiratory flow meter (PEFM) or a mini-FEV$_1$ meter
- nebulizer or metered dose inhaler (MDI) with spacer
- pulse oximeter for physicians who treat moderately severe and severe patients in their office
- an area where the patient can be observed and periodically assessed for one to two hours.

The *knowledge requirements* include:

- pathophysiology of asthma
- symptoms and signs of respiratory distress and respiratory failure
- interpretation of pulmonary function tests that measure airway obstruction
- pulmonary gas exchange impairment
- pharmacological properties of beta$_2$-agonists, corticosteroids, and theophylline.

The *skills required* include:

- use of power-drive nebulizer or MDI device to deliver beta$_2$-agonists by inhalation
- use of PEFM or spirometer
- use of pulse oximeter
- patient education in the use of PEFM and nebulizers, and MDIs with spacers.

The practice parameter includes detailed recommendations regarding initial assessment and emergency treatment, initial treatment, follow-up treatment, additional treatment and/or transfer to emergency department or hospital.

Potential for Improving Quality

There are no national estimates about the extent to which current practice is consistent with the practice guidelines available from the NHLBI and the AAP. However, increases in the death rate over a time when therapeutic interventions were improving suggests that there is a potential for improving care. Studies of practice patterns in teaching hospitals[224] and emergency rooms[225] suggest that there is considerable variability in the management of acute exacerbations. A trial of an educational intervention in Los Angeles had to be discontinued because of the poor treatment being provided to children enrolled in the study.[226] Some studies of medication regimens and self-management programs have shown reductions of greater than 50 percent in attack rates, emergency room use, and lost school days.[227]

Cost Effectiveness of Interventions

No formal cost effectiveness analyses were found. Certainly, improved management of asthma in the outpatient setting that contributes to reductions in emergency room and hospital use will be more cost-effective than strategies that lead to uncontrollable exacerbations. There are likely to be cost differences among the different medical therapies, but there is not much variation in the recommended strategies, suggesting that cost effectiveness may not be much of a consideration in chronic management.

Health Plan Role in Providing Intervention

The health plan has a role in the assessment and treatment of children with asthma. Perhaps as importantly, however, teaching parents and children how to manage this disease is likely to make a substantial contribution to improved outcomes. When a significant patient role is required, there is often a debate about the appropriate level of attribution to the health plan. Because parents and children cannot be expected to learn about self-management on their own, testing knowledge, attitudes, and beliefs of families and children with asthma may provide an indicator of the success of the health plan in communicating the necessary information.

RECOMMENDATIONS

Based on the above review of the seven conditions considered for inclusion in the HEDIS quality measures, the NCQA steering committee decided to focus its efforts on childhood asthma, coronary artery disease, diabetes, and major depression. With funding from The Robert Wood Johnson Foundation, performance measures will be developed for these four conditions.

Promising areas for measurement development include:

Coronary Artery Disease

1. Rates of cholesterol screening within the past five years by age and gender.

2. Adequacy of follow-up for elevated cholesterol levels (e.g., dietary counseling, drug therapy).
3. Proportion of persons in the plan with coronary artery disease who have elevated cholesterol levels.
4. Proportion of persons in the plan with hypertension whose blood pressure is outside the normal range.
5. Proportion of persons in the plan who smoke who have not received a smoking cessation intervention in the past two years.
6. Proportion of persons with myocardial infarctions who appropriately receive thrombolytic therapy.

Breast Cancer

1. Proportion of women over age 52 who received a screening mammography in previous two years (existing HEDIS measure).
2. Proportion of women with an abnormal mammography who had a diagnostic workup within one month of the abnormal finding.
3. Proportion of women who have documented evidence (e.g., history) of their relative risk of developing breast cancer.
4. Among women with breast cancer diagnosis, distribution by stage at presentation.
5. Among women with breast cancer diagnosis, evidence that options for treatment were explained and patient preferences taken into account in determining therapeutic regimen.

Colorectal Cancer

1. Proportion of enrolled population that has had risk factors for developing colorectal cancer assessed.
2. Among individuals at high risk for colorectal cancer, proportion receiving an annual screening examination.
3. Among individuals at average risk for colorectal cancer, capacity to identify timing of next routine screening examination (e.g., every five years).

Low Back Pain

1. Proportion of persons presenting with low back pain who receive appropriate education about symptoms, treatments, and prognosis.

2. Proportion of persons with acute low back pain who receive inappropriate medications.
3. Proportion of persons with acute low back pain who receive inappropriate diagnostic or surgical interventions.
4. Proportion of persons with acute low back pain who have extended bed rest (i.e., more than four days) recommended in the first month.

Major Depression

1. Appropriateness of medications prescribed (type, dose, duration) for persons with major depression.
2. Knowledge and skill of primary care physicians to detect and treat major depression.

Diabetes Mellitus

1. Proportion of persons with diabetes mellitus whose most recent HbA_{1c} levels are within the normal range.
2. Proportion of persons with diabetes mellitus who have an annual retinal examination (existing HEDIS measure).
3. Proportion of persons with diabetes mellitus and hypertension whose blood pressure is within the normal range.
4. Proportion of persons with diabetes mellitus who have a competent annual foot examination.

Childhood Asthma

1. Appropriateness of medications prescribed for chronic management of asthma.
2. Proportion of children and families with asthma who have adequate knowledge about the disease, control of symptoms, elimination of environmental triggers, and a plan for dealing with an acute exacerbation.
3. Adequacy of office resources for management of an acute exacerbation.
4. Appropriateness of hospitalization and emergency room visits for asthma.

These potential areas for measurement development are offered as a starting point. The above quality indicators were purposely written to draw on multiple sources of data: administrative, clinical, and patient-centered. No single source of data exists that can capture all of the important domains of quality. As greater emphasis is placed on disease management and quality assessment, the incentives to develop automated clinical information systems and routine patient surveys will increase. Better data will facilitate a process for improving the understanding of the critical elements that define a high-quality health care system.

REFERENCES

1. Lohr, K.N., et al. "Chronic Disease in a General Adult Population: Findings from the RAND Health Insurance Experiment." *Western Journal of Medicine* 145 (1986):537–545.
2. Ibid.
3. Siu, A.L., et al. *Choosing Quality-of-Care Measures Based on the Expected Impact of Improved Quality of Care for the Major Causes of Mortality and Morbidity.* Publication No. JR-03. Santa Monica, CA: RAND, 1992.
4. "Prevalence of Adults with No Known Major Risk Factors for Coronary Heart Disease—Behavioral Risk Factor Surveillance System, 1992." *Morbidity and Mortality Weekly Report* 43(4) (1994):61–63.
5. Davis, D.L., Dinse, G.E., and Hoel, D.G. "Decreasing Cardiovascular Disease and Increasing Cancer Among Whites in the United States From 1973 Through 1987." *Journal of the American Medical Association* 271(6) (1994):431–437.
6. "Public Health Focus: Physical Activity and the Prevention of Coronary Heart Disease." *Morbidity and Mortality Weekly Report* 42(35) (1993):669–672.
7. Holme, I. "An Analysis of Randomized Trials Evaluating the Effect of Cholesterol Reduction on Total Mortality and Coronary Heart Disease Incidence." *Circulation* 82(6) (1990):1916–1924.
8. U.S. Preventive Services Task Force. *Guide to Clinical Preventive Services.* Baltimore, MD: Williams and Wilkins, 1989.
9. U.S. Public Health Service. *Healthy People 2000: National Health Promotion and Disease Prevention Objectives.* DHHS Pub. No. (PHS) 91-50212. Washington, D.C.: Department of Health and Human Services, 1990.
10. Poulter, N. "Management of Multiple Risk Factors for Coronary Heart Disease in Patients with Hypertension." *American Heart Journal* 121(1) (1991):246–249.
11. U.S. Preventive Services Task Force, *Guide to Clinical Preventive Services.*
12. Department of Health and Human Services. *The Health Consequences of Smoking: A Report of the Surgeon General.* DHHS Publication No. (PHS) 82-50179. Rockville, MD: Department of Health and Human Services, 1982.
13. Centers for Disease Control, U.S. Department of Health and Human Services. "Cigarette Smoking in the United States, 1986." *Morbidity and Mortality Weekly Report* 36 (1987):581–585.
14. U.S. Public Health Service. *Healthy People 2000.*
15. U.S. Preventive Services Task Force, *Guide to Clinical Preventive Services.*
16. Kottke, T.E., et al. "Attributes of Successful Smoking Cessation Interventions in Medical Practice: A Meta-analysis of 39 Controlled Trials." *Journal of the American Medical Association* 259 (1988):2883–2889.

17. Oster, G., et al. "Cost-Effectiveness of Nicotine Gum as an Adjunct to Physician's Advice Against Cigarette Smoking." *Journal of the American Medical Association* 256 (1986):1315–1318.
18. Kottke et al., "Attributes of Successful Smoking Cessation."
19. Hubert, H.B., et al. "Obesity as an Independent Risk Factor for Cardiovascular Disease: A 26-year Follow-up of Participants in the Framingham Heart Study." *Circulation* 67 (1983):968–977.
20. Posner, B.M., et al. "Healthy People 2000. The Rationale and Potential Efficacy of Preventive Nutrition in Heart Disease: The Framingham Offspring-Spouse Study." *Archives of Internal Medicine* 153(13) (1993):1549–1556.
21. Van Itallie, T.B., and Kral, J.G. "The Dilemma of Morbid Obesity." *Journal of the American Medical Association* 246 (1981):999–1003.
22. Stunkard, A.J. "Conservative Treatments for Obesity." *American Journal of Clinical Nutrition* 45 (1987):1142–1154.
23. Ibid.
24. U.S. Preventive Service Task Force, *Guide to Clinical Preventive Services.*
25. Eaton, C.B. "Relation of Physical Activity and Cardiovascular Fitness to Coronary Heart Disease. Part II: Cardiovascular Fitness and the Safety and Efficacy of Physical Activity Prescription." *Journal of the American Board of Family Practice* 5(2) (1992):157–165.
26. Mittleman, M.A., et al. "Triggering of Acute Myocardial Infarction by Heavy Physical Exertion—Protection Against Triggering by Regular Exertion." *New England Journal of Medicine* 329 (1993):1677–1683.
27. Willich, S.N., et al. "Physical Exertion as a Trigger of Acute Myocardial Infarction." *New England Journal of Medicine* 329 (1993):1684–1690.
28. Ibid.
29. Mittleman et al., "Triggering."
30. Curfman, G.D. "Is Exercise Beneficial—or Hazardous—to your Health?" *New England Journal of Medicine* 339(23) (1993):1730–1731.
31. Hambrecht, R., et al. "Various Intensities of Leisure Time Physical Activity in Patients with Coronary Artery Disease: Effects on Cardiorespiratory Fitness and Progression of Coronary Atherosclerotic Lesions." *Journal of the American College of Cardiology* 22 (1993): 468–477.
32. U.S. Preventive Service Task Force, *Guide to Clinical Preventive Services.*
33. Woods, S.E. "Primary Prevention of Coronary Heart Disease in Women. Should Asymptomatic Women 50 Years of Age Take Aspirin Regularly?" *Archives of Family Medicine* 3(4) (1994):361–364.
34. Blankenhorn, D.H., et al. "Beneficial Effects of Combined Colestipol-Niacin Therapy on Coronary Atherosclerosis and Coronary Venous Bypass Grafts." *Journal of the American Medical Association* 257 (1987):3233–3240.
35. Strauss, W.E., and Parisi, A.F. "Combined Use of Calcium-Channel and Beta-Adrenergic Blockers for the Treatment of Chronic Stable Angina. Rationale, Efficacy, and Adverse Effects." *Annals of Internal Medicine* 109 (1988):570–581.
36. Theroux, P., et al. "Aspirin, Heparin, or Both to Treat Acute Unstable Angina." *New England Journal of Medicine* 319 (1988):1105–1111.
37. Eisenberg, M., Bergner, L., and Hallstrom, A. "Paramedic Programs and Out-of-Hospital Cardiac Arrest. II. Impact on Community Mortality." *American Journal of Public Health* 69 (1979):39–42.
38. Wilcox, R.G., et al. "Trial of Tissue Plasminogen Activator for Mortality Reduction in Acute Myocardial Infarction. Anglo-Scandinavian Study of Early Thrombosis (ASSET)." *Lancet* 1(8610) (September 3, 1988):525–530.

39. International Study of Infarct Survival (ISIS) Steering Committee. "Intravenous Strep-tokinase Given Within 0–4 Hours of Onset of Myocardial Infarction Reduced Mortality in ISIS-2." *Lancet* 1(8531) (February 28, 1987):502.

40. "Randomized Trial of Intravenous Streptokinase, Oral Aspirin, Both, or Neither Among 17,187 Cases of Suspected Acute Myocardial Infarction: ISIS-2." *Lancet* 2(8607) (August 13, 1988):349–360.

41. Gruppo Italiano per lo Studio della Streptochinasi Nell'infarto miocardico (GISSI). "Effectiveness of Intravenous Thrombolytic Treatment in Acute Myocardial Infarction." *Lancet* 2(8564) (February 22, 1986):397–401.

42. Gruppo Italiano per lo Studio della Streptochinasi Nell'infarto miocardico (GISSI). "Long-Term Effects of Intravenous Thrombolysis in Acute Myocardial Infarction: Final Report of the GISSI Study." *Lancet* 2(8564) (October 17, 1987):871–874.

43. Yusuf, S., et al. "Beta Blockade During and After Myocardial Infarction: An Overview of the Randomized Trials." *Progress in Cardiovascular Diseases* 27 (1985):335–371.

44. Goldman, L., et al. "Costs and Effectiveness of Routine Therapy with Long-Term Beta-Adrenergic Antagonists After Acute Myocardial Infarction." *New England Journal of Medicine* 319 (1988):152–157.

45. Oldridge, N.B., et al. "Cardiac Rehabilitation After Myocardial Infarction." *Journal of the American Medical Association* 260 (1988):945–950.

46. Dubois, R.W., and Brook, R.H. "Preventable Deaths: Who, How Often, and Why?" *Annals of Internal Medicine* 109 (1988):582–589.

47. Yusuf, S., Wittes, J., and Friedman, L. "Overview of Results of Randomized Clinical Trials in Heart Disease. I. Treatments Following Myocardial Infarction." *Journal of the American Medical Association* 260 (1988):2088–2093.

48. Doorey, A.J., Michelson, E.L., and Topol, E.J. "Thrombolytic Therapy of Acute Myocardial Infarction: Keeping the Unfulfilled Promises." *Journal of the American Medical Association* 268 (1992):3108–3114.

49. Yusuf, Wittes, and Friedman, "Overview of Results."

50. Chassin, M.R., et al. "Does Inappropriate Use Explain Geographic Variations in the Use of Health Care Services?" *Journal of the American Medical Association* 258 (1988):2533–2537.

51. Winslow, C.M., et al. "The Appropriateness of Carotid Endarterectomy." *New England Journal of Medicine* 318 (1988):721–727.

52. Bernstein, S.J., et al. "The Appropriateness of Use of Coronary Angiography in New York State." *Journal of the American Medical Association* 269 (1993):766–769.

53. Leape, L.L., et al. *Coronary Artery Bypass Graft: A Literature Review and Ratings of Appropriateness and Necessity.* Pub. No. JRA-02. Santa Monica, CA: RAND, 1991.

54. National Cholesterol Evaluation Program Expert Panel. "Report of the National Cholesterol Education Program Expert Panel on Detection, Evaluation, and Treatment of High Blood Cholesterol in Adults." *Archives of Internal Medicine* 148 (1988):36–69.

55. National Committee on Quality Assurance. *Report Card Pilot Project.* Washington, D.C.: NCQA, 1994.

56. Siu et al., *Choosing Quality-of-Care Measures.*

57. U.S. Public Health Service, *Healthy People 2000.*

58. Stockwell, D.H., et al. "The Determinants of Hypertension Awareness, Treatment, and Control in an Insured Population." *American Journal of Public Health* 84 (1994):1768–1774.

59. Ibid.

60. Kottke et al., "Attributes of Successful Smoking Cessation."

61. U.S.P.H.S., *Healthy People 2000.*

62. Kosecoff, J., et al. "General Medical Care and the Education of Internists in University

Hospitals: An Evaluation of the Teaching Hospital General Medicine Group Practice Program." *Annals of Internal Medicine* 102 (1985):250–256.
63. Siu et al., *Choosing Quality-of-Care Measures.*
64. Pashos, C.L., et al. "Trends in the Use of Drug Therapies in Patients with Acute Myocardial Infarction: 1988 to 1992." *Journal of the American College of Cardiology* 23 (1994):1023–1030.
65. Siu et al., *Choosing Quality-of-Care Measures.*
66. Kinlay, S., et al. "The Cost-Effectiveness of Different Blood-Cholesterol-Lowering Strategies in the Prevention of Coronary Heart Disease." *Australian Journal of Public Health* 18(1) (1994):105–110.
67. Goldman, L. "Cost-Effectiveness Perspectives in Coronary Heart Disease." *American Heart Journal* 119(3) (1990):733–739.
68. Stason, W.B. "Costs and Benefits of Risk Factor Reduction for Coronary Heart Disease: Insights from Screening and Treatment of Serum Cholesterol." *American Heart Journal* 119(3) (1990):718–724.
69. Goldman et al., "Costs and Effectiveness."
70. Laffel, G.L., et al. "A Cost-Effectiveness Model for Coronary Thrombolysis/Reperfusion Therapy." *Journal of the American College of Cardiology* 10 (1987):79B–90B.
71. Leape et al., *Coronary Artery Bypass Graft.*
72. Ibid.
73. Byrne, J., Kessler, L.G., and Devesa, S.S. "The Prevalence of Cancer Among Adults in the United States: 1987." *Cancer* 69 (1992):2154–2159.
74. National Center for Health Statistics (NCHS). *Prevention Profile. Health, United States 1989.* Hyattsville, MD: Public Health Service, 1990.
75. Feuer, E.J., et al. "The Lifetime Risk of Developing Breast Cancer." *Journal of the National Cancer Institute* 85(11) (1993):892–897.
76. Harris, J.R., et al. "Breast Cancer." *New England Journal of Medicine* 327(5) (1992):319–328.
77. Siu et al., *Choosing Quality-of-Care Measures.*
78. National Cancer Institute. *Cancer Statistics Review 1973–1987.* Washington, D.C.: U.S. Department of Health and Human Services, 1990.
79. Baker, L.H. "Breast Cancer Demonstration Project: Five-Year Summary Report." *CA: A Cancer Journal for Clinicians* 32(4) (1982):194–225.
80. Andersson, I., et al. "Mammographic Screening and Mortality from Breast Cancer: The Malmo Mammographic Screening Trial." *British Medical Journal* 297 (1988):943–948.
81. UK Trial of Early Detection of Breast Cancer Group. "First Results on Mortality Reduction in the UK Trial of Early Detection of Breast Cancer." *Lancet* 27 (1988):411–416.
82. Eddy, D.M., and Hasselbald, V. "The Value of Mammography Screening in Women Under Age 50 Years." *Journal of the American Medical Association* 259 (1988):1512–1519.
83. Veronesi, U., et al. "Comparing Radical Mastectomy with Quadrantectomy, Axillary Dissection, and Radiotherapy in Patients with Small Cancers of the Breast." *New England Journal of Medicine* 305 (1981):6–11.
84. Fisher, B., et al. "Five-Year Results of a Randomized Clinical Trial Comparing Total Mastectomy and Segmental Mastectomy With or Without Radiation in the Treatment of Breast Cancer." *New England Journal of Medicine* 312 (1985):665–673.
85. Tripathy, D., and Henderson, I.C. "Systemic Adjuvant Therapy for Breast Cancer." *Current Opinion in Oncology* 4(6) (1992):1041–1049.
86. Muss, H.B. "The Role of Chemotherapy and Adjuvant Therapy in the Management of Breast Cancer in Older Women." *Cancer* 74(7) Supplement (1994):2165–2171.
87. Breen, N., and Kessler, L. "Changes in the Use of Screening Mammography: Evidence from the 1987 and 1990 National Health Interview Surveys." *American Journal of Public Health* 84 (1994):62–67.

88. American Cancer Society. "Survey of Physicians' Attitudes and Practices in Early Cancer Detection." *CA: A Cancer Journal for Clinicians* 35 (1985):197–213.

89. National Cancer Institute Workshop. "The 1988 Bethesda System for Reporting Cervical/Vaginal Cytological Diagnosis." *Journal of the American Medical Association* 262 (1989):931–934.

90. Burack, R.C., and Liang, J. "The Early Detection of Cancer in the Primary Care Setting: Factors Associated with the Acceptance and Completion of Recommended Procedures." *Preventive Medicine* 16 (1987):739–751.

91. Bassett, L.W., et al. *Quality Determinants of Mammography. Clinical Practice Guideline No. 13.* AHCPR Pub. No. 95-0632. Rockville, MD: AHCPR, Public Health Service, U.S. Department of Health and Human Services, October 1994.

92. de Koning, H.J., et al. "Breast Cancer Screening and Cost-Effectiveness; Policy Alternatives, Quality of Life Considerations and the Possible Impact of Uncertain Factors." *International Journal of Cancer* 49 (1991):531–537.

93. Ibid.

94. University of Texas M.D. Anderson Cancer Center. "How Valuable are Mammograms?" *Cancer Outcomes* newsletter 1(1) (1993):5.

95. King, E.S., et al. "Promoting Mammography Use through Progressive Interventions: Is it Effective?" *American Journal of Public Health* 84 (1994):104–106.

96. Friedman, G.D., and Selby, J.V. "Colorectal Cancer: Have We Identified an Effective Screening Strategy?" *Journal of General Internal Medicine* 5(5) (supplement) (September–October 1990):523–527.

97. Eddy, D.M. "Screening for Colorectal Cancer." *Annals of Internal Medicine* 113(5) (1990): 373–384.

98. Ibid.

99. Zaridze, D.G. "Environmental Etiology of Large-Bowel Cancer." *Journal of the National Cancer Institute* 70 (1983):389–400.

100. Friedman and Selby, "Colorectal Cancer."

101. Eddy, "Screening."

102. Ibid.

103. Friedman and Selby, "Colorectal Cancer."

104. U.S. Preventive Services Task Force, *Guide to Clinical Preventive Services.*

105. Selby, J.V., et al. "A Case-Control Study of Screening Sigmoidoscopy and Mortality from Colorectal Cancer." *New England Journal of Medicine* 326 (1992):653–657.

106. Hertz, R.E., Deddish, M.R., and Day, E. "Value of Periodic Examinations in Detecting Cancer of the Rectum and Colon." *Postgraduate Medicine* 27 (1960):290–294.

107. Gilbertson, V.A. "Proctosigmoidoscopy and Polypectomy in Reducing the Incidence of Rectal Cancer." *Cancer* 34 (1974):936–939.

108. Friedman and Selby, "Colorectal Cancer."

109. Eddy, "Screening."

110. Ibid.

111. Selby et al., "A Case-Control Study."

112. U.S. Preventive Services Task Force, *Guide to Clinical Preventive Services.*

113. Ranshoff, D.F., and Lang, C.A. "Screening for Colorectal Cancer." *New England Journal of Medicine* 325 (1991):37–41.

114. Mandel, J.S., et al. "Reducing Mortality from Colorectal Cancer by Screening for Fecal Occult Blood." *New England Journal of Medicine* 328(19) (1993):1365–1371.

115. Eddy, "Screening."

116. Steele, G.D. "Colorectal Cancer." In *National Cancer Data Base: Annual Review of Patient Care.* Atlanta, GA: American Cancer Society, 1994.

117. Ibid.

118. Eddy, "Screening."
119. Ibid.
120. Loeser, J.D., and Volinn, E. "Epidemiology of Low Back Pain." *Neurosurgery Clinics of North America* 2(4) (1991):713–718.
121. Deyo, R.A., and Bass, J.E. "Lifestyle and Low-Back Pain: The Influence of Smoking and Obesity." *Spine* 14(5) (1989):501–506.
122. Andersson, G.B.J. "The Epidemiology of Spinal Disorders." In *The Adult Spine: Principles and Practice*, ed. J.W. Frymoyer. New York, NY: Raven Press, 1991.
123. Vallfors, B. "Acute, Subacute and Chronic Low Back Pain: Clinical Symptoms, Absenteeism and Working Environment." *Scandinavian Journal of Rehabilitation Medicine* 11 (Supplement) (1985):1–98.
124. Sternbach, R.A. "Survey of Pain in the United States: The Nuprin Pain Report." *Clinical Journal of Pain* 2(1) (1986):49–53.
125. Lahad, A., et al. "The Effectiveness of Four Interventions for the Prevention of Low Back Pain." *Journal of the American Medical Association* 272(16) (1994):1286–1291.
126. Bigos, S., et al. *Acute Low Back Pain Problems in Adults. Clinical Practice Guideline No. 14.* AHCPR Publication No. 95-0642. Rockville, MD: Agency for Health Care Policy and Research, Public Health Service, U.S. Department of Health and Human Services, December 1994.
127. Spengler, D.M., et al. "Back Injuries in Industry: A Retrospective Study. I. Overview and Cost Analysis." *Spine* 11(3) (1986):241–256.
128. Lahad et al., "Effectiveness of Four Interventions."
129. Ibid.
130. Bigos et al., *Acute Low Back Pain.*
131. Ibid.
132. Ibid.
133. Deyo, R.A. "Nonsurgical Care of Low Back Pain." *Neurosurgery Clinics of North America* 2(4) (1991):851–862.
134. Volinn, E., et al. "Small Area Analysis of Surgery for Low-Back Pain." *Spine* 17(5) (1992):575–579.
135. Deyo, "Nonsurgical Care."
136. Volinn, "Small Area Analysis."
137. Von Korff, M., et al. "Effects of Practice Style in Managing Back Pain." *Annals of Internal Medicine* 121 (1994):187–195.
138. Bigos et al., *Acute Low Back Pain.*
139. Von Korff et al., "Effects of Practice Style."
140. Kessler, R., et al. "Lifetime and 12-Month Prevalence of DSM-III-R Psychiatric Disorders in the United States." *Archives of General Psychiatry* 51 (1994):8–19.
141. Weissman, M.M., et al. "Affective Disorders in Five United States Communities." *Psychological Medicine* 18 (1988):141–153.
142. Kessler et al., "Lifetime."
143. Katon, W., and Schulberg, H. "Epidemiology of Depression in Primary Care." *General Hospital Psychiatry* 14 (1992):237–247.
144. Wells, K.B., et al. "The Functioning and Well-Being of Depressed Patients: Results from the Medical Outcomes Study." *Journal of the American Medical Association* 262 (1989):914–919.
145. Rice, D.P., et al. *The Economic Costs of Alcohol and Drug Abuse and Mental Illness.* San Francisco, CA: Institute for Health and Aging, University of California, 1990.
146. Greenberg, P.E., et al. "Depression: A Neglected Major Illness." *Journal of Clinical Psychiatry* 54(11) (1993):419–424.

147. Kupfer, D.J. "Long-Term Treatment of Depression." *Journal of Clinical Psychology* 52(5) (Supplement) (1991):28–34.
148. Depression Guideline Panel. *Depression in Primary Care: Volume 2. Treatment of Major Depression.* Clinical Practice Guideline, Number 5. Pub. No. 93-0551. Rockville, MD: U.S. Department of Health and Human Services, Public Health Service, AHCPR, April 1993.
149. Ibid.
150. Ibid.
151. Ibid.
152. Frank, E., et al. "Three-Year Outcomes for Maintenance Therapies in Recurrent Depression." *Archives of General Psychiatry* 47 (1990):1093–1100.
153. Depression Guideline Panel, *Depression.*
154. Maj, M., et al. "Pattern of Recurrence of Illness After Recovery from an Episode of Major Depression: A Prospective Study." *American Journal of Psychiatry* 149 (1992):795–800.
155. Blackburn, I.M., and Bishop, S. "Changes in Cognition with Pharmacotherapy and Cognitive Therapy." *British Journal of Psychiatry* 33 (1983):1479–1489.
156. Jarret, R.B., et al. "How Prophylactic Is Cognitive Therapy in Treating Depressed Outpatients?" Paper presented at the World Congress of Cognitive Therapy, Toronto, Canada, June 1992.
157. Weissman, M.M., et al. "The Efficacy of Drugs and Psychotherapy in the Treatment of Acute Depressive Episodes." *American Journal of Psychiatry* 136(4B) (1979):555–558.
158. Coppen, A., Mendelwicz, J., and Kielholz, P. *Pharmacotherapy of Depressive Disorders: A Consensus Statement.* Geneva: World Health Organization, 1986.
159. Depression Guideline Panel, *Depression.*
160. Frank et al., "Three-Year Outcomes."
161. Regier, D.A., et al. "The de facto US Mental and Addictive Disorders Service System." *Archives of General Psychiatry* 50 (1993):85–94.
162. Rogers, W.H., et al. "Outcomes for Adult Depressed Outpatients Under Prepaid or Fee-for-Service Financing." *Archives of General Psychiatry* 50 (1993):517–525.
163. Wells, K.B., et al. "Quality of Care for Depressed Elderly Pre-Post Prospective Payment System: Differences in Response Across Treatment Settings." *Medical Care* 32 (1994):257–276.
164. Katon, W., et al. "Adequacy and Duration of Antidepressant Treatment in Primary Care." *Medical Care* 30 (1992):67–76.
165. Wells et al., "Quality of Care."
166. Katon et al., "Adequacy and Duration."
167. Wells et al., "Quality of Care."
168. Olfson, M., and Klerman, G.L. "Trends in the Prescription of Psychotropic Medications: The Role of Physician Specialty." *Medical Care* 31 (1993):559–564.
169. Depression Guideline Panel, *Depression.*
170. Wells et al., "Quality of Care."
171. Wells et al., "Functioning."
172. Ibid.
173. NIH Consensus Development Panel on Depression in Late Life. "Diagnosis and Treatment of Depression in Late Life." *Journal of the American Medical Association* 268 (1992):1018–1024.
174. Kamlet, M.S., et al. "Cost-Utility Analysis of Maintenance Treatment for Recurrent Depression: A Theoretical Framework and Numerical Illustration." In *Economics and Mental Health,* ed. R.G. Frank and W.G. Manning. Baltimore, MD: Johns Hopkins University Press, 1992.
175. Sturm, R., and Wells, K.B. *Can Prepaid Care for Depression Be Improved Cost-Effectively?*

Pub. No. DRU-724-AHCPR. Santa Monica, CA: RAND, 1994.

176. Attkisson, C.C., and Zich, J.M. *Depression in Primary Care.* New York, NY: Routledge, 1990.
177. Brody, D.S., et al. "Improvement in Physicians' Counseling of Patients with Mental Health Problems." *Archives of Internal Medicine* 150 (1990):993–998.
178. Magruder-Habib, K., Zung, W.K., and Feussner, J.R. "Improving Physicians' Recognition and Treatment of Depression in General Medical Care: Results from a Randomized Clinical Trial." *Medical Care* 28 (1990):239–250.
179. Hoeper, E.W., et al. "The Usefulness of Screening for Mental Illness." *Lancet* 1(8367) (1984):33–35.
180. Badger, L.W., and Rand, E.H. "Unlearning Psychiatry: A Cohort Effect in the Training Environment." *International Journal of Psychiatry in Medicine* 18 (1988):123–135.
181. Roter, D., et al. "The Effects of Training on Physicians' Diagnosis and Management of Psychosocial Problems." In *Mental Disorders in General Health Care Settings: A Research Conference* (Pittsburgh, PA), pp. 215–217. Rockville, MD: National Institute of Mental Health, 1987.
182. Sriram, T.G., et al. "Training of Primary Health Care Medical Officers in Mental Health Care: Errors in Clinical Judgment Before and After Training." *General Hospital Psychiatry* 12 (1990):384–389.
183. U.S. Public Health Service, *Healthy People 2000.*
184. Ibid.
185. Mazze, R.S., et al. "An Epidemiological Model for Diabetes Mellitus in the United States: Five Major Complications." *Diabetes Research and Clinical Practice* 1 (1985):185–191.
186. Plotnik, L.P. "Insulin-Dependent Diabetes Mellitus." In *Principles and Practice of Pediatrics*, ed. F.A. Oski et al. 2nd ed. Philadelphia, PA: J.B. Lippincott Co., 1994.
187. Golden, M.P., and Gray, D.L. "Diabetes Mellitus." In *Textbook of Adolescent Medicine*, ed. E.R. McAnarney et al. Philadelphia, PA: W.B. Saunders Co., 1992.
188. American Diabetes Association. *Diabetes 1991 Vital Statistics*, Alexandria, VA: ADA, 1991.
189. Mazze et al., "An Epidemiological Model."
190. Garnick, D.W., Hendricks, A.M., and Comstock, C.B. "Measuring Quality of Care: Fundamental Information from Administrative Datasets." *International Journal for Quality in Health Care* 6(2) (1994):163–177.
191. Feldt-Rasmussen, B.S., Mathiessen, E.R., and Deckert, T. "Effect of Two Years of Strict Metabolic Control on Progression of Incipient Nephropathy in Insulin-Dependent Diabetes." *Lancet* 2(8519) (December 6, 1986):1300–1304.
192. DCCT Research Group. "The Effect of Intensive Treatment of Diabetes on the Development and Progression of Long-Term Complications in Insulin-Dependent Diabetes Mellitus." *New England Journal of Medicine* 329(14) (1993):977–986.
193. Rutstein, D.D., et al. "Measuring the Quality of Medical Care: A Clinical Method." *New England Journal of Medicine* 294 (1976):582–588 (2d Rev. of Tables, May 1980).
194. Plotnik, "Insulin-Dependent Diabetes Mellitus."
195. DCCT Research Group, "Effect of Intensive Treatment."
196. Kaplan, R.M., et al. "Effects of Diet and Exercise Intervention on Control and Quality of Life in Non-Insulin-Dependent Diabetes Mellitus." *Journal of General Internal Medicine* 2 (1987):220–227.
197. Herman, W.H., et al. "An Approach to the Prevention of Blindness in Diabetes." *Diabetes Care* 6 (1983):608–609.
198. Browner, W.S. "Preventable Complications of Diabetes Mellitus." *Western Journal of Medicine* 145 (1986):701–703.

199. Edmonds, M.E., et al. "Improved Survival of the Diabetic Foot: The Role of a Specialised Foot Clinic." *Quarterly Journal of Medicine* 232 (August 1986):763–771.
200. Bild, D.E., et al. "Lower-Extremity Amputation in People with Diabetes: Epidemiology and Prevention." *Diabetes Care* 12 (1989):24–31.
201. Lohr et al., "Chronic Disease."
202. Parving, H.H., et al. "Early Aggressive Antihypertensive Treatment Reduces Rate of Decline in Kidney Function in Diabetic Nephropathy." *Lancet* 2(8335) (May 1983):1175–1178.
203. Marre, M., et al. "Prevention of Diabetic Nephropathy with Enalapril in Normotensive Diabetics with Microalbuminuria." *British Medical Journal* 297 (1988):1092–1095.
204. Kosecoff et al., "General Medical Care."
205. Brook, R.H., et al. "Quality of Ambulatory Care: Epidemiology and Comparison by Insurance Status and Income." *Medical Care* 28 (1990):392–433.
206. Browner, "Preventable Complications."
207. NCQA, *Report Card Pilot Project.*
208. Browner, "Preventable Complications."
209. Carpentier, W.S., et al. "Efficacy of Diabetes Education: Classroom Versus Individualized Instruction." *HMO Practice* 4(1) (1990):30–33.
210. Taylor, W.R., and Newacheck, P.W. "Impact of Childhood Asthma on Health." *Pediatrics* 90(5) (1992):657–662.
211. Parcel, G.S., et al. "A Comparison of Absentee Rates of Elementary Schoolchildren with Asthma and Nonasthmatic Schoolmates." *Pediatrics* 64 (1979):878–881.
212. Halfon, N., and Newacheck, P. "Trends in the Hospitalization for Acute Childhood Asthma, 1970–1987: A National Study." *American Journal of Public Health* 76(11) (1986):1308–1311.
213. Weiss, K.B., Gergen, P.H., and Hodgson, T.A. "An Economic Evaluation of Asthma in the United States." *New England Journal of Medicine* 326 (1992):862–866.
214. National Heart, Lung, and Blood Institute. *The Study of a Childhood Asthma Management Program (CAMP).* Bethesda, MD: National Institutes of Health, NHLBI-HR-90-12, 1991.
215. Halfon, N., and Newacheck, P. "Childhood Asthma and Poverty: Differential Impacts and Utilization of Health Services." *Pediatrics* 91(1) (1993):56–61.
216. National Heart, Lung, and Blood Institute, *Study.*
217. Sheffer, A.L., and Taggart, V.S. "The National Asthma Education Program: Expert Panel Report and Guidelines for the Diagnosis and Management of Asthma." *Medical Care* 31 (1993):MS20–MS28.
218. Warner, J.O., et al. "Management of Childhood Asthma: A Consensus Statement." *Archives of Disease in Childhood* 64 (1989):1065–1079.
219. Halfon, N. "Perspectives from Pediatrics." *Medical Care* 31(3) (Supplement) (1993):MS30–MS31.
220. National Heart, Lung, and Blood Institute, *Study.*
221. American Academy of Pediatrics, Provisional Committee on Quality Improvement. "Practice Parameter: The Office Management of Acute Exacerbations of Asthma in Children." *Pediatrics* 93(1) (1994):119–126.
222. National Heart, Lung, and Blood Institute, *Study.*
223. AAP Provisional Committee, "Practice Parameter."
224. Daley, J., et al. "Practice Patterns in the Treatment of Acutely Ill Asthmatic Patients at Three Teaching Hospitals: Variability in Resource Utilization." *Chest* 100 (1991):51–56.
225. Canny, G.J., et al. "Acute Asthma: Observations Regarding the Management of a Pediatric Emergency Room." *Pediatrics* 83 (1989):507–512.
226. Lewis, M.A. Comments made during a symposium at RAND, Santa Monica, CA, 1994.
227. Siu et al., *Choosing Quality-of-Care Measures.*

II

Care Management

4

Components of a Successful Case Management Program

Sherry L. Aliotta

Case management is one of the most touted interventions in the health care industry, with many managed care organizations scrambling to implement such programs within their systems.

A recent study indicates that, of those HMOs surveyed, 86 percent are planning to implement or expand their case management programs.[1] However, the study also indicates that these decisions have been reached without the benefit of meaningful information to validate the financial and outcomes impacts of such programs.

FHP, Inc., is a large staff, IPA, and mixed model HMO. FHP/Quality Continuum was the subsidiary that housed the organization's case management operations. Using experience gained from being director of case management operations in FHP/Quality Continuum, and as a consultant in evaluating and assisting HMOs in implementing case management programs, the author has found that health care organizations can implement a successful program by following these basic steps:

- Define case management and organizational goals.
- Assess organizational strengths and capacities.
- Identify, assess, and select patient cases.
- Create, monitor, and evaluate outcome measures.

Source: Reprinted from S.L. Aliotta, Components of a Successful Case Management Program, *Managed Care Quarterly,* Vol. 4, No. 2, pp. 38–45, © 1996, Aspen Publishers, Inc.

DEFINING CASE MANAGEMENT AND ORGANIZATIONAL GOALS

Case management is defined as "a collaborative process which assesses, plans, implements, coordinates, monitors, and evaluates options and services to meet an individual's health needs through communication and available resources to promote quality, cost-effective outcomes."[2]

Through case management, an organization can ensure that health care services are available to meet the needs of its population. The primary focus is a coordinated dialogue between providers and patients to help guide patients through a continuum of services, rather than to "compartmentalize" their care.

Many people erroneously classify programs that are primarily utilization review/management programs as case management programs. However, there are many inherent differences between the two (Table 4–1).

Unlike case management, traditional utilization management models are designed primarily to control costs, ensure medical necessity, and identify trends. Moreover, traditional utilization management places an undue emphasis on acute care episodes where reducing length of stay and effective discharge planning are remaining options.

Using the case management, or more active approach, an organization stands the greatest chance of improving quality and reducing overall costs because of its focus on early intervention and emphasis on a continuum of care. The goal of this approach is to maintain the patient at the most appropriate level of care—preferably as far left on the continuum as possible (Figure 4–1).

The first step in implementing a case management program involves creating a case management definition such as that noted above and estab-

Table 4–1 Case Management and Utilization Management Comparison

Case management (Proactive)	Utilization management (Reactive)
Meant to be actively identifying patients at risk for exacerbation of chronic illness and intervening in a manner that has a positive effect on the outcome.	The patient presents for service. At this point there is already an illness or perception of illness. The only decision is how to treat the illness.
Focuses on the continuum of care (ideally from enrollment).	Focuses on the episode of illness.
Focuses on a small number of patients at a high level of intensity.	Focuses on a large number of patients at a low level of intensity.
Focuses on medically appropriate care.	Use of prior authorization and concurrent review to evaluate medical necessity.

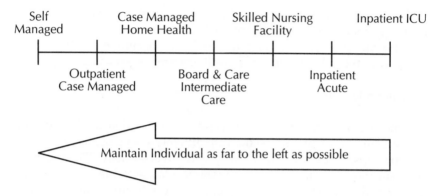

Figure 4–1. Continuum of care.

lishing program goals that fit the health plan's philosophy of care and expected outcomes. For instance, a health plan may decide its goals for a particular program or group of patients are lowering admission rates, improving clinical outcomes, reducing cost of care, or improving satisfaction. Whatever an organization's goals, they should reflect that plan's culture and philosophy of care. Moreover, senior management should be apprised of these efforts and its support sought.

In a well-structured case management program, case managers oversee this continuum, and seek to intervene early to prevent a patient's condition from progressing in severity by placing the patient in alternative settings, where appropriate. They also follow a low volume of patients at a high level of intensity. They often have contact with these patients several times per day, gaining familiarity with the patient's medical, social, and overall course of care. This approach shifts the emphasis from site of care to the patient's health care needs. Some advances, including those in home care, have increased the amount and type of services that can be safely provided in the home.

ASSESSING ORGANIZATIONAL STRENGTHS AND CAPACITIES

Many organizations have the proper resources already in place to launch a case management program, but need assistance in properly allocating them. A health plan should examine its existing utilization and case management capacities to uncover strong and weak areas. Depending on the plan's internal capacity to conduct such a review, having an independent consultant conduct an analysis is another option that could save the plan dollars and time.

The organizational assessment should focus on several key capacities: a health plan's relations with its providers; its staff, and staff training and recruitment efforts; data availability; and plan incentives. All these areas will play a role in how a plan designs its case management program.

Provider relations

A major part of the success of this effort is the relationship between the health plan and its providers. Because different providers have different relationships, models and focus vary with organizations. The case management model is most effective when it addresses the organization's quality and cost issues. For example, a medical group usually has complete control of ambulatory cost and quality, which has an impact on overall care.

Many case management programs are planned to operate independently of the physician team, which in many cases ends up alienating the very physician group and clinicians needed to achieve the case management program's goals. At FHP/Quality Continuum, managers avoided this scenario by enhancing the newly launched Primary Care Delivery System (PCDS). The PCDS is a system of care that allows patients to select their own primary care physician, and the patient and physician work together as a team to meet the patient's health care needs.

Each case management approach is designed to maximize the relationship between patient and physician, and support the physician in managing a complex panel of patients. This commitment to partnership with the physician has been successful. In a recent survey, 93 percent of FHP physicians responded that case management was of value to them in their practice. The physicians also gave high marks to the collaborative role of the case manager and the long-term health maintenance approach of case managers.

Staffing and training

Sufficient resources are necessary to implement a case management program. This may sound obvious; however, many organizations expect to achieve monumental results without investing resources, such as staff, staff training, time, and equipment. A defined plan for such investments and criteria aid this effort—and this investment does not always need to cost money. Sometimes it just means using some creativity to make the most out of current resources, including human resources. For instance, rather than insisting that all of the registered nurses (RNs) hired have previous case management experience, FHP/Quality Continuum made a decision to accept RNs who may require training in case management. Since case management was a new concept within the organization, this allowed FHP to retain RNs that were employed by FHP, but lacked case management experience.

This decision also allowed the plan to use the strong pool of internal talent within the organization, and maximize the knowledge of FHP systems this group possessed. Furthermore, these characteristics were identified as those that contributed to success as a case manager: creativity; flexibility; knowledge of community and company resources; prior nursing experience; and organizational, interpersonal, and problem-solving skills.

Once a part of the organization, the case manager must be supported with adequate training and job orientation. Even an experienced case manager benefits from an educational program that outlines the company's approach to case management. A comprehensive presentation of the company's case management philosophy and practice provides the new case managers with a common frame of reference. At FHP/Quality Continuum, an eight-hour course was created that all new case managers are required to take, regardless of prior experience.

One of the most common questions concerns the proper ratio of cases to case manager, yet this ratio will vary according to each organization's needs. At the FHP/Quality Continuum program, the ratio is 45 cases to one case manager in the ambulatory care program, and 25–30:1 for the catastrophic program. Human resources will typically be an organization's largest investment as qualified staff are essential to the success of the program.

Data availability

The availability of data will drive the design of a successful case management model; thus, data systems must be established at the onset of the program. The data collected must be consistent with the goals and objectives of the program. Currently available data are a logical starting point. There are several essential data elements an organization must have available (see Exhibit 4–1). The extent to which each item is significant will depend on the organization's goals for case management. For example, if a health plan's goal is to reduce readmissions for the same or related diagnosis, then a plan will want detailed data on the frequency for the same or related diagnosis. However, if a plan aims to reduce admission rates for a particular group of patients, plan managers should be able to readily access data on current admission rates.

Many companies undertake massive vendor searches to meet their data needs without a real understanding of those needs. FHP/Quality Con-

Exhibit 4–1 Essential Data Elements

Demographics (e.g., age, sex)	**Diagnostic data**
Utilization data (e.g., acute care days, skilled care days, office visits, home health visits)	Cost data (e.g., services unit or per diem costs of care)
Program data (e.g., referral source and reason, number of patients followed by CM)	Outcome data (e.g., clinical and financial)
Activity data (e.g., types, frequency, duration of case management activities)	Cost data (e.g., program cost, unit and aggregate)
Pharmacy data (e.g., medication usage)	Narrative data (e.g., patient level documentation)

tinuum's initial case management data capture system was a modified Paradox database. The system modifications continued as the program evolved and requirements were defined. Finally, an internally developed system was necessary to meet the expanded data needs. Many vendors were invited to submit proposals and stage demonstrations; however, none of the systems were adequate to meet the program needs. Because of FHP's initial approach to data management, staff were aware of their requirements, which enabled the plan to make the appropriate decisions.

Defining report requirements can be a complicated process. The program definition and goals will provide assistance in developing reporting guidelines. Traditional report questions must first be answered. What information is needed and who needs it? When is it needed? Where is the information available? How should it be transmitted? Who will interpret the reports and how can staff be trained to do so? In FHP's case, reporting has helped the organization identify and correct various problems and document its successes. Reporting must be a focus of continuous quality improvement.

Depending on the health plan's data availability, some organizations may need to purchase or design additional, more sophisticated data systems. Basic data systems can be developed with minimal investment to support early case management efforts while the organization more fully assesses its needs.

Financial incentives

While the case management model presented in this article (and the experiences of FHP/Quality Continuum, which uses this model) can be applied in virtually every setting, the degree to which it is effective and the way it is carried out may vary. The model is most effective when the organization's desired outcome is to reduce the number of hospital admissions and length of stay by use of outpatient and ancillary services. Despite financial incentives, the quality of care improvements make a case management program a worthwhile investment.

IDENTIFYING, ASSESSING, AND SELECTING PATIENT CASES

In order to be effective, case management must be proactive in its approach to patient care by defining the populations it will serve using statistics gleaned in the early planning phase. Once the population has been defined, individual members of that population must be selected and assessed for the appropriateness of case management intervention.

One of FHP/Quality Continuum's target populations was a group defined as "frail elderly." Characteristics of the population were developed such as age, numbers of chronic illnesses, and numbers of medications. FHP created systems that would assist in identifying members consistent with this profile for further review. One method used is the Health Assessment Questionnaire (HAQ), which is sent to new senior enrollees for FHP coverage. The returned HAQ is reviewed by a case manager to screen for high-risk indicators, and the appropriate follow-up is conducted. This procedure is being revised to incorporate a computer scored algorithm that will enhance FHP's case finding capabilities.

Assessment determines which of the patients identified through case finding are appropriate for case management. The terms screening and assessment are often used interchangeably, but are distinct. Screening is defined as the processes by which a system of managed care uses targeting criteria to select potential recipients of case management.[1] This is often accomplished by referrals from health care professionals. Assessment is the process by which the staff gathers information required to accept targeted enrollees for case management and to manage their care.[1] Methods of assessment vary, but should include a systematic approach. FHP/Quality Continuum case managers used internally developed behavioral indicators as well as standard geriatric assessment tools to complete the assessment process.

Plan managers should also accurately define the major diagnostic groups and evaluate the incidence and prevalence of disease states. In many cases, health plan managers may believe that all individuals with "high risk" diseases should be "case managed." However, approaches that manage high-risk persons on an individual or population basis, such as asthma care, enable an organization to address the typical drivers of chronic illness (Exhibit 4–2) while managing the individual outliers.

Exhibit 4–2 Drivers of Disease Cost[5]

Patient Compliance
Prevention
Rapid Resolution
Acute Flare Ups
80-20 Rule (80 percent of resources go to 20 percent of problems)

The age of the health plan's members will guide an organization's care program and resource allocation in terms of human resource investment and costs. At FHP/Quality Continuum, the management of the senior population—those patients over age 65 or disabled Medicare-eligible patients under age 65—account for 83 percent of program costs. Simply stated, the Medicare population requires more case management services than the commercial (under 65) population. The data also indicate that at any point in time 1.25 percent of the FHP Medicare risk population, and 0.25 percent of the commercial population, are being followed by case managers. Over the course of a year, approximately 10 percent of the population receives some case management intervention. Certain aged populations will require increased intensity.

Once screening and assessment are completed, case managers must identify the areas for intervention. FHP/Quality Continuum developed a problem classification system to perform this function. The system is based on behaviors that can be identified and affected by case management intervention. Each problem behavior is tied to a corresponding expected outcome. For example, if a diabetic is not taking insulin properly, the expected outcome is that the patient takes the insulin as prescribed to manage the individual's illness. Behavioral areas include: health access; safety; medications; treatment and outcomes; diagnosis; and financial. The system has helped position FHP/Quality Continuum to evaluate the impact in resolving problems, and focused the attention of case managers on goals and outcomes.

The patient care plan is the vehicle for resolving identified problems. The care planning process should be multidisciplinary, meaning that the case manager, the primary care physician, and the patient must establish the plan collaboratively. Excluding any one of those individuals is a critical error that will likely result in failure of the plan.

Once the decision to proceed with the case management program is made, and the work of analyzing systems, defining data needs, developing procedures, and hiring qualified staff is complete, the case management functions must be clearly defined. A resource for health plans is the Case Management Society of America (CMSA), which has established standards of care for case management that serve as a sound platform on which to build a program.

The CMSA standards are a guide for achieving excellence in case management. Although nonbinding, the CMSA hopes the guidelines will serve as a framework for public policy, education, practice, and research. The standards of care covered in the CMSA document include: assessment/case identification and selection; problem identification; planning; monitoring; evaluating; and outcomes.[3]

To aid a continuum of care focus, an organization can develop case management criteria as a means to create a set of quality standards and show organizational support and commitment. FHP introduced such standards to its outpatient clinic program. Part of the outpatient clinic administrator's management incentive is based on successfully meeting these standards. One of the FHP standards is that the clinic must have a case manager with an identified caseload of patients.

Written policies and procedures also help ensure consistency, and consistency allows for measurements. The benefits of procedure manuals are well known, and case management is no exception. Policies and procedures are important in conveying the program's essence to new staff, review organizations, and regulators. Many of the procedures were field tested before being included in the procedure manual. One common pitfall of the procedure manual is demonstrated by a situation in which the author was reviewing a case management program, and was presented with a very well-written procedure manual. There was only one problem. The program existed only in the pages of the manual. Obviously, there are programs that illustrate the opposite. The clear solution is somewhere in the middle, but to the extent possible existing practice should be documented to meet the requirements of licensure and demonstrate compliance with the standards of various accrediting organizations such as the National Committee for Quality Assurance (NCQA).

CREATING, MONITORING, AND EVALUATING OUTCOME MEASURES

Once the plan is crafted, the case manager is responsible for initiating the interventions and monitoring the program's effectiveness. The case manager must judge the plan's capability to meet the program's outcome goals for the patient using both objective and subjective data. It is not uncommon to modify a plan based on patient progress, or the lack of progress. A key case management responsibility involves monitoring this information with progress reports to the health care team.

Documented outcomes measurements based on objective criteria are essential to evaluating a plan's success. The establishment of expected outcomes at the onset of care planning assists the case manager in evaluating the effectiveness of case management in achieving those outcomes. At FHP the various outcomes to be measured are a part of the data system. The case managers input the data as they work with the patient; the data are then used to generate reports on individual and overall outcomes.

Case management outcomes are numerous, and measurement of the outcomes is usually an evolutionary process. In the early design phase, FHP attempted to identify not only areas of concern, but areas staff would be interested in as the program evolved. With the FHP/Quality Continuum program, the initial outcome measurement was financial savings. As the program matured, measurements became more sophisticated. In this evolution, the measurements proceeded from financial and utilization based to measurement of process outcomes. Clinical outcomes and patient satisfaction outcomes are now in the forefront of the plan's developmental activities.

Financial savings is one of the most universal measures of case management effectiveness, and frequently is the indicator that gains and sustains management support. Case management saves money even though very few companies have undertaken any accurate analysis.[4] The FHP/Quality Continuum program has consistently yielded savings. In the first year of operation the program saved nearly four million dollars.

The methodology for the calculation of savings should be presented and agreed upon in advance. The FHP savings methodology yields extremely conservative results. However, they are universally accepted within the organization. Financial results and utilization improvements are readily obtained measures of effectiveness.

The next step in FHP's evolution toward comprehensive outcomes measurement was process measurement. The organization approached process measurement by implementing "clinical trax," guidelines developed by FHP for specific high-risk diagnostic findings, such as a breast mass, to reduce fragmentation, improve continuity, and decrease the time from first discovery of the finding to treatment. These "clinical trax" improved the process times and practice variation in several areas.

In all of FHP's outcomes measurement initiatives, the ability of the case manager to achieve the identified expected outcome is documented. The next step in FHP outcomes evolution is to evaluate the effectiveness of achieving the desired process outcome in improving the clinical status of the patient. The newly implemented data system will assist us in taking the next step. Establishing the data requirements to reach this step may seem like a formidable task, but it starts with documenting the expected outcomes of the program. It is also wise for the organization to look at long-term, in addition to short-term, outcomes.

Finally, patient and physician satisfaction is another measurement of case management effectiveness. Standard tools are available to assist with this task, but consideration should be given to the development of individualized instruments, which are invaluable in measuring the specific objectives of an organization's program.

ANTICIPATING THE PITFALLS

Three basic pitfalls can reduce the effectiveness of a case management program. First is a concept referred to as *layering*. Layering occurs when an organization "layers" job duties and responsibilities on its case manager. The most common example of this pitfall is combining the concurrent review nurse duties with the case management duties. The concurrent review nurses have immediate demands on their time with inpatient activities. Active case management activities are the first casualty, and the model quickly returns to traditional utilization management.

A second pitfall is dilution. In this situation, the case manager has only case management duties, but has an overwhelming number of patients to manage. The most common cause of this pitfall is poor patient identification. The most frequent targeting problem involves poor assessment. Patients that are "screened out" are not properly assessed, and are accepted into case management when not appropriate. Often, novice case managers will continue to manage patients beyond a point where intervention is effective. Both poor assessment and inappropriate retention prevent case managers from focusing on the truly high-risk patients.

Finally, "narrowing" may occur, which involves limiting the scope of case management activities in a manner that prevents the high-risk patient from getting early intervention. This pitfall most commonly occurs in disease-specific programs. For example, one program reviewed only patients with congestive heart failure (CHF). Because CHF was the diagnosis that resulted in numerous hospital admissions, clinic managers felt it essential to case manage these patients. The result was that case managers literally declined patients with obvious problems in order to case manage less needy CHF patients. Disease management is a worthwhile initiative, but requires a separate strategic integration plan.

Clearly, case management is an effective strategy in improving health care quality and enhancing cost effectiveness. In order to achieve the maximum results, great care is required from inception to implementation. A careful analysis of a health care organization's current situation and implementation of systems based on its strengths and organizational goals will place it ahead on the success curve.

REFERENCES

1. Pacala, J.T., et al. *Case Management in Health Maintenance Organizations: Final Report.* Washington, D.C.: Group Health Foundation, 1994.
2. Case Management Association of America. *Standard of Practice for Case Management.* Little Rock: CMSA, 1995.
3. Ibid.
4. Pacala et al., *Case Management.*
5. Zitter, M. *Special Report: Disease Management.* The Zitter Group, November, 1995.

Case Management: Meeting the Needs of Chronically Ill Patients in an HMO

Ronnie Grower, Bonnie Hillegass, and Fran Nelson

Individuals who need to access numerous health care services are often faced with negotiating a complex health care delivery system. In fee-for-service models, health care services can be fragmented and disorganized, having a negative impact on the quality of care and increasing costs. HMOs may eliminate some barriers to care by providing a continuum of services. By integrating case management into health care delivery, high-risk cases can be managed to ensure that the patient receives the appropriate level of care in the least restrictive and most cost-effective setting.

By offering a spectrum of services as alternatives to hospitalization and an extensive case management system, Health Plan of Nevada (HPN) has been able to manage high risk cases effectively. On a case-by-case basis, staff propose care plans based on desired outcomes, the least amount of invasion and restriction, and the most appropriate care setting.

The following article describes the Health Plan of Nevada's case management program, how it has evolved within the corporation, how it functions today, gaps that have been identified within the system, and a proposed model to better meet the needs of the chronically ill.

ORGANIZATIONAL OVERVIEW

Sierra Health Services, a managed care holding company, operates several subsidiaries that compose a vertically integrated health care delivery

Source: Reprinted from R. Grower, B. Hillegass, and F. Nelson, Case Management: Meeting the Needs of ChronicallyIll Patients in an HMO, *Managed Care Quarterly*, Vol. 4, No. 2, pp. 46–57, © 1996, Aspen Publishers, Inc.

system. Health Plan of Nevada (HPN), one of SHS's wholly owned subsidiaries, is a federally qualified and state-licensed health maintenance organization. HPN currently serves over 115,000 commercial group members. Since 1985, HPN has offered a Medicare-risk product, Senior Dimensions, which currently provides coverage to approximately 25,000 senior citizens in Nevada.

HPN provides care through a mixed group/network model HMO, with most of the primary physician health care, specialty services, and extensive alternative care services provided by SHS's other wholly owned subsidiaries. This integration of medical care, case management, home health, hospice, mental health, and volunteer services enables access to comprehensive services, enhances quality, and controls costs. An extensive case management system, alternative care network, and computerized information system offers a health care delivery system that supports members through a continuum of care and ensures that members are cared for in the least restrictive, most cost efficient, safe environment.

HPN provides a full range of services including ambulatory care, subacute care, inpatient acute care, rehabilitation services, nursing home care, extensive home health services, mental health and substance abuse services, and a hospice program. To enhance services to the frail and chronically ill, several innovative programs have been developed. Highlights of these programs are presented below.

SENIOR DIMENSIONS SERVICE CENTER

One unique aspect of HPN is its Senior Dimensions Service Center, a walk-in resource center for its Medicare-risk contract members. Senior Dimensions Service Center staff recognize and assist members with their special needs, specifically supporting multiproblem patients by assisting them with accessing medical care and social services (e.g., arranging medical appointments, referrals for durable medical equipment, financial aid, and transportation), providing member service support (e.g., explaining benefits, providing health education information), and offering supportive volunteer programs. The concept of the "one-stop shop" has proven to be very successful.

With a staff of fourteen, including a social worker, a nurse, member services representatives, and administrative and clerical staff, the Senior Dimensions Service Center assists more than 1,000 walk-ins and more than 3,000 phone call requests per month. The staff is also responsible for administering the new member orientation program.

All new Senior Dimensions members are invited to attend a monthly new member orientation session. The primary focus of the orientation is to highlight member benefits, offer preventive services, and conduct risk assessments. Prior to new member orientation, members receive a packet of information that includes the following risk assessment questionnaires: Personal Health and Social History (PHSH), Drug History and Screen, and Pulmonary Screen. Approximately 85 percent of new members return these risk assessment forms, and approximately 56 percent attend new member orientation.

RISK ASSESSMENT

The PHSH form assesses activities of daily living (ADLs), instrumental activities of daily living (IADLs), comorbidity, and the need for immediate medical services, durable medical equipment, patient education, or case management. If a PHSH is not received after the initial mailing, the new member is contacted by the Senior Dimensions Service Center staff, and another PHSH form is mailed. If it is not completed and returned within 60 days, a closure letter is sent to the member, and a copy of the letter is included in the medical record. This update to the medical record serves as a notification to the physician provider that, when the member accesses service for the first time, the PHSH is still outstanding and needs to be completed. It also serves as notification to the provider of a member with potential compliance issues.

Upon receipt, the PHSH forms are reviewed by Senior Dimensions Service Center staff to identify those members responding positively to questions identifying medical and psychosocial risk factors. These members are followed up with a phone call, and if they meet predefined criteria, are referred directly to home health, durable medical equipment (DME), or complex case management. The PHSH form is then placed in the medical record for reference by the provider.

This process has proven effective in identifying high-risk patients at the time of enrollment; however, it does not "discover" those members who have experienced a change of health status. HPN has begun to develop methods to enhance its ability to identify these members.

VOLUNTEERS

HPN began its first volunteer program in 1989 to give individuals an opportunity to use their skills, contribute to their community, and assist HPN members. The volunteer program was designed to enhance the services offered to patients and customers by providing services the staff would not otherwise be able to provide. Through participation in the HPN Volunteer Program, many individuals receive needed socialization and enhanced self-esteem. HPN benefits from the involvement of volunteers who act as ambassadors within the community. More than 40,500 hours of service have been volunteered since 1989. Presently there are 55 active volunteers who have volunteered over 3,800 hours of service in the first five months of 1995.

Volunteers hold a variety of positions throughout the SHS subsidiaries. The following are examples of volunteer functions:

Friendly Companion

Assists homebound members with letter writing, paper work, reading, and other duties as agreed upon by the volunteer and the client. The volunteer may also provide limited errand running for the client within five miles of the client's home. The volunteer, however, can not transport the clients at any time while volunteering. Friendly companion visits usually last one to three hours per week. Documentation of the visit is completed following each visit and submitted to the volunteer coordinator monthly, with contact available daily.

Friendly Caller Volunteer

Calls homebound members once every couple of weeks to check on them and to provide socialization and a friendly discussion. The volunteer may also direct clients to appropriate community resources for further assistance.

"Thinking of You" Cards

Cards mailed by volunteers once a month to provide a nice pick-me-up for the client. Cards generally contain a nice greeting and friendly poem.

Health Fair Volunteer

Conducts blood pressure checks, inputs risk assessment data into health risk appraisal machine (computer program), distributes information, conducts height and weight measurement.

Senior Dimensions Service Center Volunteer

Assists at blood pressure clinics and special projects and collates and sorts items for new member orientation and health promotion clinic.

SMA Clinic Volunteer

Assists in the medical records department, the laboratory, and/or the surgery waiting area, making patient reminder phone calls and administering patient callback surveys, organizing the physician's library, filing and collating papers, and greeting and directing patients.

Wheelchair Repair

Wheelchairs are repaired by volunteers for low-income members upon request.

HOME HEALTH

HPN extensively utilizes its home health benefits to support the multi-problem patient to remain in or return to his or her home. Family Healthcare Services (FHS), a wholly owned subsidiary of SHS, is the primary provider of home health services to HPN members. FHS is a full service home health care agency licensed by the state of Nevada and certified by Medicare and Medicaid.

HPN has taken a liberal approach to interpreting the Medicare-risk contract in its provision of home health services. The following are some examples of how HPN utilizes the home health benefit:

1. Skilled nursing for IV therapy. When patients are unable to learn procedures and do not have a caregiver, skilled nursing visits can be made at a frequency necessary to administer IV medications. These medications are a covered benefit paid for under a capitated arrangement FHS has with HPN.

2. As an alternative to hospitalization, skilled nursing visits may be provided for round-the-clock care.

3. Respiratory therapy services to evaluate patients' pulmonary needs and to make recommendations, as needed, to physicians.

4. Home health aide services for limited respite care (for patients requiring assistance with two or more ADLs).

5. Home health aide services for extended hours (8 to 12 hours) for a short period of time until the patient improves, or until other arrangements are made (i.e., placement or private hire).

6. Home health services can be provided to members residing in group homes. In these instances, HPN monitors the patient's environment, health status, and services provided by the group home.

SUBACUTE AND REHABILITATIVE CARE

HPN has been an innovator in the management of patients in the subacute setting. HPN uses subacute and skilled nursing facilities for medical or rehabilitative treatment as an alternative to acute facility stays. Therapy services are offered that are over and above the standard Medicare-risk program to avoid extended hospitalizations and institutionalization. HPN case managers determine whether rehabilitation is appropriate, regardless of the Medicare three-day hospital stay requirement. In addition, rehabilitation services may be authorized when strengthening is required to recover from acute functional loss following hospital admission; however, the patient may not have a "typical" rehabilitation diagnosis.

In 1990, HPN was the driving force in the development of a subacute facility in the Las Vegas area. HPN determined that *medical* as well as rehabilitative care could be delivered safely in a less restrictive, lower-cost setting than the acute hospitals. What makes HPN's subacute unit unique is that other programs admit primarily rehabilitative patients, while HPN's subacute facilities provide care to medical as well as to rehabilitative patients.

HPN's subacute program was developed in partnership with a skilled nursing facility, Shadow Mountain Transitional Care and Rehabilitation Center. Placement of the services at this level of care presented several challenges to HPN as well as to the facility. For instance, patients admitted to a subacute level of care had more complex medical problems and required more intense care than patients who typically were cared for in a skilled nursing facility. To manage appropriately the care of the subacute patient, HPN undertook a major staff development effort to provide the facility staff with necessary skills. Additional equipment needs and staffing were evaluated, and admission criteria were developed. In return, the skilled nursing facility supports patient and caregiver education and affords family members more time with the patient, including overnight stays and weekend passes when appropriate. This practice prepares patients for their return to the community.

CASE MANAGEMENT PROGRAM

A major innovation for HPN has been its case management program, which HPN uses to evaluate, monitor, and treat members with multiple problems. A brief description of its evolution may help the reader understand why and how the current case management model works for the multiproblem patient in an HMO. A timeline is presented in Table 5–1, highlighting HPN's steps in the development of a case management program.

In 1985, HPN contracted with an independent home health agency, traditionally serving the fee-for-service and Medicare market, to provide case management for its members. Initially, a medical case management approach was used to care for HPN's Medicare-risk patients who were hospitalized. Soon after, Family Healthcare Services (FHS) was purchased by SHS

Table 5–1 Health Plan of Nevada Case Management Timeline

Year	Event
1985	• Contracted with Family Healthcare Services (FHS) for case management—medical model.
1986	• Included social component to case management.
	• Established task force to design case management model.
1988	• Added complex case management for community-based clients.
1989	• Expanded case management to skilled nursing facilities and group homes.
	• Established Senior Dimensions Service Center.
1990	• Segregated hospital and alternative care management components.
1992	• Consolidated hospital and alternative care of case management components.
	• Established subacute unit and introduced case management.
	• Established case management program for AIDS patients.
1994	• Awarded grant by The Robert Wood Johnson Foundation to integrate case management in the ambulatory care setting.

and became the primary provider of home health services for HPN and the vehicle for delivering case management to frail elderly members in the community.

In 1986, FHS recognized that case management was lacking a social component and hired two social workers to manage the social issues such as support systems, financial management, and environmental deficits, and to help design a new model of case management for HPN. During this time, HPN established a task force to develop a case management model to better serve the needs of its Medicare-risk members who had complex medical and social problems. The task force included a family practitioner, with strong interests in geriatrics, a geriatric nurse practitioner, a social worker, a physical therapist, and then Chief Operating Officer of FHS.

After an extensive literature search and on-site visits to several model case management programs, the task force concluded that a medical/social case management system was the model that best met the needs of HPN's frail geriatric members. An outcome of this task force was the statement of philosophy and its interpretation that continues to be the foundation for providing case management services throughout HPN today:

Philosophy

We believe that case management is a critical element of our health care delivery system which allows us to truly manage care, to avoid fragmentation of services, and use our resources in the most effective manner. The goal of case management is to provide the continuity necessary to move the client along the continuum of care towards the least restrictive, safe, cost effective environment possible.

Interpretation

In accepting the challenge of this philosophy, we understand and support all aspects of case management. Rigid, fragmented, disorganized, unbalanced health care arrangements have a negative impact on the quality of the care provided and tend to increase cost. We accept the responsibility to bring providers and members to a fuller understanding of managed care by educating them in case management principles. Appropriate care decisions are based on quality, the least amount of invasion and restriction and the best fiscal environment on a case by case basis. In the interpretation of benefits, alternatives must be available that lead to health preservation and illness prevention in a cost-effective approach.

In 1988, case management services were adopted for community-based clients with multiple and complex problems. In 1989, case management was expanded to include residents of group homes and skilled nursing facilities. Further expansion of HPN's case management program included the establishment of the Senior Dimensions Service Center in 1989 to identify high-risk cases, and to provide simple case management and the "one-stop" resource center for the Medicare-risk enrollees.

In 1990 HPN modified its case management process by segregating the hospital and nonhospital case management components. With this reorganization, case managers in the hospital functioned alongside utilization reviewers and discharge planners, each carving out a separate piece of the process; this reorganization resulted in a regression back to the classical utilization management model. Recognizing the intensity of labor, duplication of effort, service fragmentation, and increased bed days caused by this process, in 1992 HPN reengineered to consolidate case management within one department, under the leadership of a geriatric nurse practitioner. Under this new organization, the role of the institutional case manager was redefined to incorporate case management, utilization review, and discharge planning. This model has been successful and is discussed under the heading "Institutional Case Management."

March 1992 marked the opening of a network of subacute units. Case management was introduced in the subacute setting to ensure coordination of medical services, patient advocacy, and utilization management. A case management program designed to meet the special needs of the AIDS and HIV-positive population was also established in 1992 and currently functions as a separate program within Family Home Hospice, a wholly owned subsidiary of Sierra Health Services.

From 1992 to 1995 the HPN case management program continued to be refined. Policies and procedures were developed that specified types of case management and associated service levels. Specialty services were designed for high-risk pregnancies and chronic pulmonary disease. Efforts during this time also focused on building an understanding of case management services throughout the corporation. In January 1995, a separate corporate department of Case Management Services was created.

CURRENT PROGRAM CHARACTERISTICS

Case management services are offered at varying levels of intensity throughout HPN and are outlined in Table 5–2. For example, simple case management (Level I) is demonstrated in the Senior Dimensions Service Center where staff assist members with arrangements for transportation and durable medical equipment. The Utilization Management Department identifies high-risk cases such as patients requiring transplants or dialysis. Home health and hospice provide a higher level of Case Management (Level II) by coordinating care for patients within their homes. Institutional case managers coordinate care for hospital discharge. In the ambulatory care setting, case management is provided by clinical nurses who instruct patients on disease process and medication usage.

A higher level of case management intensity is offered in the various institutional settings and through HPN's complex case management program. As the patient's needs become more complex and require intervention by professional staff, the case management services are provided by nurses and social workers specifically trained in complex case management. Levels III and IV involve medical, social, and psychological interventions and may require coordination of care across multiple sites of service and providers.

A typology of case management within HMOs was defined based on an index of intensity.[1] However, the complexity and depth of HPN's case management programs make it difficult to fit a single category. The characteristics of HPN's case management program can be better categorized by the setting in which these services are provided. Table 5–3 outlines the case management characteristics described within each setting: acute institutional (in-area), acute institutional (out-of-area), subacute/skilled nursing facility, custodial, and complex case management. In all settings, the case management staff performs the initial assessments on the enrollees and arranges services regardless of location.

Institutional Case Management

Throughout the various levels of institutional care, primary care physicians are teamed with nurse case managers. In the subacute/acute facilities, the physicians are internists; for skilled nursing facility patients, the physician is a family practitioner with extensive geriatric experience. Within the teams, clinical case managers specialize in areas such as geriat-

Table 5-2 HPN Case Management Levels of Intensity

Level of intensity	Description	Examples	Provided by
Level I	Very simple One episode or contact Case finding	Arrange transportation Arrange durable medical equipment Arrange provider appointments Provide Friendly Caller services	Prior Authorization staff Member Services staff Senior Center staff Clinic Office staff
Level II	Simple One episode or contact Case finding Risk assessment Requires intervention of professional staff	Coordinate care for hospital discharge Serve as liaison between client and medical services Teach patient disease process and medication usage Coordinate community-based programs	Physicians/physician extenders Clinical RNs Institutional case managers Home health providers
Level III	Complex Short-term Medical, social, or psychological interventions Requires intervention of social worker or nurse case manager	Monitor compliance of medications Coordinate care Monitor health status Coordinate financial needs with community resources Provide risk assessment and monitor safety in home environment	Social workers Nurse case managers Home health specialty care nurses Clinical pharmacists
Level IV	Complex Long-term Medical, social, or psychological interventions Catastrophic or chronic care needs Requires intervention of social worker or nurse case manager Requires coordination of care across multiple sites of service and/or providers	Coordinate medical, social, and psychological services for complex cases such as transplant, multiple trauma, end-stage renal disease, and AIDS/HIV Assist patients with substance abuse disorders Assist terminal patients with end-of-life decision making	Social workers Nurse managers

Table 5-3 Characteristics of Case Management Models

| Program characteristics | Acute institutional in-area | Acute institutional out-of-area | Institutional | | |
			Subacute/skilled nursing facility	Custodial	Complex
Location	Hospital	Corporate	Transitional care facility Long-term care facility	Transitional care facility Long-term care facility	Corporate
Case load	less than 19	20–39	20–39	100–119	60–79
Amount of face-to-face contact with enrollee	95%	0%	100%	100%	50%
Case management provided	YES	NO	YES	YES	YES
Number of case managers	20	3	7	7	10

rics, medical/surgery, subacute care, and terminal/hospice care. The case management team physicians become the exclusive attending physicians, responsible for the patient's care until the patient is discharged, at which time responsibility is returned to the PCP.

HPN's team approach to case management has been very successful for all parties because it has

- facilitated communication between the case manager and physician
- decreased delays in changing levels of care to the least restrictive care setting
- decreased fragmentation of care at discharge
- increased follow-through on postdischarge tests and appointments
- assisted skilled nursing facility staff in appropriate use of services, thus avoiding unnecessary transfers to emergency rooms.

Acute Institutional In-Area

HPN clients who are admitted to an inpatient facility have a plan of care started within 24 hours of admission. Case managers are on-site, seven days a week, to conduct initial evaluations and to develop treatment and discharge plans for the patient. Information is obtained by interviewing the patient and family, reviewing the patient chart, and consulting with the physician.

The physician/case manager teams meet every morning, seven days a week, to review their patients. During this review, they discuss the appropriate level of care, whether the patient can be in a less restrictive setting, potential home health or complex case management needs upon discharge, and any follow-up needs at discharge such as scheduling of appointments or tests.

Acute Institutional Out-of-Area

When a patient is hospitalized out of the HPN service area, an out-of-area case manager telephonically monitors the patient's care and coordinates discharge needs. The case manager works with the patient's family, provider, and the facility's discharge planning/UR staff to ensure the least restrictive, safe, cost-efficient setting for the patient. The case manager may be involved with arranging transportation, home assessments, case conferencing, and psychosocial, home health, or therapy services. If a face-to-face intervention is required, an on-site visit is made by a contracted case management provider in the area.

Subacute Skilled Nursing

A significant accomplishment of the HPN case management program was the integration of the physician/case management team with the subacute/skilled nursing facility staff. Daily rounding of the physician/case manager team and periodic assessments, based on level of care and need, contribute to the success of this program.

Custodial

In the custodial setting, the geriatric nurse practitioner supports the physician by providing medical services to the patient between physician visits. For the patient with complex issues, the geriatric nurse practitioner also serves as case manager (a model similar to that used by EverCare in Minneapolis, Minnesota). For the patient with simpler case management issues, a nurse case manager is assigned. The nurse case manager uses the geriatric nurse practitioner on a consulting basis.

Complex Case Management

All patients who are identified as high-risk are referred to HPN's Complex Case Management (CCM) Program. Complex case management is the coordination of care and monitoring of health status for these high-risk, complex, or catastrophic cases. Most of these patients remain in the community, the primary goal being to delay institutionalization and inappropriate access of care. Approximately 70 percent of the HPN CCM caseload is the Medicare-risk product enrollees. The CCM Program is designed to manage large or complex cases alone, or in conjunction with other divisions of SHS. Complex case managers can be either RNs with experience in case management or social workers. The complex case manager has overall responsibility for the case, regardless of setting.

Complex cases have the need for medical, social, and/or financial case management. Indicators for referrals to HPN's complex case management services include:

- *Medical* indicators such as hospital readmissions within specific time frames, noncompliance/discontinuity issues, need for specialized medical services out of the service area, or specific diagnostic groups such as AIDS/HIV, dialysis, transplant, progressive severe neurological disorders, end-stage/terminal disease process, high-risk pregnancy.
- *Social* indicators such as unsafe home environment, abuse and neglect, inability to perform IADLs, inability to access medical care on an ongoing basis, or family assistance with long-term care placement.
- *Financial* indicators such as inability to pay for long-term custodial care or medications exceeding plan limitations.

After an initial assessment by the complex case manager, which may be conducted either in person or telephonically, the frequency and type of contact are determined:

High Intensity

Typically crisis intervention that requires contact until the crisis is resolved, then weekly home visits until the situation stabilizes (example: potential client abandonment by family, working on alternative placement).

Moderate Intensity

Requires a home visit one to two times per month. Typically services clients with chronic "unstable conditions" such as coronary obstruction pulmonary disease (COPD) and diabetes or those more stable requiring in-person assessments such as patients with Alzheimer's disease. This intervention would also be appropriate for patients recently discharged from the hospital.

Low Intensity

Requires at least monthly telephone contact. Clients may require follow-up on services that were arranged and possible Friendly Caller services. Members residing in group homes are typically served under this category. In these cases the case manager coordinates services with the group home to ensure that the member receives the appropriate medical care and necessary social services to prevent hospitalization or institutionalization.

Oversight

This level of service is provided when other case management services are involved in the case. In these instances, the case manager works closely with other care providers to offer continuity and coordination. Patients served by home health or hospitalized would fall into this category.

Table 5–4 describes examples of the management of different types of cases that are referred to complex case management.

CURRENT MODEL

Health Plan of Nevada has succeeded in both integrating case management services throughout its alternative care network and in identifying high-risk Medicare patients when they initially enroll in the HMO. However, for those members of the plan who age-in-place or develop chronic illnesses after enrollment, the need exists to work within the primary care setting to identify and serve these individuals who could benefit from case management. Often, patients are first seen by nurses or case managers in the hospital or alternative care settings in a crisis situation, inappropriately accessing care or not complying with treatment regimens.

The distribution of complex case management referral sources confirms that a large proportion of members are referred at the time of crisis (Table

Table 5–4 Complex Case Management Issues and Interventions

Client identified problems	Interventions
No primary care physician and chronic medical problems require ongoing medical supervision	Case manager (CM) to make initial PCP appointment and work to ensure follow-up visits.
Noncompliance with medication usage	RN CM to conduct home visit to provide education and follow-up for medication compliance on a weekly basis.
Difficulty accessing or understanding HMO system of care	CM to explain how to access the system for medical/social services and to assist with referral process. CM to serve as liaison between client and medical services, if needed.
Lack of understanding of medical problems, disease process, and medication	RN CM to teach and monitor effects of noncompliance upon body, side effects, and exacerbation of disease processes until patient is stable.
Difficulty coordinating services for multi-problem patients with psychosocial and medical needs	Team of RN CM and social worker to conduct initial comprehensive assessment and develop treatment plan that focuses on psychosocial and medical problems with appropriate interventions and follow through.
Need for coordination of community-based assistance programs and insurance benefits	Medical social worker to coordinate treatment to avoid duplication of service providers.
Financial difficulties	Medical social worker to coordinate client's financial needs with available community resources.
Need for coordination of care for organ transplant patients	RN case manager to work with "Centers of Excellence" and coordinate psychosocial, financial, and physiological services.
Drug-seeking behaviors	RN CM or social worker identifies reasons for drug-seeking behaviors and coordinates resources to assist client in treatment.

Table 5–4 Continued

Client identified problems	Interventions
Substance abuse disorders	RN CM or social worker to identify diagnosis and refer for appropriate treatment (e.g., detoxification, treatment programs, counseling). CM to follow patient until stabilized and has adequate support system.
Terminal diagnosis	RN CM to follow patient during treatment to monitor deterioration and assist with end-of-life decision making.
Hospitalization	RN CM to coordinate care with hospital CM. RN CM to follow case after hospital discharge.
Chronic patients receiving home health services	RN CM to coordinate long-term care services with home health primary care nurse.
At risk in current home environment	Team approach of RN CM, social worker and occupational therapist to conduct safety evaluation, develop plan of care, and follow patient until stabilized in home environment or alternate care setting.

5–5). Twenty-five percent of all complex case management referrals are initiated when patients are in the hospital, and another 20 percent are referred once they are receiving home health or hospice. Physicians are responsible for only 11 percent of the referrals to complex case management, yet the focal point of patient care is in the primary care setting. In the absence of a systematic means for referring members to complex case management from the primary care setting, the process becomes erratic and opportunities are lost for early intervention to prevent the decline of patient functional status and to assist patients in accessing services appropriately.

These findings led HPN to transition from a case management model to a care coordination model in which the primary care staff is educated in case management, and pharmaceutical services and case management are integrated into the ambulatory care setting. The intention of this model is to impact positively the quality of care provided to at-risk individuals served by an HMO.

IMPROVED CARE COORDINATION MODEL

A multidisciplinary project team was formed representing case management, clinical nursing, pharmacy, physicians, and the Senior Dimensions Service Center. Members of the team met several times to brainstorm and develop interventions that would better serve at-risk patients who would benefit from care coordination. The case management model was redefined into a more closely coordinated system that involved the entire health care team. A variety of ideas emerged relating to early, systematic identification and case management process. Some of these ideas included:

Table 5–5 Complex Case Management Referral Sources (1994)

Referral sources	%
Institutional case managers	25
Home health or hospice	20
Senior Dimensions Service Center	12
Physician	11
Utilization management	7
Patient or member	7
Urgent care	3
Member services	2
Mental health providers	3
Other	10
Total	100

- on-site case managers assigned to the clinic setting
- training of clinic providers and staff on identification of at-risk members and availability of case management resources within all provider sites
- preventative health screening activities supported by a resource coordinator (Level I case manager) who would assist members with completion of questionnaires and coordination of preventive health needs
- ongoing risk assessment
- medication compliance screening
- software to test potential interactions and provide drug-specific information to patients
- pharmacy consultation
- patient education on medication usage for an older population

The project team expected that these interventions would improve the quality of care by increasing provider and staff knowledge of available case management resources and increasing identification of at-risk cases after enrollment and before crises. They also anticipated that the interventions would result in proper utilization of services including hospitalization, urgent care visits, and overall expenditures.

One of eight clinic sites of Southwest Medical Associates, SHS's wholly owned medical group practice, was selected as the pilot site. Approximately 80 percent of the HMO enrollees use Southwest Medical Associates, Nevada's largest multispecialty medical group. The first intervention HPN attempted to implement was the introduction of low-level case management support to improve compliance with HPN Preventive Health guidelines. This activity required the front desk clinic staff to give to each patient a Personal Health Record form that highlights age- and sex-specific recommendations for preventive services including immunizations, cholesterol testing, breast exams, and pap and pelvic exams. Once in the examination room, the nurse reviewed the recommendations with the patient and suggested the appropriate tests, counseling, or health education classes. Patients needing or requesting classes or additional literature were referred to a resource coordinator, a case manager (Level I), who is knowledgeable in accessing resources.

Efforts to implement the intervention met with resistance and confusion from the clinic staff. The project team met again to review staff feedback on the new process. It was clear that without influencing the culture in the clinic and without "buy-in" from all levels of the clinic staff, the expectations for the project would not be met. Rather than simply applying new resources to the clinic setting, the project team decided it was necessary to truly integrate those who provide case management by making them part of the clinic team and physically locating them at the clinic site. These were the initial steps in implementing the care coordination model. It was proposed that the ambulatory care coordination team would include the primary care provider, clinic nurse and/or nursing supervisor, office manager, case manager, social worker, resource coordinator, and clinical pharmacist. This team would be charged with coordinating the patient's care and service needs at the ambulatory care site.

To address the resistance issues expressed by the clinic staff, the project team developed an action plan. The designated "on-site case manager" spent two weeks orienting to the ambulatory care site, learning current operations. A meeting was held with the clinic's medical director to explain the project's objectives, specific interventions, advantages to the clinic, and to introduce the case management team. This was followed by a meeting with all levels of the clinic staff and providers to present the program, identify potential barriers to implementation, explain case management, review project objectives, and outline the benefits of having additional resources at the clinic site.

As part of the effort to identify potential barriers to implementation, the project team developed a staff questionnaire designed to assess the clinic staff's case management knowledge and to identify areas in which on-site case management could assist the staff with their current workload.

Moving the model to a care coordination delivery system and implementation of the ambulatory case management model began in July 1995.

LESSONS LEARNED

Although HPN is in the early stages of implementing the integration program at one clinic site, the following issues have already surfaced that may be helpful to other HMOs struggling with similar scenarios:

- Center care coordination in the primary care setting. The physician's office is the focal point of patient care and provides the greatest opportunity to intervene and therefore prevent or forestall functional decline and institutionalization of at-risk patients.
- Identify and include all disciplines who have a role in care coordination (e.g., front desk staff, physicians, nurses). Each member of the team has potential contact with the patient at different times during the office visit and each of these encounters offers another reference point from which to determine the patient's needs. Patients may tell the front desk staff about medical transportation problems that they would never discuss with a physician.

- Define the care coordination model with participation from all involved disciplines. To ensure that the model is comprehensive and addresses all of the patient's medical, social, and psychological needs, input is necessary from all areas, including mental health, nursing, social work, therapies (e.g., physical, occupational, speech), and pharmacy. This process also ensures "buy-in" from all participants.
- Communicate expectations and roles to all levels of staff that will be affected by the model. Allow opportunity to discuss and address potential barriers for implementation or misunderstandings regarding roles and responsibilities.
- Do not put resources in place until it is understood how proposed interventions will work with existing processes.
- Do not develop an organizational chart before testing the intervention. Too much attention to reporting structure can interfere with the creation of a successful model.
- Do not look at case management in isolation. All integrating components need to be considered in developing a care coordination model.

HPN continues to test and modify its evolving care coordination model. The company believes that educating the primary care staff in case management, integrating case management and pharmaceutical services into the ambulatory care setting, and conducting ongoing risk assessments will positively impact the quality of care provided to their chronically ill, multiproblem patients. The feasibility of this model is currently being evaluated by HPN under a grant from The Robert Wood Johnson Foundation. Should the results prove positive, HPN will be expanding its study to include additional clinic sites as well as network providers.

REFERENCE

1. Pacala, J.T., et al. "Case Management in Health Maintenance Organizations, Final Report." In *Chronic Care Initiatives in HMOs*. Washington, D.C.: Group Health Foundation, 1994.

6

The Role of Health Organizations in Integrating Care for Persons with Special Health Care Needs

David Siegel and Nancy Combs Habel

CHANGES IN SPECIALIZED HEALTH CARE

Integration of care for persons with special health care needs increasingly is recognized not only as the honored, traditional domain of the personal care physician, but also as a key emerging role for the patient's sponsoring health organization, whether services are based in public health, a health system, a managed care plan, or a collaboration among agencies.

Important roles coexist for individuals capable and motivated in self-care, including adult children, parents, and other lay caregivers. The collaboration of patient, provider, sponsoring health organization, and lay support networks is critical to effective health service integration for all individuals—but is most acutely important for those with special needs.

Individuals are likely to pass through life stages where they will experience special health care needs. For some, such conditions will be temporary; for others, the chronicity of impairment will be life-changing.

In this article, *persons with special health care needs* refers to those who face extraordinary life challenges, particularly those who have identifiable health impairments that compromise their activities in more than one functional dimension. *Integrated care,* known in some settings as *coordinated care,* denotes a complement of services that are aligned by common protocols and collaborative practices to enhance the efficiency, effective-

Source: Reprinted from D. Siegel and N.C. Habel, The Role of Health Organizations in Integrating Care for Persons with Special Health Care Needs, *Managed Care Quarterly,* Vol. 4, No. 3, pp. 1–5, © 1996, Aspen Publishers, Inc.

ness, comfort, convenience, and outcomes associated with specific conditions or diseases.

In Detroit a number of approaches have been developed to integrate care for a variety of populations ranging from seniors to school children, from the unborn to the chronically ill. The following discussion suggests opportunities that health care organizations are starting to implement to maximize the health potential of persons with special needs.

PUBLIC OR PRIVATE? THE DISTINCTION BLURS

One of the nation's most comprehensive regional health systems, Henry Ford Health System (HFHS) was established in 1915 when auto pioneer Henry Ford founded Henry Ford Hospital, today a 903-bed urban tertiary care teaching and research center. Four community hospitals, joint-venture management of four additional hospitals, and two nursing homes complete the HFHS inpatient service component. Outpatient services are provided through a multispecialty group practice of more than 1,000 physicians operating out of 36 ambulatory care sites and other locations. The managed care component, Health Alliance Plan (HAP), contracts with more than 2,000 additional independent providers throughout southeastern Michigan and through its Toledo subsidiary, Medical Value Plan.

With a managed care membership of over 500,000 and 250,000 more persons seeking care through fee-for-service channels, HFHS has a combined patient base larger than the population of many cities. In many respects, HFHS sees itself as a public health agency because the organization faces many common challenges with public health, including disease management for persons with special needs.

SERVING THE FEW WHILE MANAGING THE MANY

HMOs often are better at managing costs than at managing care. One of capitation's great vulnerabilities is how to serve the acute, particular needs of the few while also efficiently managing the more common needs of the many. An average or better-than-average case mix is stereotypically thought to be optimal; and outside of research circles there may be little perceived reward in taking care of high-risk patients whose needs confound the benefit summary and tax the utilization management program.

Yet the opposite is true. Providing effective integrated care to those with special needs will not only optimize the outcomes of the few but actually improve the health of the many, and the effectiveness of the health system itself. In fact, a system's ability to care for special needs populations can be a chief indicator of organizational care competence, and may provide as well a template for building the infrastructure capable of serving the population at large.

These care strategies fall into three functional areas which by their very nature, are cross-cutting:

1. Strategies that *inform and validate,* providing data about the patient, risk group, or efficacy of the chosen intervention.
2. Strategies that *intervene, educate, and empower,* providing tools for effective care management and patient self-management.
3. Strategies that *catalyze change and build consensus,* imbuing a sense of mission among all participants.

To succeed, strategies within these three functional sets depend on well-designed communications, and the nurturing of collaborative partnership at all levels including the patient, lay caregivers, physician and nonphysician providers, and sponsoring health agency, system, or managed care organization.

Strategies that Inform and Validate

Research and evaluation strategies run the gamut from health status inventories, to finding best practices, to development of specific programmatic evaluation designs. However, evaluation should be begun by understanding and disaggregating meaningful categories of risk within various communities and populations. Strategies can include the use of population-based surveys or indicators such as health risk assessments, functional status surveys, sentinel health or disease indicators, and a search of pharmaceutical or other encounter databases in order to identify at-risk individuals.

In addition to the requisite subscriber contract, managed care organizations should be welcoming new members with an assessment of their needs, preferences, and health status. They should also routinely ask questions such as, "Do you smoke?" "Are you using more than one prescription drug?" "How many times have you been to see your doctor in the past year?" and "Do you or a dependent have special health care needs?" Members' responses can provide baselines for individual coordination of care, and guide organizational priorities for risk reduction in our populations at large.

Individuals and subgroups not seeking service, long an organizational blind spot, require special outreach strategies. A good place to start is to identify barriers to care, including access problems, referral patterns, transportation, language, and cultural differences. One pervasive barrier may be the personal value of health itself, which is not a motivator to some to the same degree as more immediate concerns like adequate housing, income, and personal safety. Health care organizations need to explore the psychosocial and environmental factors that influence health behaviors, and then test nontraditional venues of care which may be more readily received.

Along with patient and member health status, organizations need to measure as well the strength of their own care competencies. System performance can be tracked using criteria including effectiveness, efficiency, and client satisfaction. For specific conditions, key quality measures may include frequency of preventive services; adequacy of and access to a continuum of care; comprehensiveness of screening and follow-up programs; and outcomes related both to individual and categorical health status. The National Committee for Quality Assurance (NCQA) and Health Plan Employer Data Information Set (HEDIS) have presented unprecedented opportunities for health plans to begin to collect much of such data on more common conditions, and report it in a publicly accountable manner. But the work should not stop there.

Many health systems are redesigning information systems to support decision making, facilitate analysis, and report information back to individual practitioners and their peers so that they can judge their own effectiveness. Particularly when addressing the needs of high-risk populations, such data-driven provider feedback has the potential to favorably impact admissions, emergency visits, and adherence to clinical guidelines.

Finally, continuous research of best practices—benchmarking other health agencies that are addressing comparable opportunities—provides a veritable learning lab for service accountability and redesign. External data can be used in conjunction with internal best-practice information by quality improvement teams convened around condition- or process-related goals.

Strategies that Intervene, Educate, and Empower

Whether directed at persons or populations, patient interventions need to be guided by both research and an understanding of individual preferences.

Clinicians often envision patient demand as inexorable, and respond by managing what they can immediately control: the supply of medical services. Now new questions are being asked: "How can the value of physician encounters be offered in alternate ways?" "How can patients be supported in their interest to function with maximum independence?" Health care organizations are learning to manage demand, as well as supply.

Many health systems, HMOs, and independent companies, including (notably) some pharmaceutical firms, are developing targeted programs tailored to meet the needs of persons and subgroups with categorical risk profiles. These risk groups may include subpopulations of persons failing to obtain preventive health services, patients with a specific common chronic disease, or individuals with a common functional impairment or vulnerability. No doubt new at-risk categories will emerge as medical science matures in fields of genetics, behavioral medicine, and prevention. Prescreening for risk factors and genetic counseling in at-risk populations can be neighborhood-based to broaden participation and further impact community health.

Case management is widely recognized as a central tool to screen, assess, plan, and evaluate the care of those with specific disease conditions or functional impairments. Interdisciplinary case management teams may include (in addition to attending nurses) primary and specialty physicians, a health educator, social worker, home health provider, or others who regularly influence or deliver care. Often, the participation of a behavioral medicine specialist can help patients and families recognize and ameliorate stresses in the home that could have an impact on health status.

Certain conditions may best be addressed by multidisciplinary clinics that cluster services around the patient, or centers of excellence, providing high-quality subspecialty services at a lower cost. Health care organizations should be working to include such "essential community providers" in their delivery systems when the value of such services is demonstrable.

To the greatest extent possible, organizations need to design interventions that empower the patient and caregiver with knowledge, self-care tools, and a heightened sense of responsibility for their health. Giving patients a choice among a set of qualified providers may enhance a sense of personal autonomy and facilitate relationship-building. Patient support groups, facilitated by nonphysician providers, can promote peer learning and treatment compliance.

Clinical support systems can help patients and caregivers better manage their health issues. Features of such systems may include phone-based nurse advisors, audio health libraries, interactive shared decision making programs, computer links with other patients or pertinent health information, and audience-appropriate printed or audiovisual materials.

Automated patient registries are dynamic tools that do much more than simply record information. A computerized registry can facilitate upstream intervention for at-risk individuals and groups by providing clinical prompts for appropriate services as well as tracking mechanisms that are accessible, up-to-date, and user-friendly for providers and support staff.

Dentists, veterinarians, auto dealers, and lawn services understand the efficacy of direct mail to increase compliance with preventive care. Some physician practices, too, are learning to combine their patient registries with communication technologies to "build business" for preventive services by issuing postcard reminders for immunizations, screenings, and other preventive care services.

Marketing science increasingly allows disaggregation and segmentation, with media and messages tailored to individual and subgroup preference, age, literacy level, and cultural setting. Health care organizations should test a variety of media to determine the most effective communication vehicles, which can range from simple brochures and newsletters to videocassettes, mobile health units, and the World Wide Web.

Most managed care plans quietly and unofficially apply principles of segmentation to their benefit design, reaching beyond medical necessity to extend benefits on a case-by-case basis for those with special needs. In continuing this practice we need to monitor adjudication turnaround time, to ensure that our patient's health is not compromised by administrative red tape.

Strategies that Catalyze Change and Build Consensus

Research, evaluation, management, and communication competencies are critical to effective integrated programs of care for persons with special needs. But a third set of strategies must be engaged as well if these programs are to have more than a random impact on individual or group health. A sustainable program of integrated health services requires a core organizational commitment to the program mission.

Communication and provider education strategies can create opportunities for innovation, and facilitate input into care-path planning and implementation. Interest is heightening among many clinicians toward the antecedent, familial, environmental, and genetic causes of disease. Further, an increasing body of knowledge on the cognitive aspects of disease and health is drawing the attention of traditional medical circles. Health care organizations will be able to capitalize on the current focus in the literature by building timely internal awareness of their own best practices and capabilities. They may be able to engage even the most disaffected parties with these approaches:

- Use data to prove effectiveness, build resources, change minds.
- Offer continuing medical education–accredited programs to enhance interest.
- Encourage interdisciplinary dialogue in the identification, prioritizing, and design of prevention and disease management programs.
- Use explicit decision analysis and multidisciplinary teams to develop the assumptions inherent in common, momentous, and difficult decision making. Be willing to set priorities and to use best available empiric data to estimate outcomes of contemplated actions, accounting for confidence boundaries.

- Promote the benefits that clinicians will experience as the result of patient self-care education, shared decision making, and nonphysician-provider initiatives (e.g., increased patient compliance and self-responsibility, more "quality time" in the clinic setting, and evidence of better patient outcomes).
- Find physician "champions" for specific initiatives to stimulate interest and build consensus among diverse provider groups.

Consensus building need not be limited to inside institutional walls. All who compete in a community, which is virtually everyone, should do so with great mindfulness of the impact of such activity.

Whenever possible, organizations need to identify and collaborate with others in having an impact on causes of health and disease that occur in the community—those causes that are generally too widespread to be affected by a single agency alone. Teen pregnancy happens in neighborhoods, not in the clinician's office. Organizations should save competition for more closely held strategies that differentiate their unique competence in circumscribed areas of practice.

The interdependency of the strategies cited here is highly evident. Research and evaluation determine need, approach, and effectiveness. Intervention, education, and empowerment strategies help to optimize health status by improving self-care and caregiver competencies. Consensus building with organizational and community partners is a catalyst for change, creates integrated care paths and guidelines, and furthers the paradigm of prevention in substantive ways for all.

At the heart of any program of integrated services is the patient. Regardless of the level of chronicity, debilitation, or special need, the patient and lay caregiver should be regarded as full partners—indeed, the primary partners—in the process of care. Professional caregivers can learn to complement these natural care teams.

The most demanding clients can offer organizations a source of strength. If health plans truly wish to be providers of health, not strictly providers of medicine, they must integrate services first around populations with special needs. This is not to say that health systems should retreat from upstream education and prevention for the well, or for those at lower-than-average risk of disease. Their efforts must be strategic and comprehensive, identifying and engaging individuals at all levels of risk. But it is from those persons with special needs that organizations can learn the most: not only about their patients' particular needs, but also about the organization's own capacity to effectively improve the health of the various communities they serve.

III

Reorganizing Primary Care

7

Improving Outcomes in Chronic Illness

Edward H. Wagner, Brian T. Austin, and Michael Von Korff

Chronic illnesses confront patients and their caregivers with the dread of a restricted and uncertain future, and the burdens associated with controlling the disease. The care of patients with chronic illnesses has become a priority for managed care organizations, which are increasingly recognizing the importance of developing organized systems of care for all their patients with chronic illness. Large purchasers are demanding evidence of an effect on outcomes, and most organizations realize that this will not be achieved by their historical tendency to offer a smattering of individual components, a case manager here or a patient education class there, that reach only a small percentage of patients. Many HMOs and other large managed care systems have begun to construct integrated care management strategies for common chronic illnesses. Current efforts appear to be based more on intuition and benchmarking or copying other organizations than on a scientific foundation or explicit conceptual model. For example, some organizations are building integrated systems based in and supportive of primary care while others are developing highly focused, specialized "carve-out" systems for various patient groups. Both approaches are being pursued by integrated health care systems at present, sometimes even within the same system.

In this article, we consider the demands placed on patients and families by chronic illness and the difficulties that medical care faces in trying to help patients meet these challenges. We then review literature that suggests

Source: Reprinted from E.H. Wagner, B.T. Austin, and M. Von Korff, Improving Outcomes in Chronic Illness, *Managed Care Quarterly*, Vol. 4, No. 2, pp. 12–25, © 1996, Aspen Publishers, Inc.

promising strategies for optimizing outcomes in chronic illness, and propose a conceptual model for an integrated approach to improving care. Finally, we discuss the questions and challenges health care organizations face in trying to design and implement care improvement programs for chronically ill patients.

THE NEEDS OF PATIENTS WITH CHRONIC ILLNESS

Patients facing the discomforts and self-management demands of chronic illness struggle to maintain a productive, hopeful life. The management of their illness requires that they accomplish a series of tasks[1]:

- Engage in activities that promote health and build physiologic reserve, including exercise, nutrition, social activation, and sleep.
- Interact with health care providers and systems and adhere to recommended treatment protocols.
- Monitor physical and emotional status, and make appropriate management decisions on the basis of symptoms and signs.
- Manage the impacts of the illness on ability to function in important roles, on emotions and self-esteem, and on relations with others.

The achievement of optimal outcomes in chronic illness requires the successful accomplishment of these tasks; and effective health care for chronic illness should support patients in accomplishing these tasks.

THE DEFICIENCIES OF CURRENT CHRONIC ILLNESS CARE

High-quality medical care for chronic illnesses must accomplish three objectives:

1. assure the delivery of those interventions (evaluations and treatment, medical and psychosocial) that have been shown by rigorous evidence to be effective;
2. empower patients to take responsibility for the management of their condition[2,3]; and
3. provide information, support, and resources to assist patients in self-management tasks.

Deficiencies in the medical care of patients with chronic illness have been recognized. Surveys and audits have documented failures of practitioners to comply with well-established guidelines for the clinical aspects of care for patients with hypertension,[4] diabetes,[5] asthma,[6] frailty in the elderly,[7] and other chronic conditions. In addition, provider surveys indicate that many professional caregivers feel unprepared or too rushed to be able to meet the educational, behavioral, and psychosocial needs of chronically ill patients and their caregivers.[8]

While deficiencies in training may play a role, the culture and structure of usual medical practice may be a larger problem. Medical practices, especially those in primary care, are generally oriented and organized to respond to the acute and urgent needs of their patients. The emphasis is on diagnosis, particularly ruling out serious disease, and treatment of symptoms and physiologic abnormalities. Because primary care practices and practitioners are so oriented to acute illness, there may be little difference in clinical approach to patients with acute and chronic illness. Kottke and colleagues[9] argue that the health care system gives priority to urgent problems and "encourages physicians in clinical settings to be respondents, not initiators." This priority leaves little time or intellectual energy for addressing the less urgent, but predictable needs of patients with chronic illness in managing their condition and preventing deleterious sequelae.

In a busy practice day with a mixture of acute and chronically ill patients, it is difficult for even the most motivated providers to assure the elements of care associated with good outcomes in chronic illness: systematic assessments, preventive interventions, effective education, psychosocial support, and consistent follow-up. "Dual task theory" may explain why dealing with symptoms "distracts attention from" preventive or physician-initiated actions.[10] Dual task theory suggests that when confronted with multiple tasks, individuals will first perform those that have the greatest emotional investment. Physicians appear to fear missing serious illness more than other types of errors,[11] which probably explains the behavioral preference for "symptom swatting" over routine assessment, counseling, and the other elements of good chronic illness care.

Office staff and systems are also geared to react to acute illness and urgent care. Most practice teams have no time or inclination to meet and thus have not organized themselves for chronic illness care. Nonphysician staff are occupied with managing access and patient flow, so that responsibilities for planning care, counseling, and follow-up are not delegated and, by default, fall to the physician. Information necessary for organizing or planning care is buried in a paper medical record, which for patients with chronic illness is likely to be staggeringly thick. The lack of organization and information reinforces the focus on today's symptoms and physiologic abnormalities. A focus on symptoms encourages the addition of empirical pharmacological remedies contributing to the chronically ill patient's drug burden.

We hypothesize that these deficiencies in the delivery of routine care for patients with chronic illness contribute to suboptimal outcomes because of

- delays in the detection of complications or declines in health status due to irregular or incomplete assessments or inadequate follow-up;
- failures in self-management of the illness or risk factors due to patient passivity or ignorance as a result of inadequate or inconsistent patient assessment, education, motivation, and feedback;
- reduced quality of care due to the omission of effective interventions or commission of ineffective ones;
- undetected or inadequately managed psychosocial distress.

SUCCESSFUL CHRONIC ILLNESS CARE

The literature provides useful clues about the characteristics of practices and care systems that have been associated with improved outcomes in chronic disease. For example, drug treatment trials like the Diabetes Control and Complications Trial,[12] the Systolic Hypertension in the Elderly Program,[13] or the Hypertension Detection and Follow-up Program,[14-16] which have shown improved outcomes, wrap the drug therapy in a carefully delineated care model to assure continued follow-up, compliance with the regimen, careful assessment of side effects and other outcomes, and so on. The "wrapping" may provide important clues as to successful ways of organizing and delivering care for chronic illness.

These and other successful intervention trial protocols follow an explicit plan, which includes regularly scheduled follow-up, systematic assessments, and attention to the educational needs of patients. The plan or protocol is executed largely through delegation of key care functions to nonphysician members of the practice team. The systematic delegation of major aspects of the protocol to nurses, pharmacists, and other members of the practice team is a hallmark of randomized trials and other successful efforts to improve chronic illness outcomes. The work of the team is enhanced by information systems that track key processes and outcomes. The predictability and homogeneity of care in randomized clinical trials (RCTs), for both intervention and control groups, stands in striking contrast to the variability and ad hoc nature of patient care in usual practice.

Successful programmatic efforts to improve chronic disease care have many of the same features as RCTs. Twenty-five years ago, innovators like Frank Finnerty[17] and John Runyan[18] demonstrated better outcomes for low-income patients with chronic illness by establishing clinics that provided regular, protocol-driven care with more effective use of nonphysician providers. More recently, some managed care organizations have applied these same principles in designing chronic care programs.[19] The Veterans' Administration system established hypertension clinics to better meet the needs of these patients. Clinics achieving higher rates of fol-low-up and blood pressure control had practice team members who met together and felt supported, spent more time counseling patients, and used reminders and other tools to assure follow-up.[20]

In some Western European national health systems, concerns about costs and fragmentation of care spurred efforts to improve the manage-ment of chronic illnesses in primary care.[21,22] Interventions included regis-tries of the affected populations, periodic checks, and ready access to ancil-lary services.[23-27] Chronic disease mini-clinics, used by general practitioners in Great Britain for over 20 years,[28-30] provided one structure for these interventions. "Miniclinics" or "clinic days" integrated into a GP's practice are blocks of practice time devoted to and organized for the care of patients with particular problems. These patients are identified us-ing disease registries maintained by the practice and invited to attend the clinic. The widespread adoption of miniclinics received official recogni-tion in 1990, when they became reimbursable through the National Health Service. Despite reductions in the level of reimbursements for miniclinics, their use appears to be expanding.[31]

A more educational approach was tried in Sweden.[32] The Swedish Na-tional Board of Health and Welfare developed a primary care–based dia-betes program, with special emphasis on diabetes training and education. Although a Stockholm area study demonstrated that provider education alone did not increase compliance with guidelines,[33] an organizational de-velopment effort aimed at encouraging practice team meetings and rede-signing practice systems improved compliance with guidelines and pa-tient self-management behaviors.[34]

The Germans approached the improvement of primary care for chronic illness by developing "structured teaching and treatment programs" for patients with diabetes[35] and hypertension.[36] These programs, which give emphasis to group patient education conducted by the practice, are sup-ported by an extensive provider education effort. By 1991, nearly all Ger-man insurance funds began covering physician's fees for a structured edu-cation program, as well as reimbursing the costs of teaching materials to patients.[37] This structured, multisession group education program has been well received by both patients and providers, and accompanied by significant weight reduction and increased disease control.[38-40]

A MODEL OF CHRONIC ILLNESS CARE

The elements of care described above are in fact the enhancements to usual care delivery that have been shown to improve outcomes in more focused studies of chronic illness care. Figure 7–1 provides a high-level

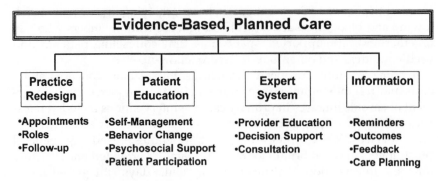

Figure 7–1 Improving outcomes in chronic illness.

overview of these elements, which have their basis in the needs of patients with chronic illness and the interventions found to be effective in meeting these needs. The following section discusses each one of these elements.

Evidence-based, planned care

Most successful chronic disease management programs reviewed for this article employ a protocol or plan which provides an explicit statement of what needs to be done for patients, at what intervals, and by whom. Usual medical care generally does not operate by protocol, and many practitioners resent the notion that care should be homogenized. They argue that patients are unique, their problems are idiosyncratic, and good care is highly individualized. Planned care, by contrast, requires an intellectual leap for the doctor from constantly thinking and worrying about specific patients, to considering all patients with specific clinical features or needs and how those needs might be met.

This leap can be bolstered by working within a care system or group practice that assists practices in their efforts to meet the needs of chronically ill patients by providing a registry of patients with the condition of interest, clear definition of the outcomes to be improved, clinical protocols or guidelines that specify the services to be delivered, provider and patient training, and other centralized resources to support service delivery and information systems to monitor care. At Group Health Cooperative of Puget Sound, the term *population-based care* describes the development and implementation of a plan for the care of all patients with specific clinical needs.[41-43] To change outcomes, population-based care planning must occur at two levels: at the level of the larger organization to assure that the necessary resources and policies are in place, and at the level of the individual practice to enable changes in care.

Population-based planning begins with the definition of the subpopulation of interest (e.g., patients with diabetes, elderly patients no longer able to ambulate) and the identification from the literature of the assessments, treatments, and services shown to improve outcomes in this group. These would be summarized and codified in evidence-based clinical policies or guidelines.

Guidelines based on clinical epidemiologic evidence of improvement in outcomes (evidence-based), as opposed to guidelines based on expert opinion, are an important advance.[44] Opinion-based guidelines tend to promulgate an academic specialty–oriented perspective on practice, emphasizing comprehensive evaluations for rare differential diagnoses and inclusion of the latest therapeutic modalities. Guidelines relying on randomized trial evidence tend to be much leaner, since few diagnostic maneuvers or treatments have been shown to improve outcomes in rigorous studies, and favor older treatments, which have been subjected to more testing. The more solid foundation of evidence-based guidelines should make them more likely to change primary care practice, although empiric evidence is lacking.

Guidelines must be considered to be relevant and credible if they are to have any impact. Recent experience suggests that even if a local organization adopts guidelines developed elsewhere, acceptance may be enhanced by local translation.[45] Then the organization and each of its practices must consider how guidelines will be implemented in practice.[46] Practice team meetings using the principles of industrial quality management may be an important step in achieving guideline-driven changes in practice style. The occurrence of regular team meetings was a significant predictor of better care and outcomes in British studies of primary care for diabetes[47] and among the VA hypertension clinics.[48] Team meetings and clinical planning, while seeming to be so sensible and obvious, are new to most practices. They need support and time to do it. Evidence suggests that the guidelines may lead to improvements in the process and outcomes of care when used as part of more comprehensive practice improvement interventions.[49] Guidelines alone have little if any impact.

Practice redesign

As discussed above, usual medical practice is not designed to meet the needs of patients with chronic illness. Successful chronic illness programs, by contrast, maintain regular contact and prevent losses to follow-up, collect critical data on health and disease status regularly, meet educational and psychosocial needs, and respond appropriately to clinical needs. To accomplish these things, health care organizations must reconsider basic ways they deliver care, such as who is the primary caregiver, and how to make appointments, allot clinic time, delegate tasks, use special resources, and manage clinical data. In this paper, planned improvements in the organization of practice to better meet the needs of the chronically ill are referred to as *practice redesign.*

Practice redesign begins with a consideration of the primary caregiver. Efforts to redesign chronic illness care range along a continuum from efforts to enhance usual primary care at one end to providing care by medical or other specialists at the other. In the middle of the continuum are models that add specialized personnel to primary care teams. Some evidence from research and demonstration programs supports specialized care such as that provided by work-site programs,[50-53] nurse-therapist clinics,[54] and specialized team care.[55] However, when usual generalist care has been compared with *usual* care from specialized providers, the results generally show little difference. For example, the Medical Outcomes Study found minimal difference in process or outcomes among diabetics or hypertensives cared for by generalists versus those cared for by specialists.[56] Several studies have examined allergist versus generalist care for asthma without consistent findings.[57-60] The cost effectiveness of case management of frail elders remains uncertain.[61,62] Usual specialized care may be no more planned or organized to meet the needs of patients with chronic illness than is usual generalist care. The discipline of the primary provider may be less important than the environment in which they practice.

Specialized programs and providers for chronic illness, while appealing, challenge basic health care values. Patients value having a single source of care for multiple needs,[63-65] and evidence supports the health and economic advantages of continuous primary care.[66-68]

The question then is whether the successful elements of special programs and clinics can be incorporated into primary care. Comprehensive changes in the way a practice organizes itself and allocates roles seem to be necessary. The need for such major restructuring was seen decades ago in now-classic studies. For example, Finnerty et al.[69] substantially improved hypertensive care for inner city residents by fundamentally reorienting clinic operations to make them more responsive to the needs of hypertensive patients through use of health aides, appointment reminders, and easier access.

The British Chronic Care Clinic or miniclinic[70] mentioned above also changes the orientation and design of primary care practice, but does so *periodically,* to meet the needs of chronically ill patients. The key features of the innovation include:

1. the invitation of a group of patients with a given condition to participate in specially designed visits with the primary care practice team at regular intervals;

2. each visit characterized by a planned set of assessments, visits with various health professionals, and a group meeting; and

3. systematic follow-up.

While the use of chronic disease miniclinics by general practitioners in Great Britain goes back over two decades,[71] they have not been rigorously evaluated. Although some observational studies have shown no positive effect of clinics,[72] more recent publications have linked diabetes miniclinics with benefits such as better glycemic control,[73,74] reduced hospitalization,[75] and improved process measures indicating better follow-up of patients.[76]

The assurance of regular follow-up seems to be a hallmark in the design of successful programs and practices. Follow-up can take the form of return visits, home visits, or telephone calls. A variety of interventions (patient reminders, outreach workers, physician reminders, patient orientation, etc.) have been shown to reduce losses to follow-up.[77] Telephone calls have important cost and logistical advantages that are only beginning to be appreciated. For example, substituting regularly scheduled follow-up phone calls for irregular follow-up visits substantially improved health status and reduced costs for chronically ill patients in one recent study.[78]

Patient self-management and behavior change

Reducing complications and symptoms from most chronic diseases requires changes in lifestyle and the development of self-management competencies by the patient and family. Interventions that facilitate behavioral change and acquisition of self-management skills are conventionally subsumed under the rubric of patient education. Essentially all successful protocols or chronic illness programs provide some sort of educational programming to meet these needs.

While the literature on the effectiveness of patient education is voluminous, the evidence is substantial that structured self-management and behavior change programs improve important outcomes in diabetes,[79-82] asthma,[83-85] hypertension,[86-90] arthritis,[91] coronary heart disease,[92] and other chronic diseases. The method of delivering the intervention (classes, one-on-one counseling, computer programs) may be less important than its ability to identify and respond to the individual needs and priorities of patients. More likely to succeed are approaches that systematically assess the patient's behaviors, readiness to change, and self-efficacy; develop a personalized improvement plan; provide feedback on progress; teach specific skills; and address some of the psychosocial demands of these illnesses.[93] Such personalized strategies need not be incompatible with system-wide interventions.

Surprisingly, the linkage between patient education for chronic illness and the patient's routine medical care has received relatively little attention.[94-97] Conversely, the role of the primary care physician in counseling for smoking and other prevention issues has been studied intensively. The prevention literature strongly suggests on the one hand that personal physicians are an important source of motivation and feedback, and their involvement enhances the effectiveness of behavioral programs.[98] On the other hand, physicians are generally not well-trained nor confident behavioral counselors. Many behavioral researchers feel that office-based, integrated programs are particularly attractive because of the influence of the physician.[99]

The impact of personal physician involvement on program effectiveness for patient education in chronic illnesses remains uncertain. In many studies of patient education, the personal physician is blinded to the intervention group of his or her patients. However, evidence from Germany, cited above, documents the effectiveness of group education taught by the primary care physician's practice staff when integrated into primary care practice.[100-102] In addition, the practice is provided teaching materials and evaluation tools. Careful study of this program for diabetes has led to its adoption by the German health care system and the provision of reimbursement for practices that participate.

Most chronic disease patient education programs target specific knowledge and behaviors associated with the disease and its treatment. Asthma and hypertension programs, for example, emphasize medication adherence and home monitoring of peak flow rates or blood pressure levels. The goals of these specific programs are increased knowledge, better adherence to the regimen, timely adaptation of the regimen to change in disease status, improved disease control, and ultimately reduced complications. The assumption underlying such programs is that knowledge facilitates behavior change, and it is changes in behavior that improve disease outcomes. Lorig and colleagues,[103] based on their influential work with patients with arthritis and other chronic illnesses, take a somewhat different view. They posit that increases in self-efficacy—the confidence or sense of mastery that one can manage the illness—may be the common medium by which self-management is improved, key behaviors are changed, and illness outcomes affected. Their interventions for arthritis patients have proven to be effective and cost effective,[104] and are now widely disseminated. They are now studying the effectiveness of a group educational intervention led by lay leaders for patients with a variety of chronic illnesses.

A critical goal in the approach of Lorig and colleagues is to help patients become more active participants in their care. Greenfield and Kaplan[105,106] have examined the impact on disease outcomes of an intervention that gives patients information, skills, and encouragement to discuss important questions and concerns with their physician. The intervention not only increased patient involvement in the interaction, but improved disease outcomes as well. Increased patient participation in care may well be a critical element of successful chronic illness care.

Clinical expertise

The debate about generalist versus specialty care for chronic illness is really about the importance to outcomes of specialized clinical knowledge or expertise. Recent evidence,[107] for example, shows that specialists have greater knowledge of effective coronary heart disease therapies than generalists. Differences in knowledge must be addressed by primary care–based models, even if clinical expertise is less important than other aspects of the care process in determining patient health and satisfaction.

Nonetheless, interventions that increase the expertise of generalist providers or increase the availability of expertise may well lead to better outcomes. Certainly the most common approach to increasing expertise has been continuing medical education in various forms. There is now general agreement that conventional didactic, lecture approaches have no enduring effects on practice style.[108] Large-scale provider education programs in Western Europe have had mixed results.[109–112] The success of the German approach[113,114] may have been more related to its emphasis on establishing a system of patient education. More personalized physician education through tutorials,[115] academic detailing,[116] consultation conferences,[117] and related interventions does seem to have some impact, although several of the more successful studies involved residents and faculty. Some training of providers, preferably using more personalized, hands-on methods, would seem to be an important initial step.

These educational strategies cannot meet the ongoing needs for expertise in the management of specific patients. Conventional referral and consultation remains the dominant source of expert assistance in managed care as well as fee-for-service practice. Referrals, however, run the potential risk of further fragmenting care, may not increase the skills of the referring physician, and contribute to increased costs. Alternatives or complements to referral have been tried. These include innovations in generalist/specialist interactions. For example, the DIABEDS program used a "hotline" to increase access of residents to diabetes expert advice.[118] Most promising are strategies that make expertise available to primary care practices through the development of a cadre of specially trained local experts or "gurus,"[119] or collaborative care whereby specialists and generalists manage patients together in the primary care setting.[120] At Group Health Cooperative, the diabetes improvement program relies on an expert team (i.e., diabetologist and nurse specialist) who spend most of their time in the primary care setting educating generalist providers and seeing difficult patients jointly with primary care teams.[121] Such models of distributed expertise may prove to be far more cost effective for common chronic illnesses than the more conventional specialty care or specialty referral models.

Finally, computer decision support systems may meet some day-to-day needs for expert advice. The evidence suggests that simple computer reminders are consistently effective in promoting recommended behaviors, while more complex diagnostic and therapeutic decision support programs have had more variable effects.[122] Work at the Regenstreif Institute,[123,124] Harvard Community Health Plan,[125] and elsewhere strongly support current efforts to develop integrated clinical information systems that incorporate guidelines in the form of "advice rules" or reminders. Randomized trials have consistently shown that computerized physician reminders increase the likelihood that patients will have blood pressure measured, receive immunizations, and other recommended maneuvers.[126]

Information

Information about patients, their care, and their outcomes is an essential ingredient of all population-based strategies to improve chronic illness care. Without a list of all patients with a condition—a registry—providers are forced to be responsive, waiting for patients to present for care. Successful strategies invite or remind patients to participate in care in accord with an explicit plan of care. The advantages of patient registries were recognized long before the computerization of medical practice.[127] The presence of a defined practice population, as in capitated care or national health plans as in Great Britain, greatly facilitates the creation of registries. The availability of a list of all patients and a few other key data elements presents opportunities to remind patients and physicians of needed follow-up or preventive interventions. The use of registries and reminders to maintain surveillance of hypertensive patients has consistently been shown to improve high blood pressure care.[128–131] Despite this, efforts to assure follow-up of hypertensive patients is not common practice, even in prepaid care, which has the advantage of a defined population.

Registries also facilitate the provision of feedback to the practice. Several rigorous studies have shown variable impacts of feedback.[132] The differences among studies may be explained by the study population (e.g., trainees may be more responsive to feedback than mature practitioners) or by the context in which the feedback is given (e.g., personal communication from an opinion leader is more potent than receiving feedback in the mail). Feedback has often been studied in isolation, as the only clinical improvement strategy being tested. It may have much greater utility when used in the context of more comprehensive approaches to improving outcomes in chronic illness.

An essential element of effective chronic illness care appears to be development of a shared plan of care, providing structure and coherence as the patient negotiates the string of care episodes that characterize chronic illness care. Patient-carried medical records or care plans have been shown to help in this regard,[133,134] and their availability in computerized clinical information systems should be even more powerful.

INTEGRATED SYSTEMS OF CHRONIC ILLNESS CARE

Research to date has tended to focus on specific components of the care model one at a time, and descriptions and evaluations of an overall plan of care are less frequent. Despite the paucity of well-tested integrated models, many HMOs and other large managed care systems are putting into place care management strategies for common chronic illnesses. Such strategies reveal genuine uncertainty among managed care leaders as to whether to enhance their primary care system's ability to provide chronic illness care, or to delegate care to specialized care providers such as medical specialists or case managers for various patient groups.

There have been no rigorously designed comparisons of an *organized* primary care management approach versus an *organized* specialty-based program. Thus, managed medical care finds itself at a crossroads, with uncertainty as to its basic care model for chronically ill patients. Specialized programs using medical specialists or case managers offer some obvious advantages. Implementation is far less complicated since such approaches involve a small number of personnel with a narrow focus and span of responsibility. Environmental pressures for this approach come from the overabundance of specialists, increasingly intense marketing of "disease management" or carve-out programs, and cultural beliefs in the superiority of specialists over generalists.

Integrated primary care models, on the other hand, may be less expensive in the long run[135] but are initially difficult to implement since they, by definition, involve large numbers of busy health professionals with varying levels of expertise and enthusiasm working in office systems that have not traditionally supported the care of patients with ongoing problems. Given these difficulties, it is easy to understand why condition-specific specialized programs are being developed and disseminated in preference to integrated primary care–based programs. But the issues of ultimate accountability for the patient's health and coordination of care among disparate providers will have to be resolved. The care of the many chronically ill patients who have multiple conditions (e.g., 50 percent or more of Type II diabetics are hypertensive, a third or more have clinically significant coronary artery disease) will challenge systems based on the specialized approach.

THE MANAGEMENT OF CHRONIC ILLNESS CARE

Managed care now refers to health systems that are widely divergent in structure, care management approach, culture, and values. In the past, traditional HMOs controlled costs by maintaining control over capacity by limiting the use of hospital beds, specialist services, and new technologies—not by actively trying to change the care being delivered.[136] Quality of care was largely assured by the hiring of qualified staff and the maintenance of a conservative clinical culture. Management, in this case, is the macromanagement of supply and culture. This strategy worked well until diagnostic related groups and competition reduced the difference in hospitalization rates between HMOs and fee-for-service care, threatening the cost advantage of HMOs.

As a result, capitated systems recognized the need to change care delivery, and approached it in two very different ways. Many systems initiated micromanagement strategies, such as preauthorization of procedures and financial incentives to limit services, in an attempt to influence clinical decisions involving individual patients. The impact of these strategies on costs has been small,[137] and the impacts on physician morale have been negative. The effect of these strategies on patient outcomes is largely unknown, but the likelihood that such approaches, whose primary objective is utilization reduction, can meet the complex needs of patients with chronic illness seems remote.

Other organizations have begun efforts to change care delivery without micromanaging individual patients. Their goal is to maximize the health outcomes of their population at an affordable cost by assuring the efficient and systematic delivery of effective interventions for defined subpopulations of patients, a strategy that has been called population-based management of care.[138-140]

HMOs have many apparent advantages in caring for patients with chronic illness, such as defined populations of enrollees, comprehensive services, information systems, a preventive orientation, and centralized resources like patient education and newsletters.[141-143] Despite these, head-to-head comparisons of the processes and outcomes of care for patients with many chronic illnesses indicate few if any differences between HMO and fee-for-service care, or between types of HMOs.[144-148] The lack of a consistent difference in process or outcomes suggests that the apparent advantages of HMOs to improve chronic illness care are not being exploited.

However, most of the published comparisons relate to care rendered many years ago, before the recent movement of many HMOs toward more organized, planned approaches to changing the care delivered to patients with chronic illness began.

Nonetheless, progress has been remarkably slow. The costs of improving care have proven to be a major barrier, whether because of limitations on reimbursement or painfully constrained fixed budgets in prepaid systems. Usual care for patients with common chronic illnesses is already staggeringly expensive. While it is tempting to suggest that better care will reduce currently high utilization and costs, there is little firm evidence to support such claims as yet. It is likely that achieving improved chronic disease outcomes will be more expensive in the short term. The cost increases can be blunted by redeploying and better using existing clinical staff rather than by adding new potentially duplicative providers. Wise health care organizations will carefully reconsider their current use of critical chronic care resources such as social workers, ambulatory nurses, nutritionists, or certified diabetes educators.

NEXT STEPS

Major experiments in the care of chronic illness are under way. Health care organizations across the country have recognized the deficiencies in care, and the costs generated by caring for chronically ill patients. In response, many are devising and piloting more comprehensive care strategies. Anecdotal evidence suggests that the pilot efforts include a broad array of models, but are only occasionally being evaluated rigorously. Despite the paucity of rigorous evaluation, the movement to "benchmark" and find good ideas in other places is leading organizations to emulate nascent, minimally evaluated programs. Systematic efforts to document the characteristics and success of care management programs for chronic illnesses are essential if we are to learn from these developments. More rigorous evaluation of current efforts and collaborative multiinstitutional testing in rigorous randomized trials of more promising strategies across multiple health care systems would advance the state of the art at a faster pace. Such multicenter trials might be facilitated by establishing a consortium of organizations interested in and capable of more formal evaluation of promising care strategies, perhaps modeled after the VA Cooperative Studies Program.[149]

There are five elements of health care systems that are likely to be maximally responsive to the needs of patients with chronic illness:

1. evidence-based protocols for managing patients;
2. reorganization of practice systems and provider roles;

3. improved patient education;

4. timely availability of relevant expertise; and

5. more organized, readily available clinical information.

The effectiveness and costs of health care services are likely to depend on how these elements of good patient care are designed and implemented.

REFERENCES

1. Clark, N.M., et al. "Self-management of Chronic Disease by Older Adults: A Review and Questions for Research." *Journal of Aging and Health* 3 (1991): 3–27.
2. Lorig, K.L., and Holman, H. "Arthritis Self-management Studies: A Twelve-Year Review." *Health Education Quarterly* 20 (1993): 17–28.
3. Funnell, M.M., et al. "Empowerment: An Idea Whose Time Has Come in Diabetes Education." *Diabetes Educator* 17 (1991): 37–41.
4. Stockwell, D.H., et al. "The Determinants of Hypertension Awareness, Treatment, and Control in an Insured Population." *American Journal of Public Health* 84(11) (1994): 1768–1774.
5. Kenny, S.J., et al. "Survey of Physician Practice Behaviors Related to Diabetes Mellitus in the U.S.: Physician Adherence to Consensus Recommendations." *Diabetes Care* 16(11) (1993): 1507–1510.
6. Perrin, J.M., et al. "Variations in Rates of Hospitalization of Children in Three Urban Communities." *New England Journal of Medicine* 3131 (1984): 295–300.
7. Hirsch, C.H., and Winograd, C.H. "Clinic-based Primary Care of Frail Older Patients in California." *Western Journal of Medicine* 156 (1992): 385–391.
8. Orleans, C.T., et al. "Health Promotion in Primary Care: A Survey of U.S. Family Practitioners." *Preventive Medicine* 14 (1985): 636–647.
9. Kottke, T.E., Brekke, M.L., and Solberg, LI. "Making 'Time' for Preventive Services." *Mayo Clinic Proceedings* 68 (1993): 785–791.
10. Litzelman, D.K., et al. "Requiring Physicians to Respond to Computerized Reminders Improves Their Compliance with Preventive Care Protocols." *Journal of General Internal Medicine* 8 (1993): 311–317.
11. Scheff, T.J. "Decisions in Medicine." In *Being Mentally Ill: A Sociological Theory.* 2nd ed. New York: Aldine Publishing Company, 1984, pp. 77–89.
12. Diabetes Complications and Control Trial Research Group. "The Effect of Intensive Treatment of Diabetes on the Development and Progression of Long-term Complication in Insulin-dependent Diabetes Mellitus." *New England Journal of Medicine* 329 (1993): 977–986.
13. SHEP Cooperative Research Group. "Prevention of Stroke by Antihypertensive Drug Treatment in Older Persons with Isolated Systolic Hypertension. Final Results of the Systolic Hypertension in the Elderly Program (SHEP)." *Journal of the American Medical Association* 265 (1991): 3255–3264.
14. Hypertension Detection and Follow-up Program Cooperative Group. "Five-Year Findings of the Hypertension Detection and Follow-up Program: I. Reduction in Mortality of Persons with High Blood Pressure, Including Mild Hypertension." *Journal of the American Medical Association* 242(23) (1979): 2562–2571.
15. Shulman, N., et al. "Correlates of Attendance and Compliance in the Hypertension Detection and Follow-up Program." *Controlled Clinical Trials* 3 (1982): 13–27.

16. Peart, W.S., and Miall, W.E. "M.R.C. Mild Hypertension Trial." *Lancet* 1(8159) (1980): 104–105 (letter).

17. Finnerty, F.A. Jr., and Shaw, L.W. "Hypertension in the Inner City. II: Detection and Follow-up." *Circulation* 47 (1973): 76–78.

18. Runyan, J.W., et al. "A Program for the Care of Patients with Chronic Diseases." *Journal of the American Medical Association* 211 (1970): 476–479.

19. Peters, A.L., Davidson, M.B., and Ossorio, R.C. "Management of Patients with Diabetes by Nurses with Support of Subspecialists." *HMO Practice* 9(1) (1995): 8–13.

20. Stason, W.B., et al. "Effectiveness and Costs of Veterans Affairs Hypertension Clinic." *Medical Care* 32(12) (1994): 1197–1215.

21. Yudkin, J.S., et al. "The Quality of Diabetic Care in a London Health District." *Journal of Epidemiology and Community Health* 34 (1980): 277–280.

22. Rosenquist, U., Carlson, A., and Luft, R. "Evaluation of Comprehensive Program for Diabetes Care at Primary Health-care Level." *Diabetes Care* 11(3) (1988): 269–274.

23. MacKinnon, M. "General Practice Diabetes Care: The Past, the Present and the Future." *Diabetic Medicine* 7(2) (1990): 171–172.

24. Gibbins, R.L., and Saunders, J. "How to Do It: Develop Diabetic Care in General Practice." *British Medical Journal* 297 (1988): 187–189.

25. Thorn, P.A., and Watkins, P. "Organization of Diabetic Care." *British Medical Journal* 285 (1982): 787–789.

26. Farmer, A., and Coulter, A. "Organization of Care for Diabetic Patients in General Practice: Influence on Hospital Admissions." *British Journal of General Practitioners* 40 (1990): 56–58.

27. Hurwitz, B., Goodman, C., and Yudkin, J. "Prompting the Clinical Care of Non–Insulin Dependent (Type II) Diabetic Patients in an Inner City Area: One Model of Community Care." *British Medical Journal* 306 (1993): 624.

28. Thorn, P.A., and Russell, R.G. "Diabetic Clinics Today and Tomorrow: Mini-clinics in General Practice." *British Medical Journal* 2 (1973): 534–536.

29. MacKinnon, M. "General Practice Diabetes Care: The Past, the Present and the Future." *Diabetic Medicine* 7(2) (1990): 171–172.

30. Koperski, M. "Systematic Care of Diabetic Patients in One General Practice: How Much Does It Cost?" *British Journal of General Practice* 42 (1992): 370–372.

31. Haynes, J. "GPs Subsidize Care of Chronic Diseases." *Pulse* (August 7, 1993): 19.

32. Rosenthal, M.M., and Carlson, A. "Beyond CME: Diabetes Education. Field-interactive Strategies from Sweden." *Diabetes Educator* 14 (1988): 212–217.

33. Carlson, A., and Rosenquist, U. "Diabetes Control Program Implementation. On the Importance of Staff Involvement." *Scandinavian Journal of Primary Health Care* Suppl. 1 (1988): 105–112.

34. Carlson, A., and Rosenquist, U. "Diabetes Care Organization, Process, and Patient Outcomes: Effects of a Diabetes Control Program." *Diabetes Educator* 17(1) (1991): 42–48.

35. Kronsbein, P., Momlhauser, I., Venhauss, A., Jorgens, V., et al. "Evaluation of a Structured Treatment and Teaching Programme on Non–Insulin-dependent diabetes." *Lancet* (December 1988): 1407–1411.

36. Muhlhauser, I., et al. "Evaluation of a Structured Treatment and Teaching Programme on Hypertension in General Practice." *Clinical and Experimental Hypertension* 15(1) (1993): 125–142.

37. Gruesser, M., et al. "Evaluation of a Structured Treatment and Teaching Program for Non–Insulin-treated Type II Diabetic Outpatients in Germany after the Nationwide Introduction of Reimbursement Policy for Physicians." *Diabetes Care* 16(9) (1993): 1268–1275.

38. Kronsbein et al., "Evaluation . . . on Non–Insulin-dependent Diabetes."
39. Muhlhauser et al., "Evaluation . . . on Hypertension."
40. Gruesser et al., "Evaluation . . . for Non–Insulin-treated Type II."
41. Voelker, R. "Population-based Medicine Merges Clinical Care, Epidemiologic Techniques." *Journal of the American Medical Association* 271(17) (1994): 1301–1302.
42. Wagner, E.H. "Population-based Management of Diabetes Care." *Patient Education and Counseling* 26 (1995): 225–230.
43. Payne, T.H., et al. "Practicing Population-based Care in a HMO: Evaluation after 18 Months." *HMO Practice* 9(3) (1995): 101–106.
44. Eddy, D.M. "A Manual for Assessing Health Practices and Designing Practice Policies: The Explicit Approach." Philadelphia, PA: American College of Physicians, 1992.
45. Brown, J.B., Shye, D., and McFarland, B. "The Paradox of Guideline Implementation: How AHCPR's Depression Guideline Was Adapted at Kaiser Permanente Northwest Region." *The Joint Commission Journal on Quality Improvement* 21(1) (1995): 5–21.
46. Gottlieb, L.K., Margolis, C.Z., and Schoenbaum, S.C. "Clinical Practice Guidelines at an HMO: Development and Implementation in a Quality Improvement Model." *Quality Review Bulletin* 16 (1990): 80–86.
47. Farmer and Coulter, "Organization of Care for Diabetic Patients."
48. Stason et al., "Effectiveness and Costs."
49. Grimshaw, J.M., and Russell, I.T. "Effect of Clinical Guidelines on Medical Practice: A Systematic Review of Rigorous Evaluations." *Lancet* 342(8883) (1993): 1317–1322.
50. Alderman, M.H., and Schoenbaum, E.E. "Detection and Treatment of Hypertension at the Work Site." *New England Journal of Medicine* 293 (1975): 65–68.
51. Fielding, J.E., et al. "Evaluation of the IMPACT Blood Pressure Program." *Journal of Occupational Medicine* 36(7) (1994): 743–746.
52. Brown, H.R., et al. "Work Site Blood Pressure Control: The Evolution of a Program." *Journal of Occupational Medicine* 31(4) (1989): 354–357.
53. Logan, A.G., et al. "Clinical Effectiveness and Cost-effectiveness of Monitoring Blood Pressure of Hypertensive Employees at Work." *Hypertension* 5(6) (1983): 828–836.
54. Schwartz, L.L., et al. "Hypertension: Role of the Nurse-Therapist." *Mayo Clinic Proceedings* 65 (1990): 67–72.
55. Peters, Davidson, and Ossorio, "Management of Patients with Diabetes."
56. Greenfield, S., Rogers, W., Mangotich, M., Carney, M.F. "Outcomes of Patients with Hypertension and Non-insulin Dependent Diabetes Mellitus Treated by Different Systems and Specialties: Results from the Medical Outcomes Study." *Journal of the American Medical Association* 274 (1995): 1473–1474.
57. Zeiger, R.S., et al. "Facilitated Referral to Asthma Specialist Reduces Relapses in Asthma Emergency Room Visits." *Journal of Allergy and Clinical Immunology* 87 (1991): 1160–1180.
58. Mahr, T.A., and Evans, R. "Allergist Influence on Asthma Care." *Annals of Allergy* 71 (1993): 115–120.
59. Freund, D.A., et al. "The Kansas City Asthma Care Project: Specialty Differences in the Cost of Treating Asthma." *Annals of Allergy* 60 (1988): 3–7.
60. Engel, W., et al. "The Treatment of Patients with Asthma by Specialists and Generalists." *Medical Care* 27 (1989): 306–314.
61. Austin, C.A., et al. *"Case Management: A Critical Review."* Report for the Administration on Aging (Grant #90AT2152/05), Pacific Northwest Long Term Care Gerontology Center, Seattle, WA, September, 1985.
62. Kodner, D.L. "Case Management: Principles, Practice and Performance." *Gerontological Topics #1.* Brooklyn, NY: Institute for Applied Gerontology, July 1993.

63. Shea, S. "Hypertension Control, 1994." *American Journal of Public Health* 84(11) (1994): 1725–1727 (editorial).
64. Hjortdahl, P., and Laerum, E. "Continuity of Care in General Practice: Effect on Patient Satisfaction." *British Medical Journal* 304 (1992): 1287–1290.
65. Wasson, J.H., et al. "Continuity of Outpatient Medical Care in Elder Men: A Randomized Trial." *Journal of the American Medical Association* 252 (1984): 2413–2417.
66. Becker, M.H., Drachman, R.H., and Kirscht, J.P. "Continuity of Pediatrician: New Support for an Old Shibboleth." *Journal of Pediatrics* 84 (1974): 599–605.
67. Ibid.
68. Starfield, B. "Longitudinality and Managed Care." In *Primary Care: Concept, Evaluation, and Policy.* New York, NY: Oxford University Press, 1992, pp. 41–55.
69. Finnerty and Shaw, "Hypertension in the Inner City, II."
70. Carlson and Rosenquist, "Diabetes Care Organization."
71. Thorn and Russell, "Diabetic Clinics Today and Tomorrow."
72. Chesover, D., Tudor-Miles, P., and Hilton, S. "Survey and Audit of Diabetes Care in General Practice in South London." *British Journal of General Practice* 1 (1991): 282–285.
73. Bradshaw, C., et al. "Work-load and Outcomes of Diabetes Care in General Practice." *Diabetic Medicine* 9 (1992): 275–278.
74. Pringle, M., et al. "Influences on Control in Diabetes Mellitus: Patient, Doctor, Practice, or Delivery of Care?" *British Medical Journal* 306 (1993): 630–634.
75. Farmer and Coulter, "Organization of Care for Diabetic Patients."
76. Koperski, M. "How Effective is Systematic Care of Diabetic Patients? A Study in One General Practice." *British Journal of General Practice* 42 (1992): 508–511.
77. Macharia, W.M., et al. "An Overview of Interventions to Improve Compliance with Appointment Keeping for Medical Services." *Journal of the American Medical Association* 267(13) (1992): 1813–1817.
78. Wasson, J., et al. "Telephone Care as a Substitute for Routine Clinic Follow-up." *Journal of the American Medical Association* 267(13) (1992): 1828–1829.
79. Padgett, D., et al. "Meta-analysis of the Effects of Educational and Psychosocial Interventions on Management of Diabetes Mellitus." *Journal of Clinical Epidemiology* 41 (1988): 1007–1030.
80. Brown, S.A. "Studies of Educational Interventions and Outcomes in Diabetic Adults: A Meta-analysis Revisited." *Patient Education and Counseling* 16 (1990): 189–215.
81. Malone, J.M., et al. "Prevention of Amputation by Diabetic Education." *American Journal of Surgery* 158 (1989): 520–524.
82. Litzelman, D.K., et al. "Reduction of Lower Extremity Clinical Abnormalities in Patients with Non–Insulin-dependent Diabetes Mellitus. A Randomized Control Trial." *Annals of Internal Medicine* 119 (1993): 36–41.
83. Lewis, C.E., et al. "A Randomized Trial of A.C.T. (Asthma Care Training) for Kids." *Pediatrics* 74 (1984): 478–486.
84. Mayo, P.H., Richman, J., and Harris, H.W. "Results of a Program to Reduce Admissions for Adult Asthma." *Annals of Internal Medicine* 112 (1990): 864–871.
85. Wilson, S.R., et al. "A Controlled Trial of Two Forms of Self-management Education for Adults with Asthma." *American Journal of Medicine* 94 (1993): 564–576.
86. Glanz, K., and Scholl, T.O. "Intervention Strategies to Improve Adherence Among Hypertensives: Review and Recommendations." *Patient Counselling and Health Education* 4 (1982): 14–28.
87. Zismer, D.K., et al. "Improving Hypertension Control in a Private Medical Practice." *Archives of Internal Medicine* 142 (1982): 297–299.
88. Morisky, D.E., et al. "Five-year Blood Pressure Control and Mortality Following Health

Education for Hypertensive Patients." *American Journal of Public Health* 73 (1983): 153–162.
89. Jones, P.K., Jones, S.L., and Katz, J. "Improving Follow-up Among Hypertensive Patients Using a Health Belief Model Intervention." *Archives of Internal Medicine* 147 (1987): 1557–1560.
90. Sawicki, P.T., et al. "Improvement of Hypertension Care by a Structured Treatment and Teaching Programme." *Journal of Human Hypertension* 7 (1993): 571–573.
91. Lorig, K.R., Mazonson, P.D., and Holman, H.R. "Evidence Suggesting that Health Education for Self-management in Patients with Chronic Arthritis Has Sustained Health Benefits While Reducing Health Care Costs." *Arthritis and Rheumatism* 36 (1993): 439–446.
92. DeBusk, R.F., et al. "A Case-management System for Coronary Risk Factor Modification after Acute Myocardial Infarction." *Annals of Internal Medicine* 120 (1994): 721–729.
93. Glasgow, R.E., Toobert, D.J., Hampson, S.E., and Noell, J.W. "A Brief Office-based Intervention to Facilitate Diabetes Self-management." *Health Education Research: Theory & Practice* 10 (1995): 467–478.
94. Kronsbein et al., "Evaluation . . . on Non–Insulin-dependent Diabetes."
95. Mulhauser et al., "Evaluation . . . on Hypertension."
96. Gruesser et al., "Evaluation . . . for Non–Insulin-treated Type II."
97. Glasgow, R.E., Toobert, D.J., Hampson, S.E., and Wilson, W. "Behavioral Research on Diabetes at the Oregon Research Institute." *Annals of Behavioral Medicine* 17 (1995): 32–40.
98. U.S. Preventive Services Task Force. *Guide to Clinical Preventive Services: An Assessment of the Effectiveness of 169 Interventions.* Baltimore: Williams & Wilkins, 1989.
99. Kottke, Brekke, and Solberg, "Making 'Time' for Preventive Services."
100. Kronsbein et al., "Evaluation . . . on Non–Insulin-dependent Diabetes."
101. Mulhauser et al., "Evaluation . . . on Hypertension."
102. Gruesser et al., "Evaluation . . . for Non–Insulin-treated Type II."
103. Lorig and Holman, "Arthritis Self-Management Studies."
104. Lorig, Mazonson, and Holman, "Evidence . . . that Health Education . . . Has Sustained Health Benefits."
105. Greenfield, S., et al. "Patients' Participation in Medical Care: Effects on Blood Sugar Control and Quality of Life in Diabetes." *Journal of General Internal Medicine* 3(5) (1988): 448–457.
106. Greenfield, S., Kaplan, S.H., and Ware, J.E. "Expanding Patient Involvement in Care. Effects on Patient Outcomes." *Annals of Internal Medicine* 102(4) (1985): 520–528.
107. Ayanian, J.Z., et al. "Knowledge and Practices of Generalist and Specialist Physicians Regarding Drug Therapy for Acute Myocardial Infarction." *New England Journal of Medicine* 331(17) (1994): 1136–1142.
108. Davis, D.A., et al. "Evidence for the Effectiveness of CME: A Review of 50 Randomized Controlled Trials." *Journal of the American Medical Association* 268 (1992): 1111–1117.
109. Rosenquist, Carlson, and Luft, "Evaluation of . . . Diabetes Care."
110. Kronsbein et al., "Evaluation on . . . Non–Insulin-dependent Diabetes."
111. Sawicki et al., "Improvement of Hypertension Care."
112. Carlson, A., and Rosenquist, U. "Diabetes Care Organization, Process, and Patient Outcomes: Effects of a Diabetes Control Program." *Diabetes Educator* 17(1) (1991): 42–48.
113. Kronsbein et al., "Evaluation on . . . Non–Insulin-dependent Diabetes."
114. Sawicki et al., "Improvement of Hypertension Care."
115. Inui, T.S., Yourtee, E.L., and Williamson, J.W. "Improved Outcomes in Hypertension after Physician Tutorials: A Controlled Trial." *Annals of Internal Medicine* 84(6) (1976): 646–651.

116. Soumerai, S.B., and Avorn, J. "Principles of Educational Outreach (Academic Detailing) to Improve Clinical Decision Making." *Journal of the American Medical Association* 263(4) (1990): 549–555.
117. Vinicor, F., et al. "DIABEDS: A Randomized Trial of the Effects of Physician and/or Patient Education on Diabetes Patient Outcomes." *Journal of Chronic Diseases* 40 (1987): 345–356.
118. Ibid.
119. Stuart, M.E., et al. "Successful Implementation of a Guideline Program for the Rational Use of Lipid-lowering Drugs." *HMO Practice* 5 (1991): 198–204.
120. Katon, W., et al. "Collaborative Management to Achieve Treatment Guidelines." *Journal of the American Medical Association* 273(13) (1995): 1026–1031.
121. McCulloch, D., et al. "A Systematic Approach to Diabetes Management in the Post-DCCT Era." *Diabetes Care* 17(7) (1994): 1–5.
122. Johnston, M.E., et al. "Effects of Computer-based Clinical Decision Support Systems on Clinician Performance and Patient Outcome: A Critical Appraisal of Research." *Annals of Internal Medicine* 120 (1994): 135–142.
123. McDonald,C.J., et al. "The Regenstrief Medical Records." *MD Computing* 5 (1988): 34–47.
124. Litzelman, D.K., et al. "Requiring Physicians to Respond to Computerized Reminders Improves Their Compliance with Preventive Care Protocols." *Journal of General Internal Medicine* 8 (1993): 311–317.
125. Barton, M.B., and Schoenbaum, S.C. "Improving Influenza Vaccination Performance in an HMO Setting: The Use of Computer-generated Reminders and Peer Comparison Feedback." *American Journal of Public Health* 80 (1990): 534–536.
126. Johnston et al., "Effects of Computer-Based Clinical Decision Support Systems."
127. Fry, J. "Record Keeping in Primary Care." In *Methods of Health Care Evaluation*. Eds. D.L. Sackett and M.S. Baskin. 2nd ed. Hamilton, Ontario, Canada: McMaster University, 1973.
128. Stason et al., "Veterans Care Hypertension Clinic."
129. Macharia et al., "An Overview of Interventions."
130. Glanz and Scholl, "Intervention Strategies."
131. Johnston et al., "Effects of Computer-Based Clinical Decision Support Systems."
132. Megford, M., Banfield, P., and O'Hanlon, M. "Effects of Feedback of Information on Clinical Practice: A Review." *British Medical Journal* 303 (1991): 398–402.
133. Turner, R.C., Waivers, L.E., and O'Brien, K. "The Effect of Patient-carried Reminder Cards on the Performance of Health Maintenance Measures." *Archives of Internal Medicine* 150(3) (1990): 645–647.
134. Dickey, L.L., and Petitti, D. "A Patient-held Minirecord to Promote Adult Preventive Care." *Journal of Family Practice* 34(4) (1992): 457–463.
135. Franks, P., Clancy, C.M., and Nutting, P.A. "Gatekeeping Revisited—Protecting Patients from Overtreatment." *New England Journal of Medicine* 327(6) (1992): 424–429.
136. Wagner, E.H. "Managing Medical Practice: The Potential of HMOs." In *The Changing Health Care Economy: Impact on Physicians, Patients, and Innovators* (IOM Workshop Proceedings), ed. A.C. Gelijns. Washington, D.C.: National Academy Press, 1992, pp. 51–61.
137. Congressional Budget Office (CBO) Memorandum. "The Effects of Managed Care and Managed Competition." February 1995.
138. Voelker, R., "Population-based Medicine."
139. Wagner, "Population-based Management."
140. Wagner, "Managing Medical Practice."
141. Wagner, E.H., and Thompson, R.S. "Cancer Prevention and HMOs." *Cancer Investigation* 6 (1988): 453–459.
142. Lawrence, D.M. "A Provider's View of Prevention Approaches in a Prepaid Group

Practice." *Cancer* 67 (1991): 1767–1771.

143. Schoenbaum, S.C. "Implementation of Preventive Services in an HMO Practice." *Journal of General Internal Medicine* 5 (1990): S123–127.

144. Horwitz, S.M., and Stein, R.E.K. "Health Maintenance Organizations vs. Indemnity Insurance for Children with Chronic Illness: Trading Gaps in Coverage." *American Journal of Diseases of Children* 144 (1990): 581–586.

145. Retchin, S.M., et al. "How the Elderly Fare in HMOs: Outcomes from the Medicare Competition Demonstrations." *Health Services Research* 27(5) (1992): 651–669.

146. Udvarhelyi, S., et al. "Comparison of the Quality of Ambulatory Care for Fee-for-Service and Prepaid Patients." *Annals of Internal Medicine* 115 (1991): 394–400.

147. Retchin, S.M., and Brown, B. "Elderly Patients with Congestive Heart Failure under Prepaid Care." *American Journal of Medicine* 90 (1991): 236–242.

148. Safran, D.G., Tarlov, A.R., and Rogers, W.H. "Primary Care Performance in Fee-for-Service and Prepaid Health Care Systems: Results from the Medical Outcomes Study." *Journal of the American Medical Association* 271(20) (1994): 1579–1586.

149. Henderson, W.G. "Some Operation Aspects of the Veterans Administration Cooperative Studies Program from 1972 to 1979." *Controlled Clinical Trials* 1(3) (1980): 209–226.

8

Kaiser Colorado's Cooperative Health Care Clinic: A Group Approach to Patient Care

John C. Scott and Barbara J. Robertson

CURRENT VISITS MODEL

Too often health care practitioners use the current model of physician office visits to care for their senior patients who have chronic conditions. This traditional model of one-on-one patient care has significant implications for health plans serving the elderly, many of whom have resource-intensive needs.

Research shows, for instance, that four out of five people over age 65 have at least one chronic condition, and that chronic disease accounts for 90 percent of all morbidity, 80 percent of all mortality, and 80 percent of all health care dollars. Moreover, the risk of disability increases with age: Among seniors 65 to 74 years of age, 6 percent are disabled; among those 75 to 84 years old, 13 percent are disabled, and among those 85 years of age and older, 40 percent are disabled.[1–7]

The question, then, has been whether providers have been trying to fit a senior population into a model of care more effectively designed for younger patients.

COOPERATIVE HEALTH CARE CLINIC EMERGES

In 1992 the Kaiser Permanente Colorado Region, which covers the Denver metropolitan area, Longmont, and Boulder, sought to change this ap-

Source: Reprinted from J.C. Scott and B.J. Robertson, Kaiser Colorado's Cooperative Health Care Clinic: A Group Approach to Patient Care, *Managed Care Quarterly*, Vol. 4, No. 3, pp. 41–45, © 1996, Aspen Publishers, Inc.

proach with a pilot project launched at the Wheat Ridge medical offices in Denver. The pilot came about when Kaiser Permanente put together a small task force made up of physicians and nurses to review the current ambulatory model of care and to recommend a more effective, alternative care approach.

From this group discussion came the creation of the Cooperative Health Care Clinic, a model that would allow the practitioners to:

- Deliver ambulatory care to seniors in such a way that they could spend more of their time on the complex aspects of their patients' conditions, such as the functional limitations and emotional issues that surround those with chronic disease.
- Expand this model to include other aspects of care influencing their patients' health, such as the physical, sociocultural, and environmental factors in their lives.
- Avoid using X-rays, lab tests, and prescriptions as "substitutes" of care, an approach that is generally less effective and more costly than most of the staff had realized.

Under the one-year pilot program, a multidisciplinary team of professionals would provide medical care to elderly patients in groups rather than on an individual physician office visit basis.

This approach not only represented a major shift in the way care is provided to senior patients with chronic disease, but it was significant in that managers and clinicians believed their care could be managed more effectively. The program's overall objective was to reduce resource use and associated costs of care and to increase the quality of care delivered.

Specifically, clinicians would aim to improve health status by enhancing preventive medicine, maintaining patients' ability to live independently, and improving their access to care. These efforts, in turn, would prevent and reduce unnecessary hospitalization, emergency room visits, use of urgent care (i.e., same day care for minor illness or injury), physician and nurse office visits, laboratory and X-ray tests, skilled nursing facility admissions, and use of home health services. Improvements in both member and physician satisfaction were also considered important measures of success.

CASE SELECTION

CHCC selected for the pilot 160 senior members over age 65 who were high users of both inpatient and outpatient resources and had one of four chronic conditions: cardiovascular disease, lung disease, diabetes, or degenerative joint disease. High utilization was defined as two or more hospitalizations and six or more office visits within a 12-month period.

A major challenge was in identifying these members on the database, for each element of selection, such as hospital, skilled nursing facility, and home health data. Likewise, encounter data, such as office visits, urgent care, and emergency room visits, were kept in a separate data file. Consequently, much of the patient profiling that follows an individual as he or she moves through the various levels of care must be done by matching information collected on each system separately. The physician and nurse care teams assisted in identifying chronic disease members over 65 years old that they felt could benefit from the group visit.

Another 161 patients over age 65 years were identified as the control group. The control group sought care in the traditional exclusively one-on-one physician-patient office visit. Members in both the control and experimental groups had been members of Kaiser Permanente for a minimum of one year.

The CHCC program was designed as follows: Patients in the CHCC experimental group met in groups of 20 to 25 every four weeks with their personal physician and nurse team and other health care professionals for a two-and-a-half-hour session. Attendance was voluntary and patients were encouraged to bring a spouse, other family member, or caregiver.

The agenda for each group session followed this general setup:

- a 15-minute introduction and welcome, where individuals meet each other and socialize, and group business and announcements are made;
- a 30-minute interactive education session, where the group selects a particular topic and educational materials are handed out;
- a 15-minute coffee break and socialization period, during which individual medical records are available and blood pressure checks are recorded in the participants' medical record and personal care notebook, and "work time" activities, such as lab and X-ray results, pharmacy refills, and questions pertaining to any individual issue, are conducted;
- a 15-minute question and answer session;
- a 15-minute session to plan future meetings; and
- a 30-minute session with the health care team, which includes one-on-one appointments with the physician for routine health maintenance checks and needed physical exams. This time was not always used, but was available should the physician or patient request a brief appointment.

Each participant received a personal care notebook which was updated at each session.

Since problems of the elderly with chronic disease are often a result of complex forces surrounding physical, psychosocial, and environmental issues, the CHCC staff focused their interventions and solutions on these particular areas. In fact, over the period of the pilot, a core curriculum evolved, which included topics not always discussed as part of a regular one-on-one office visit: nutrition and exercise; access to emergency services; living wills and advanced directives; control of chronic pain; male/female issues; allergies; stress, depression, and relaxation techniques; grief and loss; safety and prevention; and sleep disorders.

POSITIVE PILOT RESULTS

After one year, the pilot indicated statistically significant findings at the $p < 0.05$ level. With regard to overall satisfaction, CHCC patients reported that they felt their health care needs were being better met and that overall access was improved. In fact, their satisfaction rate was higher than expected, particularly, with the nurses. Physicians, too, were highly satisfied, noting that they felt the program gave them more time to deal with the patient and that patients were more informed, helping the physicians to better diagnose and treat their conditions.

Medical care utilization was lower for the CHCC patients than for the comparison patients during the pilot. Specifically, the number of patient care clinic visits was 0.87 for the CHCC group and 1.28 visits for the comparison group. The number of emergency room visits were 0.41 for the CHCC patients and 0.67 for the comparison patients. The number of X-rays were 2.15 for the CHCC enrollees and 3.26 for the comparison group. The number of internal medicine physician visits was 2.74 for the CHCC group and 3.34 for the comparison group; however, this difference was not statistically significant.

Use of inpatient, skilled nursing facility, and visiting nurse services also were lower for patients in the CHCC group compared with individuals in the comparison group. CHCC members had fewer inpatient days at 249 days, compared with the other enrollees, at 407 days; CHCC members also had fewer admissions to skilled nursing facilities at 0.03 admissions, compared with 0.07 for the other patients; and fewer CHCC enrollees received visiting nurse services, at 0.06, compared with 0.12 of the non-CHCC members.

The findings were also significant for the number of telephone calls returned by physicians and nurses. Physicians returned 1.4 calls to members of the CHCC group and 2.53 calls to the comparison group members. Nurses returned 2.9 calls to the CHCC group members and 2.26 calls to the comparison group members.

In the area of advance directives, 6 percent of CHCC members had a power of attorney, while 1 percent of non-CHCC members did; 9 percent of CHCC members had living wills, compared with 4 percent for the other members.

Regarding health prevention, 81 percent of CHCC members had influenza shots, versus 64 percent of the comparison group, and 20 percent of CHCC had pneumovax shots, compared with 4 percent of the comparison group.

LESSONS LEARNED

The pilot program offered many lessons for staff and management. Project staff learned that a project entailing a dramatic change in care approach needs the encouragement and support from senior administrators and executive medical staff to succeed.

From a clinical perspective, the staff also realized their assumptions that seniors—and their providers—hold the physician-patient relationship in complete confidence is not always true. In fact, the CHCC pilot indicated that the older patient is much more open and willing to share experiences in a group setting. In their group meetings, seniors focused on common interests and problems, creating a tremendous support system among group members with chronic disease. In fact, members were eager and willing to discuss issues such as disability and end-of-life decisions. As a result, the CHCC model actually enhanced the physician-patient relationship.

Another lesson concerned the ability of physicians and nurses to conduct group sessions. Many physicians and nurses do not need to have specific public speaking skills to act as good facilitators at the group visits; within two or three months the group office visits become a very comfortable approach for the providers. Over time, the providers realized that no significant preparation time was needed as they applied their knowledge to these new roles.

The group concept also showed members of the health care team that they needed to review the patient charts prior to the group meetings so that they have a greater understanding of their patients in the group. Moreover, they found that the psychosocial aspects of care are as important as areas that are clinically related.

For the nurses, the group care approach increased their credibility as providers and enhanced the total dimension of the care delivery team concept. Together with the physician, as a physician/nurse team, the nurses are essential to the group process being understood as an office visit and not as a health education class. In fact, the format of the group visit actually humanizes the physician in the eyes of the patient, removing some of the aura of "all knowing scientist" that leads to both poor communication and unrealistic expectations.

Over time, the task force changed some elements of the group visit which, during the pilot, appeared dysfunctional or too costly. For example, having a clinical psychologist to open each session to get the group interacting with a health care team and with each other became unnecessary. The nurses, as well as some of the physicians, became quite proficient with these techniques.

Another decision had to do with how to communicate the group concept to other physician/nurse health care teams at the Wheat Ridge medical offices. Since the group process is difficult to explain in a brief and succinct manner, a video was developed as a means of communication. This has proved to be an excellent communication vehicle and a way of promoting this concept.

EXPANDING THE PILOT TO A PROGRAM

In 1994 Kaiser Permanente expanded the program from a pilot to a regionwide program, and plans to evaluate the program using a much larger sample size over a three-year period.

The task force was reassembled to review the pilot program and determine necessary changes before applying the group concept to the other medical offices. Several approaches were improved. For example, the task force refined the approaches of selecting patients to ensure that no bias was introduced in the randomization process. Data systems had gotten better since the pilot project, improving the clinicians' and the project staff's ability to look at patient utilization patterns over an 18-month versus a 12-month period of time. Uniform procedures were adopted in areas of data collection and data management procedures to assist in evaluating the expanded program.

The task force also reviewed areas where important additional interventions could be developed. One example was the decision to add a pharmacy intervention component to the group CHCC visit. Since chronic disease patients are usually on multiple pharmaceuticals and take many over-the-counter products as well, pharmacy seemed an important area for concentration. As a result, the program would include discussions on pharmacy needs and education.

Specifically, the goals of the pharmacy intervention are to:

- identify, prevent, and resolve actual or potential drug-related problems
- ensure that members understand their medication regimen

- document drug-related utilization patterns
- measure member satisfaction
- determine compliance with medication regimen.

The task force also modified several other areas. First, the group added a few questions to the health screening form to address several issues identified during the pilot project, including questions to help staff quickly identify members who might be most interested in the group visit concept. This approach also decreased the costs of member identification. Second, the satisfaction survey was restructured to include nurses, since they were such an important aspect of the group visit. Third, the task force included in its orientation a list of "lessons learned" to help medical sites in the region apply the concept.

To build enthusiasm and interest in the CHCC model, physicians and staff who participated in the pilot project conducted the regional orientation to all primary care physician/nurse teams in internal medicine and family practice in Kaiser Permanente's Colorado region. They first described the program, invited questions from the audience, and offered their own perspectives. The senior researcher presented the data from the pilot. The same material was available in writing so that people could study it later in greater detail.

Shortly after the major orientation meetings a decision was made to produce a second video as a way of recording the results of the pilot and providing more detail on the regional orientation process. This effort also seemed to be an effective way of transferring "best practices" examples to other Kaiser Permanente regions and other health care organizations. Since the first video was basically an overview of the concept, the second video needed to more fully explain CHCC and answer the most frequently asked questions. Moreover, the second video became another way to encourage other Kaiser Permanente regions to apply the CHCC concept.

FUTURE IMPLICATIONS

Since the orientation meetings were held for the expansion to a regionwide program, the CHCC concept has been used for younger patient groups of hypertensives, diabetics, and routine well-baby visits, especially where the care and treatment regime requires periodic surveillance and monitoring. As the program becomes better known and more familiar throughout the Colorado region of Kaiser Permanente, its application will grow, even outside the Kaiser Permanente organization.

The pilot, and now the program, has assisted in defining what types of system design and data information are needed to measure the success of various interventions over a spectrum of time and care settings. Measuring outcomes for Kaiser Permanente members as they move through various levels of care will be an essential feature of suggested system design changes.

With the greater recognition of the Cooperative Health Care Clinic and resulting impacts on health care use and resources, the patient group visit approach to health care could lead to significant changes in medical and nursing education. Medical and nursing schools need to modify their curriculum and experiential focus to redefine the emerging roles of health professionals. Similar to the recognition that the one-on-one traditional model of the medical office visit does not meet the complex needs of the elderly with chronic disease, so too, the education of professionals must expand and change to a more appropriate level of knowledge that balances the psychosocial and environmental aspects of care.

The unique aspects of caring for seniors need greater visibility, as well as better definition. The excitement surrounding the potential values of CHCC in redesigning the doctor office visit has just begun to surface. Learning continues with each new CHCC group created. Learning more about ourselves as health care professionals and about our members who need counsel, direction, and care creates a new energy and enthusiasm for the future. As one care team member was heard to say, "We taught them medicine and they taught us life."

REFERENCES

1. American Medical Association. "White Paper on Elderly Health." *Archives of Internal Medicine* 150 (1990):2459–2472.
2. Dychtwald, K., and Flower, J. *Age Wave*. New York, NY: Bantam Books, 1990.
3. Freeborn, D.K., et al. "Consistently High Users of Medical Care Among the Elderly." *Medical Care* 28(6) (1990):527–540.
4. Polliack, M.R., and Shavitt, N. "Utilization of Hospital Inpatient Services by the Elderly." *Journal of the American Geriatric Society* 25 (1977):364.
5. Hibbard, J.H., and Pope, C.R. "Age Differences in the Use of Medical Care in an HMO." *Medical Care* 24 (1986):52.
6. Anderson, G., and Knickman, J.R. "Patterns of Expenditures Among High Utilizers of Medical Care Services." *Medical Care* 22 (1984):143.
7. Haug, M.R. "Age and Medical Care Utilization Patterns." *Journal of Gerontology* 36 (1980):103.

IV

Disease Management

IV

Disease Management

9

The Community Medical Alliance: An Integrated System of Care in Greater Boston for People with Severe Disability and AIDS

*Robert J. Master, Tony Dreyfus, Sharon Connors, Carol Tobias,
Zhiyuan Zhou, and Richard Kronick*

The Community Medical Alliance (CMA) in Boston has adapted principles of prepaid managed care to redesign service delivery for people with severe physical disability and with late-stage AIDS. This article discusses the policy context, the rationale for CMA, its system of care, and initial experiences of enrollment, service use, and outcomes. It concludes with a discussion of the opportunities and difficulties of expanding managed care for people with disabilities and chronic illness.

POLICY CONTEXT

For three decades millions of people with disabilities have received much of their health care through fee-for-service arrangements financed by Medicaid programs. Approximately five million people with disability under age 65 received Medicaid coverage at some point in 1993.[1] In the past decade, the growth of managed care has occurred mostly among the relatively healthy employed and AFDC populations, while only small numbers of people with serious disability have been enrolled in managed care.

Over the next decade, however, the enrollment of people with disabilities in both commercial and Medicaid managed care is likely to rise substantially. As HMO populations mature, the prevalence of chronic illness and disability will inevitably increase. New enrollment of people with dis-

Source: Reprinted from R. Master, T. Dreyfus, S. Connors, et al., The Community Medical Alliance: An Integrated System of Care in Greater Boston for People with Severe Disability and AIDS, *Managed Care Quarterly*, Vol. 4, No. 2, pp. 26–37, © 1996, Aspen Publishers, Inc.

abilities will also increase because of the continued pressures on Medicaid programs to contain costs. Medicaid programs in 14 states have applied for Section 1115 waivers that would permit statewide mandatory enroll-ment of AFDC Medicaid beneficiaries into managed care,[2] and a number of states are now discussing the inclusion of recipients with disabilities into managed care. The unrelenting pressures to contain costs will likely cause several states to act within the next few years—with more to follow the leaders.

As a consequence, HMOs must learn how to better address not only the needs of those with more disabling levels of familiar chronic illnesses but also the needs of those with less familiar causes of disability, including mental illness, developmental disability, and injury. Whether the enroll-ment of people with disabilities in managed care will improve or hurt the quality of care they receive will depend both on how fee-for-service sys-tems evolve and on how dexterously managed care can be adapted to the special needs of the population.

RATIONALE FOR COMMUNITY MEDICAL ALLIANCE

Medicaid-covered populations with severe disabilities or serious illness generally find continuous primary care, multidisciplinary coordination, and use of home and community services in lieu of the hospital or institu-tional care quite rare. In Boston, it has been the experience of clinicians and advocates that these populations generally receive care through academic medical centers, with a medical specialty and hospital dependency, con-siderable fragmentation, and little ability to coordinate or access home or community alternatives. This experience is consistent with an analysis of 1992 Medicaid claims for people with disabilities in Ohio, which showed that hospital expenditures accounted for 65 percent of expenditures (ex-clusive of oral pharmacy costs).[3] From the perspective of promoting pa-tient empowerment and a more appropriate mix of services, there is a strong imperative to innovate.

From a Medicaid policy perspective, there is also an imperative for new approaches to financing and delivery for these populations. The SSI dis-abled population represents one sixth of recipients under age 65 but ac-counts for over half of under-65 expenditures (figures do not include dis-proportionate share payments to hospitals).[4] To date, the single most important Medicaid policy reform—managed care—with rare exception has bypassed the SSI disabled population despite their expense and the apparent deficiencies in care in the prevailing fee-for-service system. Very few Medicaid recipients with disability have been enrolled in managed care because of important clinical, financial, and regulatory concerns. The

Massachusetts Medicaid-CMA experience represents one of the first attempts in the United States to adapt managed care contracting widely used for employed and AFDC populations specifically to address prevailing problems in care and cost for people with disabilities.

The Community Medical Alliance was founded in 1989 with the goal of meeting the health care needs of severely disabled or chronically ill patients in ways that would support their independence, autonomy, and empowerment through innovations in primary care and the organization of home- and community-based services. In 1992 CMA began contracting on a capitated but limited risk basis with Massachusetts Medicaid for the care of patients with severe physical disability and with late-stage AIDS. In both the AIDS and severe physical disability programs, CMA uses teams of nurse practitioners and physicians to provide total primary care and case management across a full range of settings, including patients' homes and ambulatory, long-term care and hospital sites. CMA's network includes 13 primary care sites and 8 hospitals. To support the primary care teams, CMA contracts with the following array of services:

- acute general hospital
- medical specialty services
- home health care services
- private duty nursing services
- home infusion therapy services
- day health services
- adult foster care services
- care and protection beds
- mental health and substance abuse services
- institutional hospice
- skilled nursing facility and chronic disease hospital services
- nutrition services
- medical equipment and supplies.

SEVERE PHYSICAL DISABILITY PROGRAM

The origins of the Community Medical Alliance were in the Urban Medical Group, a nonprofit physician-nurse practitioner group practice in Boston which in the 1970s developed a specialization in the care of frail elders and of adults with severe physical disability. The group pioneered the use of nurse practitioners as providers of primary care for elders who were home-bound or in nursing homes.[5]

This new approach to care attracted the attention of staff at the Boston Center for Independent Living, which asked the Urban Medical Group to create a health care program that could meet the needs of people with severe physical disability who were moving from institutions to independent living. Under arrangement with the Massachusetts Medicaid program beginning in 1982, primary care was provided on a fee-for-service basis to patients with severe physical disability, with enhanced fees for home visits and case management. The core of the system was the pairing of a primary physician with a nurse practitioner who played a central role in the provision of medical care, especially in patients' homes. The nurse practitioner or the doctor was available for routine and emergency consultation 24 hours a day, seven days a week. One evaluation of the program concluded that it had achieved reductions in length of hospital stays and in emergency room utilization for the more medically intense subset of the patient population.[6]

In 1988 Boston's Community Medical Group (BCMG) was established separately to focus exclusively on the care of people with severe physical disabilities. The program continued on a fee-for-service basis until 1992, when CMA entered a capitated contract with Massachusetts Medicaid to manage BCMG's provision of care. CMA converted the financing of BCMG's severely disabled patients to prepaid capitation. The practice has grown by purely voluntary enrollment to reach 180 patients (disenrollment for any reason is allowed at any time). At the outset, the enrolled group represented over half the people in the greater Boston area who were Medicaid-eligible and met the program criteria.

Enrollees in the program must meet *each* of the following criteria: permanent triplegia or quadriplegia; a need for personal care attendant services or equivalent to maintain independent living; and one of a number of specified diagnoses, such as spinal cord injury, cerebral palsy, muscular dystrophy and end-stage muscular sclerosis or Huntington's disease. (The need for personal care attendant services is defined by Massachusetts Medicaid and involves continuous and irreversible dependency in four activities of daily living. The inclusion of "equivalent" services in the criteria has significantly expanded the eligible group.) Medical care is provided by a clinical team that includes two physicians and four nurse practitioners, with each patient assigned to one of the nurse practitioners. Each nurse practitioner carries a caseload of approximately 50 disabled enrollees. The goal of the team approach is to provide primary care and ancillary services in the most appropriate setting (most often in the patient's home) as alternatives to specialty and hospital care.

Every enrolled patient has a primary care physician who provides medical management and coordination and is empowered to authorize inpatient admissions and most other services available in the CMA network. The physician provides medical consultation to the nurse practitioner or directly to the patient 24 hours a day, seven days a week. At weekly case conferences the clinical team focuses on cases with active medical problems or scheduled for periodic review. The primary care physician is the admitting physician of record for all hospital care and coordinates all inpatient care—an approach distinct from the prevailing practice in Boston for this population, in which inpatient care occurs on teaching services with little or no primary care management.

CENTRAL ROLE OF THE NURSE PRACTITIONER

In the CMA care system the nurse practitioner assumes a pivotal role with an unprecedented scope of practice, including comprehensive initial assessments, first response to new problems, the transfer of medical decision making to the home or alternative site, and responsibility for first call on weekends and holidays. Home visits are made frequently to monitor chronic conditions, and to provide urgent care in the home rather than in the office, clinic, or emergency room.

Beyond providing direct patient care, the nurse practitioner acts as the case manager, coordinating all needed services such as mental health, home health care, physical therapy, equipment, seating clinics, and social services. The nurse practitioner also participates in hospital discharge planning. Combining clinical and case management roles, the nurse practitioners supplement home visits with frequent phone contact to answer patient questions and offer reassurance, guidance, and support.

The case management function is clearly recognized as an essential part of the nurse practitioner's work, not merely an add-on to the home visits. Fifty percent of the day is devoted to work other than home visits. The integration of clinical care and case management functions by the nurse practitioner is substantially different from more usual approaches, in which the case manager is not a direct provider of medical care.

To provide services in the home even for urgent problems requires two capacities: the clinical ability to quickly make decisions and the management ability to promptly marshal resources. The intent of having the nurse practitioner perform both roles is to allow the integration of clinical decision making and management and the potential for more rapid response. The nurse practitioners have at their disposal an established system to assemble the needed services, for example, the infusion antibiotics, equipment and supplies, private duty nursing, and home respiratory therapy for an episode of pneumonia. As case manager, a nurse practitioner can bring into the patient's home various elements of expertise and authority, can discuss options with a patient the moment a problem is recognized, and can initiate decisions and treatments much more quickly than a less knowledgeable or less empowered case manager.

Consider the following case study as an example: Steve S. is a 32-year-old man with a C_{6-7} cervical spinal cord injury in 1986 from a motor vehicle accident. Between 1987 and 1991, with fee-for-service Medicaid coverage, he had three long hospitalizations to treat stage IV recurrent decubitus ulcers with surgical flap procedures. In 1991, prior to his last admission, his primary care nurse practitioner recommended a short-term hospital stay for intensive nursing care to be followed by a home private duty nurse and a specialized air mattress as a strategy to prevent the deterioration of his decubitus ulcer. Under the fee-for-service system, the admission was denied for not meeting the criteria of medical necessity, and the approval of home private duty nursing and the specialized mattress was delayed because of a cumbersome bureaucratic process; as a result, hospitalization for surgical reconstruction was eventually needed. In 1993, when a similar deteriorating decubitus ulcer recurred and Steve was enrolled at CMA, the care plan of a short hospitalization, home private duty nursing, and a specialized mattress was carried out, with a prompt reversal of the ulcerating process.

The close personal relationship between nurse practitioner and patient is intended to contribute to a more effective and empowering treatment of the patient. One purpose of the home visits is to foster strong communication with the patient, in order to improve the prompt reporting of incipient problems, attention to medical advice, and the ability of patient and provider to resolve together complex medical, psychological, and social problems faced by people with disabilities. Nurse practitioner visits in the patient's home are also intended to foster a relationship of greater equality and exchange than is likely when the patient sees a doctor in an office setting.

AIDS PROGRAM

The rising incidence of AIDS presents a host of challenges to managed care systems. As survival times lengthen, AIDS has become more of a chronic illness, and people with AIDS can increasingly benefit from ongoing coordination of care. Yet enormous difficulties are posed by the intensive level of care required, the rapidly changing treatment technologies, and the stigma, substance abuse, and unstable living circumstances often associated with AIDS. While the model of care developed for people with severe disability had many features that were readily transferable to the care of people with late-stage AIDS, the two programs also have some important differences.

As in the physical disability program, individuals enroll and disenroll voluntarily. They must meet the clinical criteria of CDC-defined AIDS with at least one opportunistic infection, malignancy, or other sign of advanced HIV infection. The nurse practitioners specializing in AIDS care assume the same broad array of responsibilities as described in the physical disability program.

The most obvious difference between the two programs is in the relationship between CMA and enrollees' physicians. Unlike people with severe physical disability, who are affiliated with only a few providers, people with AIDS in greater Boston can be found under the care of many physicians, health centers, and hospitals. As a result, CMA's AIDS program has more the characteristics of an independent practice association, while the severe physical disability program has more the characteristics of a staff model.

Patients with AIDS enter the CMA program under the care of doctors who have specialized in family practice, internal medicine, and infectious disease, and are located in private practices, community health centers, and tertiary hospitals. All contracted physicians are required to be board-certified in their specialty and to have demonstrated experience in the treatment of AIDS. Infectious disease specialists are encouraged to serve as primary care physicians. To compensate for the prevalent fragmented physician call system found in the Boston area and to help attract physicians to the AIDS program, CMA's nurse practitioners assume first call at night and on weekends, offering a first contact with someone familiar with the patients and their illness.

In supporting the clinicians who care for people with AIDS, a critical strategy is to facilitate the provision of care in patients' homes. Physicians order services provided in the home with a single call to the patient's nurse practitioner at CMA, whose service coordinator contacts the vendors. The nurse practitioner and service coordinator work to *facilitate* the ordering of services, not to impede them.

In teaming with physicians from different specialties, nurse practitioners must play varied roles. For physicians whose practices are not predominantly focused on the care of AIDS, the nurse practitioners can support the physician in exploring diagnosis and treatment decisions. Conversely, for patients under the care of physicians who are expert in the care of AIDS, the nurse practitioners can assist with their better knowledge of primary care and home care needs. The nurse practitioners meet weekly with the medical director of the AIDS program to discuss the most acute cases, to review periodically the condition of other patients, and to consider new approaches to challenging cases. Nurse practitioners are also responsible to facilitate enrollees' participation in clinical trials.

In the AIDS program, each nurse practitioner cares for approximately 25 enrollees.

Though patients with AIDS do not face the transportation and physical access problems of people with severe physical disability, the need for care in the home rises when patients with AIDS become more debilitated. As a substitute both for office visits and for inpatient care, home visits by nurse practitioners are critical to the management of patients with more advanced disease. Because of the complexity of AIDS, the attendant psychological and social problems, and the diversity of settings the patients move through, the nurse practitioners must be experienced and flexible in applying their knowledge. All nurse practitioners in the program have specialized in AIDS care and benefited from training with the program's senior nurse practitioner, who is a nationally recognized leader in the development of AIDS training for health care professionals.

EXPERIENCE

The following section presents information available on the program's initial experience with enrollment, satisfaction, cost and utilization, and quality monitoring.

Enrollment

Between April 1992 and December 1994, 212 individuals with severe disability and 197 individuals with advanced AIDS enrolled in CMA. In the severely disabled population during the period April 1992–December 1993, 51 percent of enrollees had stable neurologic illness (typically cerebral palsy with functional spastic quadriplegia), 30 percent had cervical spinal cord injury, and 19 percent had degenerative neuromuscular illness (e.g., Duchenne's muscular dystrophy, amyotrophic lateral sclerosis, or Friedreich's ataxia). About one tenth of the enrollees depend upon ventilators.

The enrolled population with AIDS has tended to be far along in the illness. In the period from April 1992 through December 1993, enrollees had a median CD_4 lymphocyte count at enrollment of 61, with an annual mortality rate of 50 percent. (The CD_4 counts at enrollment are summarized in Table 9–1; no comparative data for the fee-for-service population was available.) A case-mix classification based on AIDS-related diagnoses was adapted from the work of Turner and colleagues[7] to compare the severity of illness of fee-for-service Medicaid recipients with AIDS *eligible* for CMA to the severity of CMA's patients. Classified at a low level of severity were almost half of the eligibles but only one fifth of CMA enrollees; classified at a high level of severity were only 15 percent of the eligibles but 38 percent of CMA enrollees.

Table 9–1 Community Medical Alliance Enrollees with AIDS: Caseload Severity of Illness Measurement, April 1992 through December 1993

CD_4 count at enrollment	Number of enrollees	Percent of enrollees
0–50	52	46
51–100	21	19
100–200	16	14
>200	24	21

CMA enrollees with AIDS are predominantly individuals with injection-drug use as a risk factor whose attendant physical, psychological, and social problems present significant challenges to any care delivery system. Among patients in 1993, 56 percent had injection-drug use as a risk factor, 30 percent were female, and 40 percent were people of color. (Risk factors of enrollees are summarized in Table 9–2.) The program in 1994 reached average monthly enrollment levels of 85 to 90 patients. Enrollments have slightly outpaced deaths, which in the last three quarters of 1994 occurred at an average rate of four per month.

Satisfaction

In the physical disability program, a survey by Massachusetts Medicaid found a high level of satisfaction, and a review of the program by the National Committee for Quality Assurance found satisfaction "impressively high," based on discussion with a group of randomly selected enrollees[8]:

> Probably one of the most significant reflections of the effectiveness of this program was the glowing praise offered by participants in the focus group. Even when pressed to offer suggestions for improvement,

Table 9–2 CMA Enrollment—AIDS: Risk Factors, April 1992 through December 1993

Risk factor	N	%
Male sex w/male	23	20.4
Injecting drug use	61	54.0
Male/male sex and IDU	2	1.8
Heterosexual	2	1.8
Receipt of blood products	1	0.8
Pediatric	1	0.8
Unknown	23	20.4
Total	113	100.0

members were unable to think of anything that could be done to better serve them. The members themselves provided a resounding endorsement of the program.[9]

Disenrollments were few, with most resulting from enrollees moving from the greater Boston area and from death. From April 1992 to March 1994 there were 320 enrollee years and four voluntary disenrollments, mostly for dissatisfaction with the requirement to use services within CMA's network of providers.

In the AIDS program, member satisfaction was examined by a telephone survey of enrollees performed in June 1993 by Massachusetts Medicaid, which found surveyed enrollees "very satisfied."[10] Although the usefulness of the survey was limited by its small respondent group of 19 enrollees, 89 percent were satisfied with their health care and 95 percent would recommend the program—over two thirds of them strongly agreeing that they would recommend. In 1993 there were only two voluntary disenrollments, and in 1994 there were also two.

Across both programs, the rate of voluntary disenrollment from 1992 to 1994 has been two percent per year, with nine complaints made to CMA and no formal grievances.

Cost and utilization

Efforts to evaluate levels of cost and utilization have been limited by the difficulty of establishing valid comparison groups. Massachusetts Medicaid set the monthly capitation rates of $1,998 and $3,756 respectively for patients with severe physical disability and AIDS who did not also have Medicare coverage. Both rates were set at 95 percent of the estimated fee-for-service average, covering medical services exclusive of oral pharmacy, personal care attendant, and dental services. There was substantial uncertainty, however, about Medicaid's ability to define these averages accurately.

In both programs, 1993 medical care costs were substantially less than the capitation rates, about $1,300 per patient per month in the physical disability program and $2,950 in the AIDS program. The contract with Massachusetts Medicaid was written with quite limited risk, in order to provide the flexibility of capitation without imposing a large risk or profit incentive: all savings beyond 5 percent of the capitation are returned to the state. The state thus protects itself from making large overpayments because of inaccurate ratesetting or favorable selection. Most likely, some of the difference between the capitation rates and the actual costs was due to care management and some to the initial rates perhaps being set too high. (Since

August 1995, the enrollment criteria, capitation rates, and risk arrangements have been modified.)

Massachusetts Medicaid, using the case-mix classification adapted from Turner and colleagues, recently compared 1993 medical care costs of patients with AIDS enrolled in CMA to the costs of comparably ill Medicaid recipients with AIDS in fee-for-service care. With adjustments made for differences in age, sex, and location between the CMA and the statewide comparison group, CMA costs were found to be 91 percent of fee-for-service costs.[11] This apparent cost advantage of 9 percent is partially offset by CMA's higher costs for administration and case management. Work remains to establish proper fee-for-service comparison groups for CMA enrollees. For example, the comparison of CMA and fee-for-service costs did not adjust for the higher proportion of CMA enrollees with injection drug use as a risk factor, which is associated with higher medical costs even when severity of illness is controlled for by diagnostic categories.[12] We imagine that further analysis will support the contention that CMA's system with its enhancement of coordination and primary care need cost no more, and may well cost less, than traditional fee-for-service care.

Forty-eight percent of the enrollees with disabilities and 18 percent of the enrollees with AIDS were, or became, dually entitled, that is with Medi*care* as primary payer in addition to Medicaid. Medicaid capitation rates were set at $457 and $312 per month for dually entitled enrollees with physical disability and AIDS, respectively. These rates were almost certainly set too low, with the result that the apparent savings on the Medicaid-only enrollees were considerably offset by losses on the dually eligible patients. In the AIDS program, the rate for dual eligibles was far short of 1993 average medical service costs of $1,448 per month.

Comparisons of the hospital utilization of CMA patients with that of Medicaid recipients with quadriplegia in Ohio suggest that CMA has succeeded in reducing the use of inpatient hospital services. From April 1992 to June 1993, when CMA had 2,276 months of care for patients with severe physical disability, approximately 40 percent of the dollars were devoted to care in acute and subacute hospitals. Data from Ohio for 1993 Medicaid recipients with quadriplegia under fee-for-service indicate that, for a comparable benefit package, 66 percent of total dollars went to inpatient care. Ohio data are for disabled recipients eligible for at least one month in 1993 who had at least one claim with a diagnosis of quadriplegia in 1991, 1992, or 1993, and exclude the institutionalized, those with Medicare coverage, waiver services, or diagnoses of mental retardation or severe mental illness. Because comparisons of expenditures are influenced by variation across states in hospital and provider reimbursement, we have greater confidence in comparisons of utilization. For CMA patients during the period April 1993 through March 1994, average acute and rehabilitation hospital days were only 5.4 days per person per year compared with an average of 9.9 hospital days per person per year for Ohio Medicaid recipients with quadriplegia.

The service use and cost experience of CMA enrollees with severe physical disability and AIDS suggest that significant redistribution of services from hospital to home and from specialty care to primary care occurred in the CMA system. The CMA emphasis on primary care is reflected in the distribution of physician expenditures in the physical disability program, with 90 percent of physician expenditures being made for primary care and only 10 percent for specialty care. Although data for a comparable population are not available, we expect that expenditures on specialists would be a much higher proportion. A comprehensive study of costs of care for AIDS patients in ten cities found that, excluding prescription drugs, 75 percent of dollars in 1992 were for inpatient care.[13] (Hellinger gives 58 percent as the inpatient share when drugs are included.) Although neither the method nor the study populations are directly comparable, at CMA the proportion for inpatient care has been approximately 56 percent. A much greater proportion of CMA expenditures are for home health services than are reported in the ten-city study. (See Table 9–3 for a comparison of service distributions in the ten-city study and in CMA and Table 9–4 for the distribution of outpatient expenditures in the physical disability program.) Eighty-seven and 40 percent of medical encounters occurred at home for the disabled and AIDS populations, respectively—a pattern dramatically different from that found in fee-for-service care.

Table 9–3 AIDS Care Service Distribution Comparison

	Hellinger's ten-city study* 407 patients, 10 cities, 1992 21% injection drug users 51% Medicaid recipients	CMA 154 patients, 1993–1994 56% injection drug users all Medicaid recipients
Acute inpatient	75.6%	42.4%
Other inpatient	—	13.9
Physician services	15.6	11.6
Home health & therapies	6.7	26.9
Other	2.1	5.2

*Hellinger, F.J. "The Lifetime Cost of Treating a Person with HIV," *Journal of the American Medical Association.* 1993): 270(4): 476. Hellinger's distribution was modified to exclude pharmacy costs.

Table 9–4 Physical Disability Program Outpatient Expenses, April 1992 through June 1993 (2,276 Months of Care)

Service	Cost per member per month*	% Share
Primary care—home	$86.70	12.2
Primary care—office, hospital clinic	42.41	6.0
Nonvisit case management	20.58	2.9
Medical specialty care	18.93	2.7
Emergency room care	4.01	0.6
Mental health & substance abuse	58.26	8.2
Home health†—RN, PDN, ADH, infusion	179.23	25.3
Medical equipment & supplies	298.14	42.1

*Excludes dually entitled.
†Registered nurse, private duty nursing, adult day health.

Quality monitoring

Quality improvement standards specific to people with disabilities have not yet been established as they have for general populations. CMA has selected for study the incidence of Stage III and IV decubitus ulcers and pneumocystis pneumonia (PCP) in the disabled and AIDS programs, respectively, gathered baseline data on these conditions, and developed interventions for outcome evaluation. Quality monitoring studies found decreased rates of these conditions when compared to the incidence of these conditions found in the very same population in the year prior to enrollment.

Management of pressure sores was identified as an area for quality improvement in care outcomes. For patients with spinal cord injury, pressure sores are the most common cause of rehospitalization.[14] Service use and cost experiences to treat advanced pressure sores in fee-for-service and CMA's prepaid system show that inpatient days, hospital costs, and reconstructive surgical procedures declined (Table 9–5). Although the rate of hospital admission for pressure-sore management was unchanged, fewer procedures were required and lengths of stay and per member per month costs were substantially reduced. CMA plans to further reduce pressure sore incidence with new screening tools and protocols for interventions at various stages, accelerated seating evaluations, development of a specialized inpatient program at a chronic hospital for intensive nursing and education, and use of peer counselors.

A CMA quality assurance review of the incidence of PCP among CMA patients before and after enrollment suggests that the program helped reduce the incidence of PCP and promote the management of PCP episodes

Table 9–5 Comparison of Pressure Sore Incidence and Management in Spinal Cord Injured Patients in Two Reimbursement Systems: Fee-for-service and Prepaid Managed Care in the Same Primary Care Practice, 1991–1994

	BCMG experience 1991–1992 fee-for-service (n = 49 pts, 49 pt yrs)	BCMG experience 1992–1994 prepaid care (n = 45 pts, 90 pt yrs)
Hospital admissions for pressure sore management (per patient per year)	0.12	0.13
Reconstructive flap procedures performed* (per patient per year)	0.14	0.08
Average length of inpatient stays	57.9 days	27.2 days
Hospital days for pressure sore management (per patient per year)	7.1	3.6
Inpatient costs for pressure sore management including acute and subacute (per patient per month)	$491	$239

Study periods: fee-for-service, 4/91–3/92; prepaid care, 4/92–3/94.
*The rate of procedures exceeded the rate of admissions because one patient underwent two procedures in one admission.

outside the hospital. PCP is the most common pneumonia in people with AIDS and a frequent cause of hospitalization, despite the availability of prophylaxis such as daily oral trimethoprim/sulfamethoxazole or monthly aerosolized pentamidine.[15] Achieving compliance with prophylaxis can be difficult with those who are intermittently homeless, using drugs, unaware of scheduled visits, or simply averse to intervention. For injection-drug users, a study in Brooklyn found recurrent PCP as the most common specific cause of hospitalization (35 percent of all their AIDS-related hospitalizations).[16]

The review found a decline in the incidence of PCP among CMA members after they enrolled. Among 113 CMA enrollees over 977 months there were 14 PCP episodes for a rate of 17.2 per 100 patient years. By contrast, in the medical records of the 1,793 patient months for these members with AIDS *before* they enrolled in CMA, 84 episodes were identified, for a rate of 56.2 per 100 patient years (Table 9–6). Eight of the episodes were managed entirely at home, three partially in the hospital, and three totally in the hospital. The Brooklyn population over 456 patient months experienced a rate of 39.6 episodes per 100 patient years. Some caveats must be made about comparing these figures: episodes prior to enrollment were often "sentinel" or first definite indications of AIDS, prior to which patients may not have been receiving

Table 9–6 CMA AIDS Program PCP Rate Comparison

	Months of care	PCP rate per 100 patient years	PCP hospital admission rate per 100 patient years
CMA enrollees	977	17.2	9.8
CMA enrollees with CDC AIDS prior to enrollment	1793	56.2	—
New York City IVDU Population with AIDS*	456	39.6	39.6

*Bennett, C.L., and Pascal, A. "Medical Care Costs of Intravenous Drug Users with AIDS in Brooklyn," *Journal of Acquired Immune Deficiency Syndromes* 5 (1992): 1–6.

---

medical care or known of a need for prophylaxis. (Further, the Brooklyn group all were injection-drug users, versus CMA's 56 percent, and in the period of the Brooklyn study prophylaxis was recommended but did not yet have the status of standard of care.) But CMA enrollees were probably more immunocompromised after enrollment than before, and the ability to manage a majority of episodes entirely at home suggests that PCP was being identified and managed at an early stage.

EVALUATING THE DATA

Summary of strategies and principles

While CMA has used certain strategies in the development of care systems for people with severe physical disability and AIDS, these specific approaches are not always possible or desirable in other circumstances. In some states, for example, the use of nurse practitioners might need to be modified because of legal restrictions; populations with less intensive needs might alternatively receive care from registered nurses. Exhibit 9–1 lists some of the strategies used by CMA and some of the more general principles of managed care for people with disability that could be realized in other ways.

Because the CMA experience is limited with respect to time, numbers of enrollees, and clinical characteristics of the enrollees, any assertion of the efficacy of these financing and delivery approaches must be made with caution. Nevertheless, this experience seems to support the contention that prevailing patterns of care and cost for the severely disabled are determined mostly by hospital and provider requirements rather than patient need. Because of the complex needs of both populations, care has historically

Exhibit 9–1 Principles and Strategies of Managed Care for the Disabled

Principles	*Strategies*
• integrate case management with clinical decision making in new clinical roles	• use nurse practitioners as key providers of primary care and case management
• make providers who know the patient as accessible as possible	• use nurse practitioner/physician teams to provide care in the home and consultation around the clock
• create the environment in which a strong personal relationship between patient and clinician can develop	• set the caseload of nurse practitioners to allow frequent home visits, phone contact, and adequate time for case management
• help clinicians provide services in the most appropriate setting; allow prompt allocation of needed resources	• help clinicians respond to problems quickly by giving them full authority and a centralized system to order all services
• use care providers with special knowledge of patients' conditions	• require board-eligible physicians and nurse practitioners specialized in AIDS or severe physical disability
• use early interventions aggressively to limit complications of chronic conditions	• focus systematically on complications that can be reduced or cared for better at home
• use risk-adjusted capitation to allow innovation for serving people at varying levels of need	• secure financial resources needed for even the most complex cases and use the flexibility of full capitation with limited risk to shift services from hospital to home

been in the domain of the specialty physician with considerable hospital dependency. Yet the CMA experience suggests that the flexibility of prepayment can be used to substantially shift care to primary care clinicians, mostly nurse practitioners, and to home and community options with a high degree of patient satisfaction and without apparent compromise in quality.

Opportunities and dangers of managed care for people with disabilities or chronic illness

Prepaid managed care has the potential to yield great improvements in health care for people with chronic illness and disability, because it provides the flexibility needed to redesign the delivery system around the needs of the target population. Capitation allows innovative providers to fund early interventions, to coordinate services, and to develop systems specifically for people with disabilities, and it rewards them when these investments produce savings. Yet optimism must be tempered by an awareness of the shortcomings of traditional forms of managed care. For managed care to bring improvements to the health care of people with chronic illness, it must be adapted to their particular needs.

As political and financial pressures accelerate the movement of Medicaid recipients with disability into prepaid managed care, delivery systems that do not redesign services but simply use traditional strategies of utilization management and selective contracting are likely to do more harm than good. Population-specific medical specialty networks need to be developed, since people with disabilities are especially sensitive to the disruption of long-standing relationships with essential specialty providers. For those with mental retardation or chronic mental illness, traditional benefit restriction and carve-out strategies should be replaced with innovations that link case management to primary care and to the resources of state departments of mental retardation and mental health. For enrollees who draw inspiration from the independent living movement, managed care plans should promote self-care and self-management strategies. Plans will also need to establish new measures of quality and outcome, since many of the currently used measures have little relevance to people with disabilities. For these many challenges to be met and better systems developed over time, people with disabilities will need to have meaningful choice among competing health plans designed for their needs.

The reimbursement approach so widely used for the general employed and AFDC populations requires substantial modification if plans are to be rewarded for developing systems of care that are responsive to people with disabilities. First, capitation must be risk-adjusted, since there are many identifiable subgroups whose health service expenditures are well above the average expenditures for people with disabilities. Without adequate risk adjustment, plans face strong incentives, perhaps even financial imperatives, to avoid the very populations for which managed care offers the greatest promise. The adjustment of capitation rates to reflect the risks of people with disabilities has been addressed in detail in a recent article.[17]

Second, creative risk sharing and reinsurance arrangements are required. Until a credible risk-adjusted payment system is developed and tested, Medicaid programs should offer some combination of risk-sharing and reinsurance if plans are to enroll and care for the sickest and most complex subsets of the disabled.

Third, Medi*care* capitation needs to flow into plans concurrently with Medicaid capitation for SSI disabled enrollees, since about 30 percent of

Medicaid recipients with disability also have Medicare coverage.[18] Capitation for "Medicaid only" services creates perverse incentives to promote hospital care while removing from the plan the pool of hospital dollars that is essential to finance enhanced primary care and home and community options. Any large-scale effort to move SSI eligibles into managed care plans will require a new role for Medicare capitation as well.

For people with disabilities the potential pitfalls of managed care are many, with serious implications for the health of a population that includes some of the most fragile and vulnerable members of our society. Yet the potential benefits of managed care for people with disabilities certainly far surpass the benefits of managed care for the nondisabled. The authors hope that managed care can expand to serve this population, not with the haste that some managed care advocates might prefer, but with the attention required to develop a better system of health care for people who can benefit so greatly in terms of health and quality of life.

The prevalent delivery models widely seen in fee-for-service practices and HMOs enrolling employed or AFDC populations require substantial redesign if the needs of Medicaid's disabled are to be met. Such redesign involves approaches that recognize the need for an integration of acute care, long-term care, and mental health services, an enhanced role for primary care, and an integration of case management into the primary care function. The CMA experience perhaps offers some applicable models in this regard.

REFERENCES

1. Kronick, R., Zhou, Z., and Dreyfus, T. "Making Risk Adjustment Work For Everyone." *Inquiry* 32 (Spring 1995): 41–55.
2. Tanenbaum, S.J., and Hurley, R.E. "Managed Care, Disability and the 1115 Waiver Frenzy." Unpublished paper, December 1994, p. 2.
3. Kronick, R., et al. "Preliminary Analysis of Health Expenditures in the SSI Population." Unpublished Medicaid Working Group paper, March 1994.
4. Urban Institute analysis of Health Care Financing Administration (HCFA) data 1994, as reported in handbook for the conference "The Federal-State Partnership for State Health Reform: The Role of 1115 Demonstration Waivers," sponsored by HCFA, March 14–15, 1995, Arlington, Va.
5. Master, R.J., et al. "A Continuum of Care for the Inner City; Assessment of Its Benefits for Boston's Elderly and High-Risk Populations." *New England Journal of Medicine* 302 (June 26, 1980): 1434–1440.
6. Meyers, A.R., et al. "A Prospective Evaluation of the Effect of Managed Care on Medical Care Utilization Among Severely Disabled Independently Living Adults." *Medical Care* (November 1987): 1057–1068.
7. Turner, B.J., et al. "The AIDS-defining Diagnosis and Subsequent Complications: A Survival-Based Severity Index." *Journal of Acquired Immune Deficiency Syndromes* 4(10) (1991): 1059–1071.

8. National Committee for Quality Assurance. *Focused Review: Care of the Severely Disabled; Community Medical Alliance.* Unpublished paper, Washington, D.C., May 1994, p. iii.

9. Ibid., p. 8.

10. "Patient Satisfaction Survey Results." Unpublished paper, Boston, Mass., Massachusetts Division of Medical Assistance, 1993, p. 5.

11. McNulty, P. "Comparison of PMPM Costs: CMA vs. DMA." Unpublished paper, Massachusetts Division of Medical Assistance, May 1995.

12. Markson, L.E., et al. "Patterns of Medicaid Expenditure After AIDS Diagnosis." *Health Care Financing Review* 15(4) (Summer 1994): 43–59.

13. Hellinger, F.J. "The Lifetime Cost of Treating a Person with HIV." *Journal of the American Medical Association* 270(4) (July 28, 1993): 476.

14. Ditunno, J., and Formal, C. "Chronic Spinal Cord Injury." *New England Journal of Medicine* 330(8) (1994): 550–556.

15. Golden, J., et al. "Prevention of PCP by Inhaled Pentamidine." *Lancet* 1 (1989): 654–657.

16. Bennett, C.L., and Pascal, A. "Medical Care Costs of Intravenous Drug Users with AIDS in Brooklyn." *Journal of Acquired Immune Deficiency Syndromes* 5 (1992): 1–6.

17. Kronick, Zhou, and Dreyfus. "Making Risk Adjustment Work For Everyone."

18. Ibid., p. 43.

10

A Systems Approach to Asthma Care

Thomas F. Plaut, Tom Howell, Susan M. Walsh,
Mary Pastor, and Teresa Jones

Asthma is the most common chronic disease affecting children, with a prevalence rate estimated to be between 5 and 10 percent. Nationally, asthma affects nearly 11 million Americans, more than 3 million of whom are under 15 years of age. It accounts for more than $2.4 billion in direct health care costs annually.[1] The national hospitalization rate for asthma for children under 15 was 2.8 admissions per 1,000 and 9.5 hospital days per 1,000 in 1993.[2] Hospitalization and emergency room care account for two thirds of the asthma care dollars spent for children under age 18.[3]

The main goal in managing asthma is preventing acute exacerbations and providing early treatment for those that occur. Experts suggest that the major factors contributing to morbidity and mortality associated with asthma are underdiagnosis and inappropriate treatment.[4] Many hospitalizations are preventable since they are due to a failure in outpatient management.

In September 1994, Principal Health Care of Louisiana (PHCLa) launched an intervention to improve the care of children with asthma. PHCLa is a 26,600-member independent practice association (IPA) model health maintenance organization (HMO) managed by Principal Health Care with headquarters in Rockville, Maryland. Forty-six pediatricians, 13 in solo practice and 33 in seven pediatric groups, care for Principal's 6,642 members under age 15. Principal's members account for only 1 to 25 percent of each physician's patient load. Of the 18 HMOs managed by Princi-

Source: Reprinted from T.F. Plaut, T. Howell, S.M. Walsh, M. Pastor, and T. Jones, A Systems Approach to Asthma Care, *Managed Care Quarterly*, Vol. 4, No. 3, pp. 6–18, © 1996, Aspen Publishers, Inc.

pal Health Care, the Louisiana plan had the highest hospitalization rate for childhood asthma. In 1993, asthma generated 9.6 hospital days per 1,000 PHCLa child enrollees, or 101 percent of the U.S. rate for 1993. The admission rate was 3.5 per 1,000, or 125 percent of the U.S. rate. Cost for hospitalizations was $82,734, averaging $1,293 per day (Table 10–1).

Plan managers identified pediatric asthma as a likely area for improving care and saving costs if hospitalizations could be reduced. After a feasibility study confirmed this view, Principal administrators agreed that a comprehensive program could be cost-effective. A physician consultant then analyzed PHCLa baseline hospitalization data for 1993 using the HMO Data Sheet (Table 10–2). An improvement in outpatient asthma care could reduce hospital days for asthma by 33 percent during the first year of the intervention, and half that amount during the second year. This effort could lower the Principal rate for asthma hospital days to 50 percent of the national rate for 1993 and could save a total of 53 days during a two-year intervention from September 1, 1994 to August 31, 1996.

The intervention focuses on provider education emphasizing early diagnosis of asthma, early use of oral steroids, proper use of inhalation devices, objective monitoring of patient status, and use of daily preventive treatment. Patient education is an integral part of treatment. This approach supports the primary care physician as the provider and coordinator of care by supplying monitoring and treatment devices, books, diaries, home care services, and allergy consultation. It also manifests a systems approach to asthma care in its reliance on a nurse case manager who oversees patient and family support networks.

Table 10–1 Baseline Data for Principal Health Care, New Orleans 1993

Membership in IPA/HMO	26,656
Pediatric membership	6,642
Pediatric membership as a % of total	24.9%
Number of children with asthma	482
Prevalence of asthma in children	7.25%
Pediatric hospital days 1993	64
Goal: Reduce hospital days for childhood asthma by 33% from baseline in first year and 50% in second year, a total reduction of 53 days.	
Average hospital cost per day	$ 1,293
Expected savings (53 × $1,293)	68,529
Costs:	
Physician Consultant	18,000
Consultant travel and travel time	6,500
Equipment and books	8,502
Projected net saving:	35,527

Table 10–2 HMO Data Sheet

Number of child enrollees under 15 years of age on January 1, 1993: 7,671.
Number of child enrollees under 15 years of age on January 1, 1994: 5,613.

Average for 1993 is 6642.

Hospitalizations under 15 years of age after newborn discharge in 1993:

	New Orleans			U.S. 1993
	Discharges	Days	Rate per 1,000	Rate per 1,000
Asthma (ICD CM-9 493)	23	64	9.6	9.5
Acute Bronchitis/Bronchiolitis (ICD CM-9 466)	5	14	2.1	N.A.
Pneumonia (ICD CM-9 480–486)	15	63	9.5	12.6

SPECIFIC INTERVENTION ACTIVITIES

Managers accepted the physician consultant's stipulation that every admission for asthma should be considered due to failure of outpatient treatment unless proven otherwise. Patients were not to be blamed for poor asthma control.

Primary care physicians are the cornerstone of this intervention. They initiate and manage all aspects of patient care. Six asthma advocates—three pediatricians, an internist, and two allergists—were selected by the health services manager because of their interest in asthma, their good working relationships with Principal, and their membership in major practice groups. They maintain continuous dialogue with the physician consultant and communicate current asthma care practices to their colleagues.

Through this intervention the physicians can offer a broad array of essential resources at no cost to the patient: durable medical equipment (e.g., compressor-driven nebulizers, peak flow meters and holding chambers); a home care program for assessment, education, and skill building; and consultation with an allergist (see Exhibit 10–1). Principal provides a copy of the 40-page basic asthma guide, *One Minute Asthma: What You Need to Know*,[5] to the family of each asthma patient. A more comprehensive book, *Children with Asthma: A Manual for Parents*,[6] is given to families whose children have moderate or severe asthma problems. Estimated costs for equipment and books are listed in Table 10–3. Patients are managed through the entire continuum of care in a manner consistent with the National Heart, Lung, and

Exhibit 10–1 Resources for Primary Care Practitioners

Home care services
Consultation with allergist
Equipment
   Peak flow meters
   Holding chambers
   Compressor-driven nebulizers
Literature
   One Minute Asthma: What You Need to Know
   Children with Asthma: A Manual for Parents
   Asthma diaries and matching home treatment plans
Phone contact with consultant

Blood Institute (NHLBI) *Guidelines for the Diagnosis and Management of Asthma.*[7]

A two-day site visit by the physician consultant in September 1994 included two conferences for 80 physicians, office nurses, school nurses and respiratory therapists (see Exhibit 10–2). Two additional conferences were held in March 1995 during the second site visit (see Exhibit 10–3). Each of these conferences emphasized six basic points:

1. the early diagnosis of asthma
2. early use of steroids
3. proper use of inhalation devices
4. objective monitoring of the patient's status

Table 10–3 Cost Estimate for Equipment and Books per 1,000 child enrollees

Equipment or book	Distribution (%)	Number needed	Cost per item	Total cost per 1,000 enrollees
Peak flow meter	60	30	$20.00	$600
Compressor-driven nebulizer	30	15	65.00	975
Holding chamber	70	35	20.00	700
One Minute Asthma	100	50	1.50	75
Children with Asthma	40	20	4.25	85
Asthma diaries (pads of 100)	100	12.5	10.00	125
TOTAL (two years)				**$2,560**

This estimate assumes 5 percent of children in the plan have asthma. The 6,642 enrollees will need $17,004 worth of equipment and books. Since half of these materials would have been purchased without the intervention, the charge to the intervention is $8,502.

Exhibit 10–2 First Site Visit Schedule

Monday, September 26, 1994
8:30 P.M.   Meet with health services manager
Tuesday, September 27, 1994
7:30 A.M.   Asthma conference for physicians (40)
9:30 A.M.   Meet with six asthma advocates
1:00 P.M.   Asthma conference for office nurses, school nurses, and respiratory therapists (40)
4:00 P.M.   Visit pediatric office (advocate)
6:30 P.M.   Dinner with advocates, health services manager, nurse case manager
Wednesday, September 28, 1994
9:00 A.M.   Visit allergists' office (advocate)
11:00 A.M. Visit allergists' office (advocate)
12:00 P.M. Lunch with health services manager, nurse case manager, staff, home health service vendor
1:30 P.M.   Visit internists' office (advocate)
2:30 P.M.   Visit pediatricians' office (advocate)
4:00 P.M.   Visit pediatricians' office (advocate)
7:00 P.M.   Dinner with health services manager and two allergists

Throughout the two days, the consultant discussed use of home care and allergy referral, as well as details of health care organization and practice in New Orleans with health services manager and nurse case manager.

---

5. use of preventive medicines for asthma

6. the use of uniform educational material and treatment plans.

These points are emphasized throughout the consultant's conferences and visits, and in educational materials provided to physicians (see Exhibit 10–4). They are also presented in the books, diaries, and home treatment plans used by home care staff, as well as in the allergists' consultations.

Many physicians hold outdated beliefs that can hinder the implementation of this program. To address these issues, the physician consultant stated these beliefs, the corresponding facts, and their potential solutions in his meetings with physicians.

Early diagnosis of asthma

Belief: The diagnosis of asthma will frighten and upset parents.

Fact: Absence of the diagnosis will deprive parents or patients of the opportunity to learn about asthma and to intervene early in the course of an attack.

Exhibit 10–3 Second Site Visit Schedule

Wednesday, March 22, 1995	
9:00 A.M.	Meet with director of Meadowcrest Hospital Emergency Room
10:00 A.M.	Visit pediatrician's office
10:45 A.M.	Visit family practitioner's office
12:00 noon	Asthma conference, 60 physicians attend
2:30 P.M.	Meet with executive director, Principal Health Care
3:30 P.M.	Meet with Pediatric Services of America/Ambulatory Services of America (home care company) staff to get acquainted and to review procedures.
6:00 P.M.	Dinner with asthma advocates
Thursday, March 23, 1995	
8:00 A.M.	Conference at Lakeland Hospital, 30 physicians attend
10:30 A.M.	Meet with director of Doctors Urgent Care at Lakeland Hospital
1:00 P.M.	Debriefing with health services manager and nurse case manager

Solution: Describe asthma as an illness with a broad range of severity. Parents will be reassured to hear that most cases are mild.

Early use of oral steroids

Belief: Overuse may cause serious side effects.

Fact: Oral steroids are the most potent medicine available to treat inflammation during an attack. Concern with overuse leads to underuse: thus many patients who would benefit from oral steroids do not get them. As a result, they will require emergency care or admission to the hospital where they will receive high doses of steroids.

Solution: Describe the 1988 study that shows early use of steroids decreased hospitalizations by 90 percent in an experimental group.[8] Because these patients had fewer serious episodes, they used less steroids than the control group.

Use of inhalation devices

Compressor-driven nebulizer:

Belief: Home administration of an adrenaline-like medicine by compressor-driven nebulizer is dangerous because a parent might treat too often and cause toxicity.

Exhibit 10–4 Materials for Physicians' Conferences

September 1994
General:
- Letter from medical director describing intervention and resources
- Outline of talk, "Asthma 1995: Peak Flow Meters and Inhalation Devices."
- "Principal Health Care of Louisiana Pediatric Asthma Guidelines," taken from the NHLBI *Guidelines.*
- *One Minute Asthma: What You Need to Know* (revised).

Articles:
- Misdiagnosis of asthma[13,14]
- Peak flow monitoring[15]
- Asthma diaries[16,17]
- Inhalation devices[18]
- General asthma care[19–21]
- Asthma peak flow diary and home treatment plan for adults, teens, and children over four years of age
- Asthma signs diary and home treatment plan for children under four years of age.

Equipment:
- MiniWright peak flow meter
- Placebo metered dose inhaler
- Aerochamber holding chamber.

The six asthma advocates also received a copy of *Children with Asthma: A Manual for Parents* as well as a ProNeb compressor-driven nebulizer with Pari LC Jet +.

Additional material distributed at March 1995 Conference:
- *Executive Summary: Guidelines for the Diagnosis and Management of Asthma*, NAEP Expert Panel Report, NHLBI, National Institutes of Health, Bethesda, MD. Publication No. 94-3042A, reprinted July 1994.
- Home Visit Protocol for Principal Health Care by Pediatric Services of America
- Two general articles[22,23]
- Allergy referral.

Fact: The major danger of using the compressor-driven nebulizer at home is that it can mask symptoms. An inadequately instructed patient or parent will not recognize that the asthma is going out of control.

Solution: Give patients a home treatment plan based on the asthma care zones as determined by peak flow or asthma signs. This will limit the frequency of use and will direct parents at what point to see the doctor.

Holding chamber:

Belief: Most patients who use metered-dose inhalers (MDIs) will not benefit from using a holding chamber.

Fact: The holding chamber increases the benefits of inhaled steroids and decreases the side effects of all medicines delivered by MDI.

Solution: Ask physician to demonstrate proper MDI use with and without holding chamber during hands-on practice. The physician will appreciate the difficulty patients have in using the MDI alone and the ease of its use with a holding chamber.

Objective monitoring of patient status

Monitoring peak flow:

Belief: An asthma symptom diary is just as good as a peak flow diary in helping patients manage asthma.

Fact: Peak flow often drops before symptoms occur. The peak flow meter is the best tool for assessing asthma at home.

Solution: The Asthma Peak Flow Diary, which includes both peak flow scores and symptoms, can serve as an educational, monitoring, and management tool for patients over four years of age (Figure 10–1).

Monitoring asthma signs:

Belief: Parents are not competent to assess asthma symptoms in children under five.

Fact: Well-trained parents can accurately assess their child's status.

Solution: Provide asthma assessment system based on signs that parents can hear and see, using the Asthma Signs Diary (Figure 10–2).

Daily preventive treatment

Belief: Only about 10 percent of asthma patients need to take preventive medicine daily.

Fact: About 40 percent of asthma patients, practically all those with symptoms more than two days per week, will benefit from daily preventive medicine.

Solution: Encourage physicians to prescribe preventive treatment for their patients with moderate asthma while tracking them with an asthma diary. They will be impressed with the results.

Education

Belief: Prescribing medicines is much more important than providing asthma education.

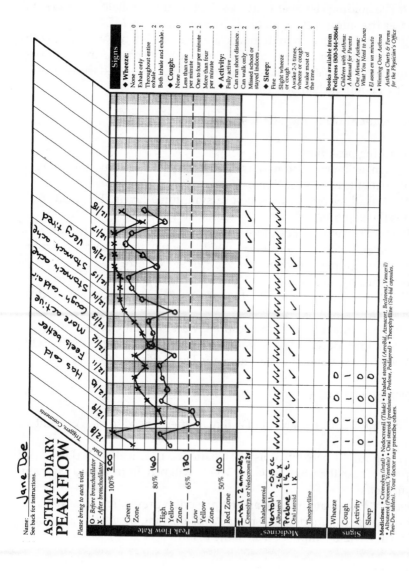

Figure 10–1 Asthma peak flow diary. *Source:* Copyright © 1995 Pedipress, Inc. From *Asthma Charts and Forms for the Physicians Office* by Thomas F. Plaut and Carla Brennan. Used with permission.

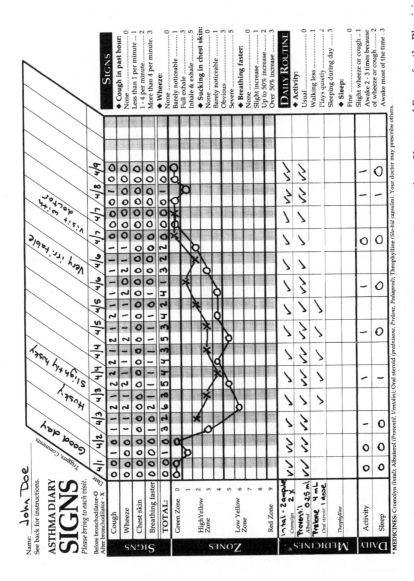

Figure 10–2. Asthma signs diary. *Source:* Copyright © 1995 Pedipress, Inc. From *Asthma Charts and Forms for the Physicians Office* by Thomas F. Plaut and Carla Brennan. Used with permission.

Fact: Many asthma patients take their medicines improperly and derive little benefit from them. Patients who do not understand what triggers their asthma attacks cannot prevent them.

Solution: Teach doctors the correct techniques for taking medicines and ways that patients can avoid their asthma triggers.

This asthma intervention is grounded in the care provided by primary care physicians and other clinical managers. At PHCLa, the essential starting point was the actions of the PHCLa health services manager, who initiated the asthma intervention and coordinated each step of the process with the various participants, including the physician consultant, nurse case manager, medical director, and the asthma advocates. Specifically, the health services manager:

- evaluated and hired the consultant
- designed a process that led to adoption of the NHLBI *Guidelines* for Principal Health Care physicians
- selected six asthma advocates
- expanded the original program to include allergy consultation and home care services
- adopted criteria for referral to an allergist (see Exhibit 10–5) and determined proper source of compensation
- decided on home care treatment guidelines and services needed and hired a vendor (see Exhibit 10–6)

Exhibit 10–5 Criteria for Allergy Referral

Consider specialty referral if:
- Patient is not responding optimally to the asthma therapy after three office visits
- Patient requires guidance on environmental control, consideration of immunotherapy, smoking cessation, complications of therapy, or difficult compliance issues
- Clinical entities complicate airway disease (e.g., sinusitis, nasal polyps, aspergillosis, and severe rhinitis); or
- Patient has had a life-threatening acute asthma exacerbation, has poor self-management ability, or has difficult family dynamics.

Source: From Care Guideline, Asthma in Children (revised December 1993). Institute for Clinical Systems Integration, One Appletree Square, Suite 1155, 8009 34th Avenue South, Bloomington, MN 55425. Used with permission.

Exhibit 10–6 Home Care Visit Plan

First visit, within one day of discharge from hospital (except weekends)
- Observation/physical assessment.
- Initial home assessment and history for possible triggers.
- Brief explanation of asthma (give *One Minute Asthma* booklet).
- Medication review and teaching including return demonstration of inhaler/spacer (Aerochamber)/compressor-driven nebulizer (ProNeb).
- Review red zone signs and plan.
- Discuss follow-up visits/when to call doctor.

Second visit
- Observation/physical assessment.
- Complete asthma teaching, give home treatment plan based on age.
- Introduce instructions on how to use a peak flow meter/introduce Asthma Peak Flow Diary.
- Return demonstration of compressor-driven nebulizer/holding chamber/inhaler.
- Completion of home assessment/instruct on how to avoid or eliminate trigger factors.
- Verify physician follow-up/discuss plan for school setting.

Third visit
- Observation/physical assessment.
- Evaluation of understanding and compliance.
- Review asthma peak flow meter use.
- Review and reinforce physician's instructions.
- Discharge instructions/review when to seek appropriate medication intervention.

Source: Asthma Program Home Visit Protocol, developed for Principal Health Care by Pediatric Services of America, 3159 Campus Drive, Norcross, Georgia 30071. Used with permission.

- broadened the scope of intervention to include adults and selected seven additional asthma advocates.

The asthma intervention is committed to case management. The plan's nurse case manager is the liaison between the health services manager, the physician consultant, and the other participants and is the key staff person during the implementation phase of the intervention. The case manager's responsibilities include:

Preparation for conferences:
— discusses materials needed with consultant
— sends literature out inviting to the conference 180 primary care physicians, emergency room physicians and staff, allergists

and pulmonologists who care for PHCLa patients as well as local school nurses
— obtains commitment to attend from physicians
— arranges facilities for meetings.

Interactions with health services manager:
— meets to review each asthma hospitalization
— reports on performance of home care vendors
— alerts health services manager if problems occur with services in hospital, emergency room, or physician's office.

Interactions with consultant:
— provides asthma hospitalization data on a regular basis
— provides additional information on various aspects of the program.

Interactions with patients:
— sees each patient in the hospital to track their status and treatment
— informally assesses patient satisfaction with program.

The physician consultant advised the plan with respect to the content, approach, and sequence of the intervention, as well as the purchase of equipment and books.

During the first year, the consultant will spend the equivalent of 12 days on the project: two two-day visits and eight days of preparation and follow-up by letter, fax, and phone. The second year, the consultant will make one two-day site visit and spend four days following up by letter and phone. Though primary care physicians almost always use the consultation services of Principal Health Care allergists in New Orleans, they are free to contact the program's physician consultant at any time with a patient or intervention-related question.

In addition to the books, home treatment plans were recommended based on peak flow (Figure 10–3) and asthma signs (Figure 10–4), which dovetail with the diaries. Together these materials allow physicians, home care staff, and family to provide a consistent approach to care.

A three-visit home care program is recommended for each patient after hospital discharge and, in some cases, after a visit to the emergency room. This program includes a patient and home assessment, basic asthma education, and review of medicines, delivery devices, and peak flow monitoring. Home management is based on the asthma diaries and home treatment plans.

In the first nine months of the PHCLa intervention, the following steps were taken and results noted:

For Adults, Teens and Children Age 5 and Over
PEAK FLOW BASED HOME TREATMENT PLAN

Name: _____   Date: _____   Best Peak Flow: _____

Green Zone

GREEN ZONE: Peak flow between _____ **and** _____ .

- **Normal activity.**
  - ❑ *Albuterol (Proventil, Ventolin):* 1 or 2 puffs 15 minutes before exercise.
  - ❑ *Cromolyn (Intal):* 2 puffs before contact with cat or other allergen.

- **Medicine to be taken every day:**
  - ❑ *Nedocromil (Tilade)* or *cromolyn (Intal):* _____ puffs _____ times a day (a total of _____ puffs daily).
  - ❑ *Inhaled steroid (Aerobid, Azmacort, Beclovent, Vanceril):* _____ puffs _____ times a day (a total of _____ puffs daily).
  - ❑ *Albuterol (Proventil, Ventolin):* _____ puffs before each *nedocromil, cromolyn* or *inhaled steroid* dose for the first month.
  - ❑ *Theophylline (Slo-bid capsules, Theo-Dur tablets):* _____ mg _____ times a day (a total of _____ mg daily).

Yellow Zone

HIGH YELLOW ZONE: Peak flow between _____ **and** _____ .

- **Eliminate triggers and change medicines. No strenuous exercise.**

- **Medicine to be taken:**
  - ✓ *Albuterol:* _____ puffs by holding chamber. Give three to six times in 24 hours. Continue until peak flow is in the *Green Zone* for two days.
  - ✓ Double *inhaled steroid* to _____ puffs daily until peak flow is in the *Green Zone* for as long as it was in the *Yellow Zone.*

- -

LOW YELLOW ZONE: Peak flow between _____ **and** _____ .

Follow this plan if peak flow does not reach *High Yellow Zone* within 10 minutes after taking inhaled albuterol, or drops back into *Low Yellow Zone* within four hours:

- ✓ Continue *albuterol* treatment as above.
- ✓ Add *oral steroid** _____ mg immediately. Continue each morning (8:00 A.M.) until peak flow is in the *Green Zone* for at least 24 hours.

*If your condition does not improve within two days after starting oral steroid, or if peak flow does not reach the *Green Zone* within seven days of treatment, see your doctor.

Red Zone

RED ZONE: Peak flow less than _____ .

Follow this plan if peak flow does not reach *Low Yellow Zone* within 10 minutes after taking inhaled albuterol, or drops back into *Red Zone* within four hours:

- ✓ *Albuterol* _____ puffs by holding chamber.
- ✓ Give *oral steroid* _____ mg.
- ✓ Visit your doctor.

Figure 10–3. For adults, teens, and children age 5 and over: peak flow–based home treatment plan. *Source:* Copyright © 1995 Pedipress, Inc. From *Asthma Charts and Forms for the Physicians Office* by Thomas F. Plaut and Carla Brennan. Used with permission.

- 1993 Principal rate of hospital days for asthma was 9.6 per 1,000 members, or 101 percent of the 1993 U.S. rate (9.5 per 1,000), a total of 64 days for children under fifteen.
- Summer 1994: Consultant reviews Principal's hospitalization data. Based on previous interventions, he believes asthma hospitalization could be reduced by 50 percent during a two-year intervention.

For Children Under Age 5
SIGNS-BASED HOME TREATMENT PLAN

Name: Date:

Green Zone

GREEN ZONE: Absolutely no cough, wheeze, breathing faster, or sucking in of the chest skin.

- **Normal activity.**
- **Medicine to be taken every day:**
  - ❑ *Cromolyn (Intal):* _____ ampules in _____ doses.
  - ❑ *Albuterol (Proventil, Ventolin):* _____ cc by compressor-driven nebulizer with each *cromolyn* dose for the first month.
  - ❑ *Theophylline* (Slo-bid capsules): _____ mg _____ times a day (a total of _____ mg daily).

Yellow Zone

HIGH YELLOW ZONE: Total asthma sign score 1 to 4 measured before taking inhaled bronchodilator.

- **Eliminate triggers and change medicines.**
- **Medicine to be taken:**
  - ✓ *Cromolyn:* as above.
  - ✓ *Albuterol:* 0.___ cc in 2 cc cromolyn or saline by compressor-driven nebulizer. Give three to six times in 24 hours. Continue until signs score is 0 or 1 for 48 hours.

LOW YELLOW ZONE: Total asthma sign score 5 to 8.

Follow this plan if sign score does not reach *High Yellow Zone* within 10 minutes after taking inhaled *albuterol,* or drops back into *Low Yellow Zone* within four hours:

- **No strenuous exercise.**
- **Medicine to be taken:**
  - ✓ Continue *albuterol* and *cromolyn* as above.
  - ✓ Start *oral steroid** _____ mg, _____ cc immediately. Continue each morning (8:00 A.M.) until sign score is 0 or 1 for at least 24 hours.**

*Liquid prednisolone: Prelone is 15 mg per 5 cc and Pediapred is 5 mg per 5 cc.
**If condition does not improve within two days after starting *oral steroid,* or if your child does not reach the *Green Zone* within seven days of treatment, see your doctor.

Red Zone

RED ZONE: Total asthma sign score 9 or more.

Follow this plan if sign score does not reach *Low Yellow Zone* within 10 minutes after taking inhaled *albuterol,* or drops back into *Red Zone* within four hours:

- ✓ ***Albuterol:* 0.___ cc by compressor-driven nebulizer.**
- ✓ ***Oral steroid* _____ mg.**
- **Visit your doctor.**

Figure 10–4. For children under age 5: signs-based home treatment plan. *Source:* Copyright © 1995 Pedipress, Inc. From *Asthma Charts and Forms for the Physicians Office* by Thomas F. Plaut and Carla Brennan. Used with permission.

- September 1994: Intervention begins. Asthma advocates are selected. First on-site consultation and conferences for physicians and other health professionals are held. Consultant visits practice sites of the six asthma advocates.
- November 1994: Criteria for allergy referrals are established and home care program is initiated.

- March 1995: Second on-site consultation is held with family practitioners, internists, and pediatricians totaling 90 physicians. Adult care asthma advocates selected in preparation for expansion of the intervention to adults.
- April 1995: Addition of adult patients quadruples size of the intervention population and more than triples the number of primary care physicians.

DATA COLLECTION AND ANALYSIS

In order for a health plan to compare its data across sites and programs with accuracy it must use identical definitions and demographic criteria.

Data. Hospital days and admission/discharge data should be collected automatically by the financial planning and analysis department in the corporate office. Data should also be collected locally as a control.

Age range. National Center for Health Statistics data show that the younger the child, the higher the admission rate for asthma. This intervention includes children from newborn discharge to the 15th birthday. A similar program that excludes infants or includes teenagers after their 15th birthday will have a lower discharge rate.

Hospital days versus discharges. Hospital days are a better indicator of the care children receive for asthma than hospital discharges. They distinguish between the child who needs short rescue therapy and a child whose poor outpatient management necessitates a prolonged stay. They also are not confounded by transfer from one hospital to another.

Diagnosis of asthma. Misdiagnosis has been recognized as a problem since 1978, and physicians were urged to diagnose asthma in most patients they had previously labeled as having bronchitis, wheezy bronchitis, or bronchospasm.[9] In addition, asthma was recognized as the major cause of recurrent pneumonia in 1982.[10] It is likely that 100,000 of the 300,000 children hospitalized for bronchitis, bronchiolitis, and pneumonia in 1988 should have been diagnosed with asthma.[11] If asthma is not diagnosed it cannot be treated optimally.

Diagnostic transfer. Hospital days for asthma are the major outcome measure for this intervention. However, PHCLa monitored and analyzed asthma hospital admissions and collected data for pneumonia, bronchitis, and bronchiolitis to achieve a fuller understanding of results. The misdiagnosis of asthma as pneumonia or bronchitis is a common problem, particularly in children under five years of age, and can skew data positively or negatively.[12] For example, physicians who improve their diagnostic ability will shift a diagnosis from pneumonia to asthma, worsening their asthma statistics. Conversely, physicians who want to improve their asthma statistics might shift a diagnosis from asthma to pneumonia. Finally, an epidemic of viral pneumonia might lead to a rise in rates for asthma, as well as bronchitis, bronchiolitis, and pneumonia.

Emergency room. The PHCLa intervention has not yet reviewed data on patient visits to the emergency room. Data will be monitored to see whether emergency visits increase as hospital days decrease.

IMPLEMENTATION ISSUES

Consistency is an essential component of any asthma intervention, and educational materials help ensure a true systems approach at PHCLa. The NHLBI *Guidelines* provides clear protocols for the important aspects of patient care. After PHCLa adopted them, the *Guidelines* became the common basis for the plan's discussion of asthma care. All the primary care physicians use the same books, monitoring tools, and medical equipment, and refer patients to allergists and home care providers who use them as well. Thus, patients receive a consistent message that uses the same words, whether coming from their regular physician, on-call physician, consulting allergist, home care staff, or emergency room physician, and from all educational materials.

The New Orleans intervention is distinctive in that it focuses on the practices of the primary care physicians who continue to improve their asthma care. All the equipment, materials, information, and referral services are designed to support the physician in providing effective asthma care, which will become an integral part of practice at all levels at PHCLa.

The asthma advocates, in turn, worked within their own practices to use and teach current concepts and techniques for asthma care to their colleagues. Through the conferences, physicians and nurses learned about and gained hands-on experience with peak flow meters and inhalation devices. During his visits to physicians' offices, the consultant discussed current asthma treatment and observed staff techniques for using equipment and educational materials.

Home health care staff are a significant unifying factor in the intervention. They ask physicians to prescribe home treatment plans based on the zones of the asthma diaries (see Figures 10-1 and 10-2). They teach patients to assess the severity of asthma, how to use equipment, and how to follow their own progress. They report both to the primary care physicians and to the nurse case manager.

Success factors

The health services manager and the physician consultant agreed that each admission for asthma would be considered a failure of outpatient management by the physician or by the HMO unless proven otherwise. Providers are responsible for identifying problems that should be remedied to prevent a future admission. This is more productive than blaming the patient and avoids endless discussion of patient noncompliance.

This entire intervention is grounded in the experience of the health services manager, the nurse case manager, and the physician consultant. At least one of the three had experience in every major area of the program. The health services manager was experienced in initiating and implementing other programs that called for partnerships among physicians, vendors, and Principal staff. The nurse case manager had worked in utilization review and case management for several years. The consultant had guided or advised a dozen asthma interventions in practice settings and has assisted in creating asthma programs in schools, medical institutions, and Medicaid programs.

Pitfall

The biggest concern the intervention faced was staff time. No one dropped other duties to participate, no staff were added, and the nurse case manager has been overextended. This is a problem that all similar interventions will face. The nurse case manager assigned to an intervention should be allotted an adequate amount of time to see each patient in the hospital, and sometimes the emergency room, and to coordinate their care thereafter.

Adaptation

This intervention took place in an IPA model HMO. The general principles and concepts can be applied to any HMO or managed care practice, although it will be easier to implement in a staff model HMO, where patients and physicians are more concentrated and the manager's control is greater. This systems approach is also suitable for improving care of adults with asthma; PHCLa has recently expanded it to include the entire adult population at the plan. *One Minute Asthma,* the basic text for patients, is written at the sixth grade level and is available in Spanish.

Projection

At the nine-month mark, most elements of the intervention are in place. PHCLa will soon begin analyzing inpatient care, emergency room care, physician prescribing habits, patient drug profiles, and patient satisfaction. Currently, some primary care physicians are taking full advantage of the resources offered. Within two years the majority of the physicians will be carrying out the entire program.

This systems approach to asthma care offers health plans a means for improving care and reducing unnecessary hospitalization. Most important, it provides health professionals with the knowledge, the tools, and the support they need to provide appropriate and current care for their asthma patients. It empowers the patients to play a significant role in improving the quality of their life.

REFERENCES

1. Weiss, K., Gergen, P.J., and Hodgson, T.A. "An Economic Evaluation of Asthma in the United States." *New England Journal of Medicine* 366 (1992): 862–868.
2. Graves, E.J. *1993 Summary: National Hospital Discharge Survey.* Advance data from vital and health statistics, no. 264. Hyattsville, MD: National Center for Health Statistics, 1995.
3. Weiss, Gergen, and Hodgson, "An Economic Evaluation."
4. Plaut, T.F. "Childhood Asthma: A Missed Diagnosis." *HMO Practice* 5 (1991): 102–105.
5. Plaut, T.F. *One Minute Asthma: What You Need to Know.* Rev. ed. Amherst, MA: Pedipress, 1995.
6. Plaut, T.F. *Children With Asthma: A Manual for Parents.* 2nd ed. Amherst, MA: Pedipress, 1988.
7. National Heart, Lung, and Blood Institute. *Guidelines for the Diagnosis and Management of Asthma,* National Asthma Education and Prevention Program (NAEP) Expert Panel Report. Bethesda, MD: National Institutes of Health, 1991.
8. Brunette, M.G., Lands, L., and Thibodeau, L.P. "Childhood Asthma: Prevention of Attacks with Short-term Corticosteroid Treatment of Upper Respiratory Tract Infection." *Pediatrics* 81 (1988): 624–629.
9. Speight, A.N.P. "Is Childhood Asthma Being Underdiagnosed and Undertreated?" *British Medical Journal* 2 (1978): 331–332.
10. Eigen, H., Laughlin, J.J., and Homrighausen, J. "Recurrent Pneumonia in Children and Its Relationship to Bronchial Hyperreactivity." *Pediatrics* 70 (1982): 698–704.
11. Plaut, "Childhood Asthma."
12. Ibid.
13. Ibid.
14. Plaut, T.F., et al. "Is Asthma Misdiagnosed?" *Journal of Asthma* 23 (1986): 23–24.
15. Plaut, T.F. "What a Peak Flow Meter Can Do for Children with Asthma." *Contemporary Pediatrics* (Technology Issue) (1989): 33–52.
16. Plaut, T.F. "Asthma Signs Diary." Amherst, MA: Pedipress, 1994.
17. Plaut, T.F. "The Peak Flow Diary." *American Journal of Asthma & Allergy for Pediatricians* 7 (1994): 37–39.
18. Plaut, T.F. "Helping Asthma Patients Breathe Easier." *Contemporary Pediatrics* (Technology Issue) (1989): 59–76.
19. Stevens, M.A., and Weiss-Harrison, A. "Program for Children with Asthma." *HMO Practice* 7 (1993): 91.
20. Plaut, T.F. "Comprehensive Asthma Care Reduces Hospitalization" (letter). *Pediatrics* 78 (1986): 542.
21. Plaut, T.F. "Why Don't Pediatricians Give Better Asthma Care?" (letter). *Contemporary Pediatrics* 11 (1994): 15.
22. Plaut, T.F. "Your Patient Has Asthma Symptoms?" *Advance for Managers of Respiratory Care* 3 (1994): 57–60.
23. Plaut, T.F. "Discharging of Asthma Patients" (letter). *Chest* 96 (1989): 953.

11

The Treatment of Chronic Benign Pain Syndrome in Capitated Health Care

Jaylene Kent

An estimated 15 million Americans suffer from low back pain, and another 25 million suffer from recurring headache.[1] This article describes the efforts at Santa Teresa Hospital, a Kaiser Permanente Medical Center, to respond to the clinical and organizational challenges presented by caring for members with chronic benign pain syndrome (CBPS). The Santa Teresa Medical Center/Kaiser has 52,000 enrollees with cross-over utilization from adjacent Kaiser facilities of 10,000 enrollees.

A decision to provide targeted services for individuals with CBPS was made in 1989 by the physician-in-charge of Santa Teresa Hospital/Kaiser. At the outset, a part-time psychologist, a part-time social worker, and a part-time anesthesiologist staffed the program. These resources formed the foundation for the development of two organizational entities: Behavioral Medicine/Health Psychology within family practice, and the Pain Clinic.

Appreciating a medical center administrator's decision to dedicate scarce resources to this population requires some understanding of CBPS, its impact on utilization in a health care delivery system, and how system and provider factors affect the syndrome's management. CBPS is a condition that occurs on a continuum of severity, and is characterized by pain in excess of six months and a lack of or minimal physical findings on examination or medical studies.

In addition, CBPS is usually associated with elevated clinical scales on the Minnesota Multiphasic Personality Inventory (a standardized person-

Source: Reprinted from J. Kent, The Treatment of Chronic Benign Pain Syndrome in Capitated Health Care, *Managed Care Quarterly,* Vol. 4, No. 2, pp. 77–83, © 1996, Aspen Publishers, Inc.

ality test used by psychologists), sleep disturbance, reliance upon pain medications, deconditioning, depression and/or anxiety, pain behavior, and physical dysfunction disproportionate to medical findings. Typically, the condition has not responded to treatment modalities such as medication, surgery, psychotherapy, or physical therapy. Frequently, functioning deteriorates and utilization increases over time. In fact, a dysfunctional relationship often develops among the patient, the health care providers, and the system.

PROVIDER AND SYSTEM INFLUENCES

Many variables have an impact on CBPS. This discussion focuses on those aspects of relevance to the primary care provider and the health care delivery system.

Management complications

Management of CBPS is complicated when the primary care provider fails to remain the "captain of the ship." Primary care should maintain responsibility for coordinating care with appropriate specialists, making appropriate referrals, assuring completion of necessary behavioral/psychological and medical work-ups, monitoring of medications, providing and discussing a diagnosis, and initiating discussions of management versus cure. Failure to carry out this responsibility can lead to patients feeling abandoned, and believing "it is all in their head." This can precipitate a downward spiral of depression, erosion of personal responsibility for taking control of their pain, and increased hostility toward the health care system.

Attitudes in primary care providers

Primary care providers may treat these individuals as "crocks," and believe their pain is "all in their heads," thus complicating the management of CBPS. This attitude reveals itself within the health care system with repeated referrals to specialists, limited office time, and over-reliance on the "quick fix" of prescriptions. Referrals may be made to mental health departments, even though research and clinical experience has demonstrated traditional mental health care to be ineffective with this population.

Chronic versus acute pain

Providers treat chronic pain as if it is acute pain, for example, prescribing "rest if it hurts," encouraging the use of medications "as needed" rather than on a scheduled basis, and encouraging time off from work, hobbies, and other meaningful activities and roles. This approach generally fosters dependency on the system, promotes the idea that the body requires further healing to correct the pain problem, and sets the stage for further depression, anger, and disappointment with the provider and the health care system. It may also lead to a rupture in the therapeutic alliance between the physician or health care provider and the patient.

Problems in health care delivery

Specific demands of the health care delivery system may make it difficult for providers to work collaboratively in consultation, diagnosis, management, and treatment of individuals with time-consuming problems. Most commonly, this arises because provider schedules are too full, appointment times are too short, and time is too limited to respond in an informed, coordinated fashion to multiple phone calls expressing complex complaints, or to evaluate fully past treatments and failures.

Lack of expertise

Primary care providers often have a biomedical orientation and lack expertise in basic behavioral management. Consequently, they may inadvertently provide powerful reinforcements for disability and suffering, undermining patients' motivation to take responsibility for managing their chronic pain.

Primary care providers need support

A health care delivery system's failure to provide some level of expertise in the management of chronic pain deprives the primary care physician of the consultation and referral resources required to manage these patients. Most important, the primary care provider must know when to refer to a chronic pain specialist for consultation and must have access to a treatment program for chronic pain available within the system.

CBPS has a large impact on any health care delivery system, but it presents special problems for a capitated system like Kaiser. Patients with CBPS use medical services at a high rate and respond poorly to the traditional services that are offered. Frustrated patients may demand services outside of the system and seek reimbursement from the capitated health care organization. Consequently, the resulting impact on provider morale is negative because these patients often fail to improve.

The benefits of recruiting and allocating specialized resources for the care of CBPS include reduced health care costs, improved and more effective patient care, enhanced provider morale, and improved patient functioning and satisfaction. If return to work is achieved, the appeal of the health plan in the marketplace is greatly increased.

Pioneering work has determined that the most effective treatment approach for CBPS begins with a multidisciplinary evaluation by pain specialists from both psychology and medicine and appropriate referral to a multidisciplinary program.[2] At Santa Teresa Hospital/Kaiser, the multidisciplinary "Skills Not Pills" program was initially developed. This spawned the Behavioral Medicine/Health Psychology Department, which now offers a range of services to members with a variety of chronic medical conditions.

BEHAVIORAL MEDICINE/HEALTH PSYCHOLOGY

The Department of Behavioral Medicine/Health Psychology is a division of family practice directed by a health psychologist. Health psychology is a specialty area within psychology characterized by specialized knowledge and training in disease prevention and health promotion. Significantly, health psychologists' advance training is provided in medical departments, rather than psychiatry departments.

The department's clinical staff is multidisciplinary, and currently includes Ph.D. health psychologists (total of 1.75 FTE [full-time equivalent]), two family practice physicians and one internist (.8 FTE), a licensed clinical social worker (.25 FTE), two registered nurses (1 FTE), and a biofeedback specialist (three hours weekly). The department receives approximately 45 referrals per month. Currently, there is a 3-month wait for a Kaiser enrollee to obtain an evaluation appointment in the department. All group programs run to capacity, with an ideal group size ranging from six to eight participants.

The professional staff was selected for their interest and expertise in the behavioral and emotional aspects of medicine and health, outcomes research, and program development. The staff provides evaluation, consultation, and treatment on an outpatient basis for a variety of chronic and stress-related medical problems. A partial listing would include somatic complaints, hypertension, diabetic neuropathies, fibromyalgia, myofascial pain, centralized pain, and Reynaud's disease. Treatment plans for these conditions include education, physical reconditioning, appropriate management of psychotropic medications, systematic withdrawal from narcotic and other addictive medications, biofeedback, relaxation training, stress management, cognitive-behavioral therapy, and brief dynamic therapy.

Referrals are received primarily from medicine, the pain clinic, spine clinic, occupational medicine, and neurology. All referrals are screened and triaged by a staff nurse who is cross trained to provide nursing support for the psychologists and physicians on the staff.

If an individual evaluation appointment is needed, the nurse collects preliminary information in a brief clinical interview, administers a Minnesota Multiphasic Personality Inventory-2, and schedules a return appointment with staff health psychologist.

The health psychologist comprehensively reviews health records, conducts an in-depth clinical interview, interprets any psychological tests, and completes a consultative report on the patient, which includes an analysis of findings, a clinical impression, and a recommended disposition. This evaluation is designed to document as completely as possible the nature of each patient's conditions and goals. Copies are sent to the referring provider, to the medical chart, and to the Behavioral Medicine/Health Psychology chart. The evaluation may result in one of several dispositions:

- Referral to another resource within the medical center when appropriate, such as the department of psychiatry or health education.
- Referral to outside private or public resources in the community, such as long-term psychotherapy setting or highly specialized services such as those for incest victims.
- Referral for individual treatment within the Behavioral Medicine/Health Psychology Department, as for brief psychotherapy, hypnosis, biofeedback, medication tapering or adjustment.
- Referral to one of the three chronic pain group treatment programs offered in the Behavioral Medicine/Health Psychology Department.

SKILLS NOT PILLS PROGRAM

"Skills Not Pills" is Santa Teresa/Kaiser's most comprehensive treatment program for CBPS. Participants who graduate with a sense of control over their pain without the use of analgesic medications are considered treatment successes. Individuals eligible for this program must have completed all appropriate medical and surgical evaluations and treatments for their pain problem prior to participation. Most important, the individual must believe all medical options have been exhausted, "nothing medical has been missed," and a medical "cure" will not be sought for their pain.

The program is a 10-week, multidisciplinary, cognitive/behavioral outpatient service. The program concept relies heavily on learning theory with an operational focus on the behavioral reinforcers of pain. To optimize control of the dysfunctional behaviors that limit the patient's adjustment to the pain, the multidisciplinary treatment team of "Skills Not Pills" assumes all responsibility for psychological and medical care during the 10-week program.

The treatment plan typically focuses on reduction of behaviors associated with pain (e.g., rubbing the affected body part, groaning, pain-focused conversation), appropriate treatment of psychological symptoms (primarily anxiety and depression), tapering contraindicated analgesic and sedative/hypnotic medications, and reconditioning. Skill building, specifically in the areas of pacing (learning appropriate levels of activity), assertiveness, communication, psychological strategies (attitude, attention, cognitions, affect), stress management, and reconditioning are emphasized. Group support and process are also key therapeutic elements of the program.

Patients attend the clinic twice weekly for three and one half hours on each visit. On nonclinic days, daily homework includes twice daily stretching and strengthening exercises, relaxation, and a walking program. Charting of homework is completed on an honor system. The team nurse monitors participants' daily logs to ensure the homework has been completed.

Because of the demanding requirements of the program, all candidates must be evaluated by a staff psychologist prior to participation. Once this evaluation is completed, the candidate and the candidate's support person (most often a spouse) must also be screened by the "Skills not Pills" treatment team (a psychologist, physician, and social worker). This team interview serves a variety of purposes.

First, the interview allows staff to assess the individual's motivation. Experience has shown that pain management requires a commitment to mastery of a particular skill set, to attitudinal and life style changes (including exercising regularly, relaxing regularly, pacing), and maintaining a positive outlook. If the member is not adequately motivated, the potential benefit from the program is limited.

Second, because several disciplines are represented, the concept is communicated that pain is a complex phenomena involving psychological and behavioral aspects as well as physical events. The team interview also builds confidence that specialized expertise is available to address any clinical problem that may arise during the 10 weeks.

Third, the team interview allows the physician to determine a schedule for appropriate medication tapering during the course of the program. All analgesics used for symptomatic relief are weaned. Other medication trials may be initiated or adjustments may occur at this time also. These medications typically involve antidepressants for adequate management of depression and sleep dysfunction.

Fourth, the interview provides the opportunity for the staff to screen the support person, most often a spouse, who usually plays a significant role in the experience of the individual with CBPS. It is important to determine during the team interview that the support person is appropriate for a group setting, and understands and accepts the program goals and philosophy. Without this interaction support persons may undermine the "Skills Not Pills" experience and sabotage the program if they are not understanding and cooperative of the program, its objectives, and their role in supporting the program participant.

Fifth, the team interview is an opportunity for patients to "tell their story" and ask any questions regarding their participation. Certain aspects of the program are reviewed, such as being unable to see other providers when in the program except in the case of a medical or psychological emergency or upon referral. The patient is also told the goal is not to cure his or her pain but rather to gain control over it.

Sixth, on rare occasions, a physical examination may be conducted for clarification of physical limitations (e.g., fused ankle, artificial hip).

Once the 10-week, intensive portion of the program has been completed, responsibilities for the medical and psychological care return to the primary care providers and a 10-month follow-up program begins. In this phase, graduates of the 10-week intensive portion of the program come to the clinic for a monthly meeting with a health psychologist.

The goal is to encourage participants to solidify gains made in the first 10 weeks, and to provide ongoing support, structure, and encouragement.

RESULTS

Outcome measurements from the "Skills Not Pills" program have demonstrated its effectiveness. Satisfaction is high for the participants and the referring providers alike. Outpatient medical utilization by graduates of "Skills Not Pills" was reduced by 57 percent, based on a measurement of utilization one year before and one year after graduation. When only pain-related visits were measured, the decrease of utilization was found to be 84 percent. Positive gains have been found on psychometric instruments as well, including both the Beck Depression Inventory and the McGill Pain Questionnaire.

PAIN EDUCATION GROUP

This is an eight-week program that relies heavily on a psychoeducational structure but also includes some group process and support. The program is led by a staff psychologist and physician. An evaluation by a staff psychologist is not required for participation in this open-ended program. Individuals may self-refer or be referred by any provider. This program is versatile in its utilization and is often used as adjunctive support for patients on a drug taper or in brief psychotherapy in the Health Psychology/Behavioral Medicine Department. The program also serves as an immediate resource for physicians in primary care or the spine, pain, or occupational medicine clinic whose patients need to learn more about one of the topics covered in the curriculum.

Each class is one hour in length and may be attended by 6 to 12 participants. Because the structure is set up as an ongoing, rotating series of classes, patients can start at any time. Subscribers may come to one class or all eight classes. The topics covered include: neurophysiology of pain, pain medications, pacing and the use/disuse syndrome, relaxation and pain, depression and pain, cognitive strategies for managing pain, assertiveness, and family dynamics.

CHRONIC DAILY HEADACHE PROGRAM

The Chronic Daily Headache Program is a group program that meets for eight sessions on a weekly basis. The program is appropriate for people with a diagnosis of chronic daily headache, characterized by headaches that occur more than 15 days a month and in which the patient takes analgesic medications on a daily or near-daily basis. These regularly used substances may be narcotic or nonnarcotic, prescription or nonprescription, or even caffeine. Treatment consists of helping the patients taper medications, teaching management strategies, and teaching a stress-reduction relaxation technique called Autogenic Training. Treatment does not target intermittent acute headaches such as migraine, which is a common concomitant with chronic daily headaches.

This program is led by a physician and a licensed clinical social worker. Consult requests must contain a diagnosis (e.g., chronic daily headache), identification of the analgesic medication responsible for the rebound headache, and a medication regimen for the intermittent severe headaches (most often migraine). Participants remain under the care of their primary care provider during and after this program.

Preparation of the participant by the referring provider is important. This is an educational process by the physician, most often a neurologist, and informs the patient that:

- The role of medications is in fostering rather than alleviating headache.
- The program is not a cure, but rather, the goals are reduced frequency of headache, decreased pain level, and increased sense of support.

- There is a necessary commitment to the endeavor, as the program is eight weeks, 1.5 hours each week plus homework when not in the clinic (e.g., maintaining logs and doing autogenics).
- The pain is real, not "in their heads," and they are not "crazy."

CHALLENGES

Establishing these kinds of multidisciplinary, innovative departments are challenging. Several key principles will enhance the likelihood of a successful implementation:

1. There needs to be an identified lead expert in health psychology who is respected by the referring physicians.
2. The services offered must be cost-efficient and meet the needs of a busy primary care provider as well as the clinical needs of the patients served. This requires an understanding of the time constraints and clinical demands of the primary care physicians and developing treatment services and programs accordingly. In most cases, primary care physicians want help with patients who overuse medications, are depressed and preoccupied with pain, and overuse the health care system.
3. The clinical work must be high quality. CBPS does not have a cure. Thus, the primary care physician is responsible for the long-term management of the CBPS patient. Having patients return to the primary care physician with a brighter affect, free of medications, and resuming a more normal life "sells" the physician on the treatment services of the Behavioral Medicine/Health Psychology Department.
4. Orienting the primary care physicians is crucial. They need education not only on CBPS but also how best to use services offered in a department of Behavioral Medicine/Health Psychology. Equally important, they need instruction in assisting patients in accepting these services. Most physicians and patients associate psychology and psychologists with mental illness and departments of Mental Health and not with the medical conditions that are the expertise of the health psychologist. Health psychologists' training and expertise is in parameters of normal personality, physical health/disease, and the behavior of medical patients. Education of physicians and other providers can occur in many ways: grand round presentations, patient feedback, publications, informal dialogues, and physician visits to programs.
5. Establish and maintain close working relationships with primary care providers. The primary care providers, along with the health

plan subscribers, are the "customers" of the Behavioral Medicine/ Health Psychology Department.

6. Ask for feedback. What services are still missing? What expertise has not yet been offered or fully utilized? What patients are most problematic in the system?

7. Determine how the services are impacting the health care delivery system's "bottom line." Can it be done in a more cost-efficient way? Know the bottom line objectives of the health care delivery system.

8. Provide outcome measurements demonstrating the clinical efficacy and cost reduction of services offered.

Creating successful behavioral medicine programs is exciting; the rewards are potentially far greater than the challenges. These kinds of integrative, innovative services have improved patient care and established productive and close working relationships between psychology and medicine as well as the other involved disciplines such as nursing and social work. The need for cost-effective, quality care will continue to grow and there is every reason to believe that this need provides a compelling rationale for psychologists and physicians to collaborate on biobehavioral interventions.

REFERENCES

1. Tulkin, R., et al. "Management of Chronic Benign Pain in Prepaid Practice." In *Managed Mental Health Care*, eds. J. Feldman and R. Fitzpatrick. Washington, DC: American Psychiatric Press, 1992.
2. Fordyce, W. *Behavioral Methods for Chronic Pain and Illness*. St. Louis, MO: CV Mosby, 1976.

12

Physician Attitudes Toward Computerized Practice Guidelines

Ellen Aliberti and Timmothy J. Holt

Experts in guideline development and outcome measurement note that electronic information and decision support systems are crucial elements of any long-term strategies for promoting the implementation, evaluation, and maintenance of clinical guidelines. Moreover, they claim that only through applying technologies to health care delivery can dramatic improvements be achieved in outcomes measurements, such as cost, quality, accessibility, and service capabilities.[1]

They also agree that without a computerized system for collecting and analyzing baseline data on all patients, the ability for any clinical guideline to influence patient care and improve the effectiveness of health care is limited. Most suggest that patient-centered online clinical information would present a reasonable approach for the application of technology.[2]

But clearly, provider acceptance is critical for applying automation to practice guidelines. Research indicates that providers' willingness to accept or use a new technology is not only based on their knowledge and past experience, but also on whether the technology is able to integrate the "cues" from the medical environment, such as a medical history, physical and medical records, and any other patient information that assists in medical decision making. Moreover, factors such as administrative structure or process, education, feedback, incentives, and regulations can affect behavior and could be used to influence change.[3]

Source: Reprinted from E. Aliberti and T. Holt, Physician Attitudes Toward Computerized Practice Guidelines, *Managed Care Quarterly,* Vol. 4, No. 2, pp. 70–76, © 1996, Aspen Publishers, Inc.

With the support of a Robert Wood Johnson grant under the Chronic Care Initiatives in HMOs program, in fall 1994 several organizations researched physicians' views about clinical guidelines for chronic conditions and their opinions concerning automated information systems to direct guidelines: St. Mary's Medical Center, an acute care hospital in Long Beach, California, a local IPA provider, and PacifiCare of California, a managed care organization.

The team chose to examine the use of automated clinical guidelines for coronary obstructive pulmonary disease (COPD) and congestive heart failure (CHF) in particular because these conditions accounted for significant utilization among the study's patient population. Furthermore, with continued threats of decreasing health care dollars and rising numbers of older adults in whom chronic diseases are common, the team has a great interest in improving chronic disease management.

This article discusses the project's study findings regarding operational issues, success factors, and issues of concern that surround automated clinical guidelines for chronic conditions in a managed care setting.

STUDY STRUCTURE AND ISSUES

Most physicians agree that the body of knowledge and available cues concerning their patients is either too immense to comprehend, or so disorganized and unavailable that its use is minimal at best and futile at its worst. The project, through automated clinical guidelines, would prioritize the essential information needed for physicians to make decisions while still having the total medical record available.

The model targets improving the availability of such environmental "cues" and information by better information systems management. Motivation is also influenced by decreasing the paper "hassle factor" and supporting the physician's desire to provide the best quality care possible for their patients.

At the time the physician study was conducted, St. Mary's, PacifiCare, and the IPA provider each had already begun to invest time and capital in improving their information systems. Electronic data interfaces between systems would increase their capabilities to manage patients, resources, and health care dollars, and improve both patient and provider satisfaction. Currently, St. Mary's Medical Center is placing its patient care pathways "online"; the management company of the IPA is exploring the use of an information system to ease the authorization process; and PacifiCare is developing a computerized case management system to manage its chronically ill members.

SITE VISITS

By examining the existing literature and using the PacifiCare experience, the project team from the three health care organizations developed the following assumptions regarding chronic disease guideline development and physician attitudes toward computerized guidelines:

- Physicians will support clinical guidelines if they decrease the hassle factor of managed care regulations.
- A computer-based guideline will prove to be more efficacious and therefore increase physicians' compliance and satisfaction.
- Clinical guidelines can be useful in managing chronic diseases and can be successfully developed and applied in an IPA model of health care delivery.
- Simply knowing the key data elements necessary in providing care without adequate information systems would be no help to physicians in managing chronically ill patients.

The two assumptions involving physicians' ability to identify key elements of disease progression and their attitudes toward applying computerized technologies to direct clinical guidelines were explored in two ways: by on-site interviews conducted with health systems staff that had dedicated resources to guideline development and by focus groups held with managed care physicians of the IPA.

Site visits were made to two different health care systems, one an Illinois hospital-based health system, and the other a Michigan multispecialty physician group affiliated with a closed provider panel managed care system.

Hospital system

The hospital system, which had formal contractual relationships with several skilled nursing facilities, a home health agency, and two provider groups, had been successfully using patient care—but paper-based guidelines—internally for many years. The organization wanted to extend its patient care pathways for those patients requiring nursing home placements or home health care after discharge from the acute care setting. By including these additional sites, the hospital system aimed to enhance communication along the entire health care continuum and improve patient outcomes.

The system currently has more than a dozen extended care pathways in effect. Patients must meet certain eligibility criteria to be put on a clinical pathway and can be removed from a pathway if their condition warrants alternative treatment modalities, for example, if a total hip replacement patient who was receiving physical therapy in a skilled nursing facility suffered a disabling stroke. Prior to the addition of this system, the organization noted that most of the clinical practice variation occurred when these sites worked with ancillary providers.

In reviewing implementation issues, the site representatives noted two major issues to be considered in designing and implementing automated practice guidelines: the current paper-based status of its guidelines and physician input. Because the hospital system's guidelines are paper-based and data collection for reporting and outcomes measurement are currently being hand tabulated, they are limited in their capabilities to measure the success and variation in guideline use.

Physicians did not initially contribute to the development of the guidelines. Yet, once contacted, they had difficulty in giving support for something they had no input in. The project manager at the hospital made the following recommendations: that physicians be involved in the process from the beginning and that the hospital system invest in an information system so that computerized communication linkages take place among sites of care. The physicians admitted that computerized guidelines would solve many of their current communication disconnects between sites of care, as well as improve efficiencies in resource utilization.

Multispecialty group

The multispecialty group has been providing health care services to managed care beneficiaries for the past few years. A progressive medical director realized that practice guidelines had great potential in reducing unnecessary and inappropriate utilization, but physicians needed to be better educated on managed care principles prior to developing the practice guidelines. Their efforts gave rise to a managed care college in 1993 that provides courses to physicians on managed care concepts, chronic disease management, and outcomes measurement. Two-thirds of their physicians have completed the first phase of course work. The second phase of the college curriculum will focus on developing clinical guidelines for use in their daily practice.

Similar to the hospital system site visits, the multispecialty physicians rely on paper-based information systems to direct patient care decisions, although they are planning to invest in a computerized information system. Techniques they employed to give incentives for physicians to participate in the managed care college included obtaining support of senior administrators, providing continuing medical education (CME) credits for course work, reimbursing physicians for their time spent in class, and using individual practitioners' data on resource utilization and treatment patterns.

The project team noted several lessons from this effort that are major factors to be considered when implementing automated clinical guidelines: physician "buy-in" is critical; baseline data must be collected; physicians should be adequately educated about basic managed care principles; and physicians should be told what they will gain in return for their efforts. Furthermore, project leaders noted that developing a plan for implementation and program analysis needs to be given as much thought and resources as the developmental phase of guidelines.

The medical group's approach is very practical, but the course work involved with phase one was over 80 hours, a luxury that most medical groups and IPAs cannot afford. However, the basic education on managed care principles is an essential first step for physicians who are just beginning to enter the managed care marketplace.

FOCUS GROUPS

In addition to the site visits, four focus groups were with primary care and specialty care physicians that belonged to the IPA. The group facilitator was a health care researcher and not a clinician. This individual was selected because of her expertise in group facilitation and program evaluation and the fact that she had no vested interest in the outcomes of the group activity.

As mentioned previously, the chronic conditions of COPD and CHF were chosen because of the significant prevalence of these conditions among the patients served by this IPA.

At the first session, the physicians received an overview of the evolution of practice guidelines and discussed the various uses for guidelines in medical care. The group also discussed how and why the management of chronic conditions could benefit from clinical guidelines. They noted several reasons:

- Many markers of disease progression are easily discernible in the treatment of COPD and CHF, for example, peak flow meter readings in COPD patients and EKG changes in cardiac patients.
- Chronic diseases are managed across the entire continuum of care, and instituting practice guidelines could enhance the communication between sites and reduce duplication in care delivery. The emergency room physician could access the diabetic patient's home health records as well as the last blood sugar report in the primary care physician's office.

- Health care dollars are shrinking, and different methods for decreasing inappropriate utilization are necessary, particularly in chronic disease management. In many cases, for example, home care settings may be more appropriate for certain discharged patients, especially those who can be taught to self-manage chronic conditions.

IDENTIFYING KEY MARKERS FOR CHRONIC DISEASE MANAGEMENT

The goal of the remaining sessions of the focus groups was to answer several questions related to clinical guidelines for chronic diseases: What are the essential data elements necessary to determine disease stability or progression in treating COPD and CHF? Would physicians value computer technology that could direct the utility of a practice guideline? What additional factors would influence a physician to adhere to guidelines?

The participating physicians were asked to identify key markers of disease progression and stability that are necessary in determining treatment decisions. They were able to identify key variables for both chronic conditions. Once this task was completed they were then asked to further delineate between variables by discerning which elements were essential or nonessential to making treatment decisions. Table 12–1 displays their recommendations.

The number of variables shown in Table 12–1 is somewhat smaller than what was initially anticipated and identified by the focus group. However,

---

Table 12–1 Elements Essential to Treatment Decisions

Essential elements of care for COPD	Essential elements of care for CHF
Medications (including affordability)	Medications (including affordability)
Patient self report of health	Patient self-report of health
Comorbidities	Functional status changes
Spirometry (peak flow)	Weight changes
Functional status changes	Edema
Support system	EKG
	Chest x-ray
	Chem 7
	Support system

Source: Reprinted with permission from Schwartz, J.S., and Cohen, S.J. "Changing Physician Behavior." In *Primary Care Research: An Agenda for the 90s,* edited by J. Mayfield and M. Grady. Washington, D.C.: Dept. of Health and Human Services, Public Health Service/Agency for Health Care Policy and Research, 1990: 45–53.

the second meeting of each disease session was spent comparing the importance of each data element with each other to arrive at a hierarchical stratification in the event all data elements could not be captured in a computer-based guideline. Participating physicians felt that they could always refer to the complete medical record to check on these secondary variables when necessary. Interestingly enough, research shows that in a chronic disease database model a limit of 10 variables per module would yield most of the power realized in much more elaborate systems of outcomes measurements.[4]

Also of interest was how strongly the physicians felt about patient self-reported data regarding health status and functional capabilities. Physicians also indicated equal interest about the psychosocial aspects of disease management and their awareness of the impact of financial constraints on patient compliance. They were interested because these factors indicated whether a family or other caregiver was involved in the chronic patient's care and whether patients were able to afford proper foods that have an impact on a person's overall well-being.

Overall, it was found that the focus groups could identify key markers of disease progression and arrived at the same variables identified in published guidelines. This indicated that it was possible to use published guidelines with some allowance for local practice patterns as a foundation for guideline development within a health care system. The feeling among the research team is that managed care physicians are very interested in streamlining care delivery to chronically ill patients, and they can easily appreciate the inherent value in reducing variation through the implementation of practice guidelines.

ACCEPTANCE ISSUES

Considerable research has shown that the ideal approach to gaining physician acceptance and compliance with treatment guidelines is to include physicians at the local level in both the development and implementation phases. Peer-developed and peer-accepted guidelines are more influential than simple scientific studies and clinical trials.[5] Moreover, physician involvement should extend into all aspects of guideline development: review, endorsement, and adaptation to actual physician practice.[6] Physician education can also affect the degree of acceptance of practice parameters.

The findings from the site visits and focus groups revealed that physicians are willing to use clinical guidelines under the following conditions:

- The guidelines are not totally prescriptive and allow for deviation when appropriate.

- The guidelines are easy to use and are incorporated into their daily routine of administering patient care.
- The guidelines do not significantly increase the workload for themselves or their office staff.
- The guidelines will improve patient outcomes, including patient satisfaction.
- The guidelines will reduce overall cost of care.
- The guidelines will decrease the "hassle factor" associated with the managed care authorization and administrative processes.

Generally, physicians overwhelmingly supported a computerized format for using clinical guidelines. Specifically, they were interested in the flexibility of the system and whether it could provide patient trend data over time, such as functional status, and present this in a chart form for their interpretation.

Physicians also wanted timely, accurate information that was accessible across all sites of care and that incorporated patient information from community-based agencies and other services. For example, the information system should be able to verify the prescribed medication covered under the health plans formulary or provide physicians with the patient's benefit information regarding home health care. Their ideal system would be user-friendly and ultimately decrease the "hassle factor" of providing patient care.

The guideline technology would warn them of abnormal lab values and allow them to access historical pieces of the medical record on an ad hoc basis. The ability to abstract various data elements from patient records is extremely important as the demands on physicians to produce this type of information grows from such organizations as the National Committee for Quality Assurance (NCQA) and national and local performance measurement efforts. Equally important to physicians is having the ability to opt out of or modify guideline recommendations when necessary. Focus group participants raised issues of confidentiality and questioned where the "collective data base" would reside.

The physicians also suggested a potential incentive to encourage compliance with guidelines: create in the guideline an authorization for certain procedures and treatments. Physicians who choose not to follow the guideline would still need to call the health plan or administrative body for approval, a step back to the "hassle factor" that many physicians dislike.

They also indicated that computerized information that was timely and current and if possible to trend overtime would significantly reduce the time to retrieve lab data, review patient records, and ultimately improve the patient-doctor encounter dramatically. The group reached a consensus that the most important attribute of a clinical guideline is its capability of assuring their patients receive the "best practice," highest quality care. Their sense was that computerized practice guidelines and outcome measurements would enable them to achieve this.

OVERSIGHT AND VENDOR CAPABILITY

A major objective of the research was to investigate computer system technologies to determine their current scope of capabilities for clinical guideline application. Prior to the evaluation of systems these components of the "ideal" system were identified:

- Ability to manage the following data points: clinical data; insurance eligibility; authorization and claims; and patient treatment plans.
- Capability to perform these functions: acuity/severity ratings; coding schemes (e.g., ICD-9 and CPTs); billing functions; report generation; outcome measurements; real time clinical data; decision support with practice guidelines; and notification process.

In searching for a comprehensive system to fulfill the team's objective, the team discovered an industry still in its infancy. While the technology exists to meet a plan's expectations, most systems in operation today fall very short of providing all but the most rudimentary capabilities for two major reasons: financial issues of who should pay for the system if organizations such as hospitals, medical groups, and health plans are affiliated, and the staffing requirements of who is responsible for warehousing and maintaining an interactive, multisite clinical system. Other obstacles facing interactive, multisite systems are patient confidentiality issues and the lack of standardization among individual systems in how and what data they collect.

The team was unsuccessful in locating a single vendor that was able to meet all of its system requirements. Current large commercial vendors are unwilling to provide a core set of functions to the general medical community. Instead their systems consist of a tightly integrated set of modules relying on each other to perform generalized functions. Organizations must begin to look beyond this narrow focus to a model that allows for inclusion of third party system connectivity without major cost penalties. Through its research the team has realized that smaller, innovative companies, educational institutions, and companies that have reengineered their work force have shown the greatest willingness to be involved and pursue such a vision. They are more willing to be part of a universal clinical resource for each other, using interactive media to provide a core set of functions, such as eligibility, authorization, claims processing, clinical data collection and dissemination, treatment decision support, and clinical guidelines.

FUTURE ISSUES

The findings and conclusions presented here have great potential in different models of health care delivery. From a disease management perspective, the focus in the St. Mary's, PacifiCare, and HMO effort was very broad and looked at markers for disease progression as a starting point to begin guideline development in these systems' settings of care. Moreover, the team's initial thoughts were to design guidelines to help physicians more easily manage chronically ill members.

The study feedback indicated that the guidelines will not only help as tools to assist with precertification and automatic authorization, and to advise providers of the next steps in disease management across the health care continuum, but that they also will help providers evaluate these activities as part of an overall quality improvement effort.[7] In fact, the focus group participants were very interested in collaborating with one another on how to treat a chronic heart or lung patient. They were also able to identify important areas for assessment with chronically ill members regardless of their funding source. Clearly, physicians are more than willing to use practice guidelines when they have significant input into their creation, if the incentives are appropriate, and if the environment is supportive.

From an organizational structure perspective, providers in a managed care setting may be more accepting of automated clinical guidelines than providers in sole fee-for-service arrangements because payment is not an issue in a capitated environment. Also, ancillary providers that contract with managed care organizations would also support guidelines because they, too, are being capitated for services provided. This is an important factor when developing a guideline for a chronic disease where the site of care delivery varies greatly and changes frequently.

The team's assumptions regarding computer technology to drive the guideline application were also on target. The feedback indicated that physicians are interested in the capabilities of computers and can easily see how a centralized database shared by all caregivers can have a significant impact on their current practices. Physicians had no problem noting the potential improvements in communication, cost efficiencies, early treatment of exacerbations, and increased patient and provider satisfaction made possible by applying technology to health care delivery. Physicians saw computerized guidelines as a way of comparing costs with clinical effectiveness of different treatments for like conditions or symptoms.

A major lesson learned through the planning grant is that senior management's support is essential to the overall success of such a program. Senior management can approve the incentives such as "automatic authorizations" and create a corporate culture that supports collaboration and continuous improvement efforts. Furthermore, their support is vital for securing the capital expense required to invest in information technology.

Finally, health systems that pursue guideline development as their vehicle to improve care delivery must develop methods for educating key personnel and evaluating the utility of the guideline for clinical and cost effectiveness. Information systems allow for integration of the entire delivery system across all continuums of care and assist in outcome measurement. Information technology is key to achieving quality and cost effectiveness.

REFERENCES

1. Fries, J.F. "The Chronic Disease Data Bank Model: A Conceptual Framework for the Computer-Based Medical Record." *Computers and Biomedical Research* 25 (1992): 586–601.
2. Eddy, D.M. *A Manual for Assessing Health Practices and Designing Practice Policies.* Philadelphia, PA: American College of Physicians, 1992.
3. Schwartz, J.S., and Cohen, S.J. "Changing Physician Behavior." In *Primary Care Research: An Agenda for the 90s,* edited by J. Mayfield and M. Grady. Washington, D.C.: Dept. of Health and Human Services, Public Health Service/Agency for Health Care Policy and Research, 1990.
4. Fries, "The Chronic Disease Data Bank Model."
5. Gates, P.E. "Think Globally, Act Locally: An Approach to Implementation of Clinical Practice Guidelines." *Journal of Quality Improvement* 21(2) (1994): 71–85.
6. Kelly, J.T., and Toepp, M.C. "Development, Evaluation, and Implementation of Medical Practice Parameters." *The Medical Staff Counselor* 6(4) (1992): 45–49.
7. National Quality of Care Forum. "Bridging the Gap Between Theory and Practice: Exploring Clinical Practice Guidelines." *Journal on Quality Improvement* 19(9) (1993): 384–400.

V

Children with Special Needs

13

Enhancing Preventive and Primary Care for Children with Chronic or Disabling Conditions Served in Health Maintenance Organizations

Margaret A. McManus and Harriette B. Fox

GROWING NUMBERS OF CHILDREN WITH CHRONIC CONDITIONS

Health maintenance organizations (HMOs) provide care to a substantial number of children, many of whom have chronic or disabling conditions. In 1993, an estimated 20 percent or 12 million children nationwide received their care through HMOs.[1] This percentage is expected to increase in light of states' growing reliance on HMOs for Medicaid recipients, at least half of whom are children. Since 1993, ten states have been awarded waiver demonstrations which allow for the statewide enrollment of Medicaid recipients into fully capitated managed care arrangements. An additional nine states have statewide applications pending.[2]

Unfortunately there are no reliable estimates of the number of children with chronic conditions who are enrolled in HMOs. In a recent analysis of national survey data (shown in Tables 13–1 and 13–2), however, little difference was found between the prevalence of chronic childhood conditions or disability among privately insured children enrolled in HMOs and those enrolled in indemnity plans.[3] It is reasonable to assume, therefore, that national prevalence estimates of chronic conditions among children would apply to privately insured children in HMOs. For the Medicaid child population, there is no comparable data set. However, it is

Source: Reprinted from M.A. McManus and H.B. Fox, Enhancing Preventive and Primary Care for Children with Chronic or Disabling Conditions Served in Health Maintenance Organizations, *Managed Care Quarterly*, Vol. 4, No. 3, pp. 19–29, © 1996, Aspen Publishers, Inc.

Table 13–1 Prevalence of Chronic Childhood Conditions Seen in Commercial Indemnity and HMO Plans, 1992

Chronic Condition	Indemnity	HMOs
Selected skin and musculoskeletal conditions:		
—Arthritis	1.8	1.7
Selected impairments:		
—Visual impairments	9.5	4.3
—Hearing impairments	13.4	8.0
—Speech impairments	17.6	16.0
—Orthopedic impairments/		
deformity	36.9	35.3
Selected conditions of the genitourinary, nervous, endocrine, metabolic, or blood systems:		
—Diabetes	—	2.0
—Epilepsy	2.0	1.5
—Migraine headaches	14.0	13.0
Selected circulatory conditions:		
—Heart disease, total	17.3	17.8
—Heart rhythm disorders	14.2	10.2
—Congenital heart disease	1.6	4.5
—Other heart disease	1.6	3.0
—Hypertension	0.9	1.1
—Cerebral vascular disease	0.5	—
Selected respiratory conditions:		
—Chronic bronchitis	65.1	53.8
—Asthma	58.9	67.0

important to note that children in the Medicaid program have a higher incidence of chronic disabling conditions than their counterparts in the private sector (as shown in Table 13–3) and these children are increasingly being included in states' HMO-enrolled population groups.[4]

According to current national estimates, 31 percent of all children have one or more chronic physical conditions.[5] In addition, an estimated 20 percent of children have experienced developmental delays, behavioral and emotional problems, and learning disabilities.[6] No national data exist to estimate the combined prevalence of chronic physical and mental conditions among children.

Overall, chronic conditions affecting children include a few very prevalent conditions. These are respiratory allergies, repeated ear infections, asthma, eczema and skin allergies, frequent or severe headaches, speech

Table 13–2 Prevalence of Limitations of Activity Among Children Seen in Commercial Indemnity and HMO Plans, 1992

	Indemnity	HMOs
Activity Limitations		
—Percent without limitation	95.2	94.4
—Percent with limitations:	4.8	5.6
——Unable to perform major activity	0.3	0.6
——Limited in kind/amount of major activity	3.0	3.4
——Limited in other activity	1.5	1.5

Adapted from *Health Affairs*, Volume 14:1, Spring 1995, exhibits appear on pages 238, 239, and 240. "Do HMOs Care for the Chronically Ill?", by Fama, T., Fox, P.D., and White, L.A. *The People-to-People Health Foundation, Inc.*, Project HOPE, All rights reserved.

defects, attention deficit disorder, and depression. Most chronic conditions among children are rare conditions such as diabetes, cerebral palsy, sickle cell disease, and spina bifida. This is in stark contrast to the adult chronic illness profile, which is essentially composed of a small number of prevalent conditions.

Importantly, however, only a small number of children with chronic physical and mental conditions—6 percent, or four million in 1992—suffer from limitations in their usual activity or disability. The leading causes of childhood disability are respiratory system diseases, principally asthma; mental retardation; mental and nervous system disorders; and orthopedic impairments.[7] While the number of affected children remains relatively

Table 13–3 Prevalence of Activity Limitation Among Children by Insurance Coverage, 1992

Degree of Activity Limitation	Private Insurance Only	Public Insurance Only	Both Public and Private	No Insurance
Children with activity limitations	51.5%	30.6%	3.7%	14.2%
Unable to conduct major activity (severe)	41.8	43.4	5.3	9.6
Limited in amount or kind of activity	50.2	31.6	3.7	14.4
Limited in other activities (mild)	58.2	23.3	3.0	15.5
Children without activity limitation	65.4	18.6	1.9	14.5

Adapted to special tabulations from unpublished data of the 1992 National Health Interview Survey prepared by Paul Newacheck of the University of California, San Francisco.

small, there is evidence that the number of disabled children is increasing. Specifically, over the last 30 years, the prevalence of limitation of activity has more than tripled.[8] This increase is due to real increases in the incidence and duration of chronic childhood conditions, aging of the child population, improved access to health care services, expanded screening programs in schools, and changes in the survey questions.[9]

All children with chronic or disabling conditions require routine preventive and primary care services, but often at a level that exceeds the requirements of children without these ongoing conditions. These children may require more regular and lengthy physician visits for routine preventive, acute, and chronic care management. They may also require specialized physician and hospital services, greater use of prescription medications, ancillary therapies, mental health counseling, home health services, and equipment and supplies. They may require family support services, such as family counseling and education, and comprehensive case management. They may also require early intervention, special education, and social services.

Managing the care of children with chronic or disabling conditions is of particular concern to HMOs because such children use more services than their healthier counterparts. In 1988, children with chronic physical conditions were estimated to have made 92 million ambulatory physician contacts (about five contacts per child), in addition to visits made for routine preventive care and services obtained in treating acute conditions like colds, the flu, and minor injuries. An estimated 690,000 children were hospitalized for a total of nearly 7.2 million days for treatment of chronic physical conditions. The cost of physician and hospital care related to childhood chronic conditions alone was estimated to be approximately $7.5 billion in 1988.[10] The total cost of care would be significantly higher were data available for children with chronic mental conditions.

The disparity in service use is particularly dramatic for chronically ill children with limitations of activity. Children with activity limitations or disability made almost three times as many physician visits as children without activity limitations (11.2 visits versus 4.1 visits). In addition, an almost tenfold difference was found in the number of hospital days among these two groups of children (1,445.5 days per 1,000 children with limitations of activity versus 157.5 days per 1,000 children without limitations of activity).[11]

Providing effective preventive and primary care to children with chronic conditions will be challenging because it requires more comprehensive and intensive strategies than are traditionally pursued for healthy children in most health maintenance organizations. Equally challenging will be the need to address so many rare conditions. HMOs will want to consider their current policies regarding pediatric staffing and organization; scope of commercial and Medicaid covered benefits; linkages with pediatric specialists and related education, public health, and social service programs; and quality performance measures.

This chapter describes seven recommended design elements for enhancing preventive and primary care for children with chronic conditions:

1. specially trained primary care providers
2. improved screening and risk assessment
3. multidisciplinary teams for evaluation and diagnosis
4. individual and group health education
5. flexible gatekeeping arrangements
6. comprehensive case management services
7. coordination with public health, education, and social services.

The seven design elements were identified through a variety of research activities, including a review of the literature on managed care and children, a survey of 22 managed care plans, and an examination of state Medicaid HMO contracts. These activities gave us a picture of current HMO practices, including their strengths and weaknesses in serving children with chronic conditions and their families, and also provided us with considerable information about efforts under way to improve the primary and preventive care services that children with chronic conditions receive in HMO arrangements.

Although it may appear that some of the suggested design elements stretch beyond conventional preventive and primary care, they do not represent a paradigm shift for HMOs. The features are a natural extension of HMOs' already integrated approach to care. In fact, the design elements were derived from existing HMO practices in many cases. Taken together, they offer HMOs a comprehensive strategy for improving their preventive and primary care services for children with chronic or disabling conditions.

FEATURES FOR ENHANCED PREVENTIVE AND PRIMARY CARE

Element 1: Specially Trained Primary Care Providers

Definition and purpose

Specially trained primary care providers for children with chronic conditions are those who have knowledge and experience in chronic illness management and behavioral-developmental pediatrics. During this century, the leading causes of childhood morbidity have shifted from infectious diseases to chronic conditions. Increasingly pediatricians are finding developmental, behavioral, and environmental causes and consequences of these conditions. Consequently, a growing need has emerged for primary care providers educated and experienced in treating children with more complex problems at different stages of childhood development. Unfortunately, the supply of pediatricians and family physicians trained in these areas still remains quite limited. Thus, to the extent that specially trained primary care providers are not available, HMOs can identify pediatric subspecialists or multidisciplinary teams to furnish backup consultation.

Implementation issues

Many primary care providers in HMOs, as in other financing and delivery arrangements, report a reluctance to treat children with chronic conditions. However, as primary care physicians assume a greater role in the care of children with chronic physical or mental health problems, HMOs may want to explore the following issues. What opportunities exist to improve the training of existing plan physicians in the areas of chronic care management and behavioral-developmental pediatrics? Should new multidisciplinary team or consultative arrangements be created to support the plan's primary care physicians? What financial arrangements or incentives should be offered to encourage the use of specially trained primary care providers and to allow for pediatric specialty consultation?

Examples

- Arizona IPA has contracted with Phoenix Pediatrics, a group that receives a higher capitation amount to serve children with various types of special needs, many of whom are severely disabled. To care for this population, the staff at Phoenix Pediatrics pursued additional training in outpatient care, including how to change gastrostomy tubes and tracheostomies. They also expanded their training in routine gynecologic exams for special-needs adolescents and young adults because the local obstetricians were reluctant to care for these children.[12]
- The Florida state Medicaid agency requires that its HMO contractors have specific staffing requirements for certain subgroups of children with special needs. The primary care team must include a minimum of a primary care provider or specialist willing to provide primary care, a registered nurse with two years of experience in pediatrics and one year of experience working with the state's program for children with special needs, a health educator, and a nurse or social worker case manager. The specialist care team must include the primary care provider, case manager, specialty physicians, and others as needed, such as dietitians, genetic counselors, health educators, speech therapists, and psychologists.[13]

Element 2: Improved Screening and Risk Assessment

Definition and purpose

Improved screening and risk assessment requires an examination of the interrelationship of multiple factors—biological, environmental, and behavioral—to identify children who are at high risk for various kinds of health problems, with the ultimate result being a definitive evaluation and appropriate treatment, as necessary. To be effective, it also requires an understanding of the cultural values and norms of families. The concept of screening children for health-related risks is not new. It is a cornerstone of pediatric preventive care and has long been a covered benefit offered in commercial HMOs and under the Medicaid program. What is new is the expansion of the screening process to focus not only on physical health but also on developmental, behavioral, and emotional health, and to provide increased attention to peer relationships and family needs, resources, and strengths.

Many instruments exist that assess specific components of child health (social, emotional, developmental, and intellectual disabilities, for example), but no single instrument has yet been developed or tested that reliably assesses multiple, interactional risks. Several different guidelines or instruments, however, have been developed.

- Bright Futures, a new set of pediatric preventive care guidelines, has defined a set of health supervision standards for infants, young children, school-aged children, and adolescents. During the preventive care visit, these pediatric guidelines call for a family interview; a physical examination; an observation of children and family; psychosocial, educational, developmental surveillance; and vision screening. Hearing and metabolic screening may also be performed.[14]
- The National Early Childhood Technical Assistance System (NEC*TAS), a resource center created to provide expert consultation to help states and communities establish a comprehensive system of early intervention services for chronically ill children from birth to three, has developed a set of guidelines for screening and assessing young children at risk of developmental problems. It includes a wide range of demographic, parental characteristics, and child health status and functioning components.[15]

Implementation issues

HMOs have led the way in offering preventive benefits for children. However, their providers, like many other private providers, have tended to rely only on medical histories, physical examinations, and results from single screening instruments or developmental scores to identify potential health problems in children.

An HMO interested in improving the use of risk assessment and screening tools will need to consider several additional issues. What risk assessment and screening tools are its pediatric providers currently using as part of a clinical preventive visit? Are these sufficient to identify the large and growing number of children exposed to serious biological, environmental, and behavioral problems? What additional tools should be used? What referral protocols should be established? To what extent can primary care providers perform more sophisticated screening and risk assessments or will the plan need to contract with a specialized provider for the service?

Examples

- Group Health of Puget Sound (the Northwest Division), in the state of Washington, has developed a screening questionnaire for use by its adolescent enrollees to predict risk of physical and mental health problems. This questionnaire is called HEADS-SET (Home, Education, Activities, Drugs, Sexuality, Suicide risk, Eating disorder, and Total)—"a kind of behavioral Apgar score." This survey is used to determine the need for preventive interventions or case management.[16]
- Northern California Kaiser Programs, in 18 facilities, have designed a Temperament Program. Parents are asked to complete a temperament questionnaire when their infant is four months old. A temperament profile is prepared and placed in the child's medical record and used to provide anticipatory guidance as part of the clinical preventive visit. Parents requesting written feedback will receive guidance materials and referral to a temperament counselor.[17]
- In Florida, the state Medicaid agency requires its HMOs to use a Healthy Start Postnatal Screen to identify high-risk infants. The provider uses this screen with each newborn and those identified at risk are referred to the local county public health unit.[18]

Element 3: Multidisciplinary Teams for Evaluation and Diagnosis

Definition and purpose

Multidisciplinary teams for evaluation and diagnosis would include two or more health care professionals with different expertise who can be used to perform comprehensive medical, developmental, psychological, and social assessments of children with or at risk of chronic conditions. Such children may suffer from multiple problems that are often complex and difficult to diagnose, necessitating coordinated and state-of-the-art approaches. Depending on the needs of the child and family, a multidisciplinary team may include (in addition to the primary care provider) pediatric subspecialists, mental health professionals, developmental specialists, ancillary therapies, nurses, or others. Multidisciplinary teams have historically been based at tertiary care medical centers, but they also operate at regional referral centers, child development centers, or specialized clinics and can be formed on an ad hoc basis as well.

Implementation issues

Most HMOs have relied almost exclusively on children's hospitals and other tertiary medical centers for multidisciplinary evaluations and diagnoses, and these have been essentially for children with complex physical problems. In general, HMOs have been less likely to use multidisciplinary teams for children who are experiencing emotional, behavioral, and neurological problems. These children are often referred for multidisciplinary evaluation through the schools, which take a limited view of the child's health and functional status, focusing only on school performance.

HMOs may want to consider the following implementation issues: What is the capacity of participating plan providers to offer multidisciplinary team evaluations for children with developmental, behavioral, and emotional problems? Are these arrangements linked in any way to the schools? What kind of teams will be needed in the plan to address the various problems and different ages of children with chronic conditions? What referral mechanisms and financial incentives will be needed to encourage appropriate and timely referrals to multidisciplinary teams for evaluation and diagnosis?

Examples

- The Harvard Community Health Plan in Massachusetts uses multidisciplinary teams for diagnosis and treatment planning for certain children with chronic or disabling problems.[19]
- Medica, in Minnesota, offers multidisciplinary teams for diagnosis and treatment planning for some children with chronic or disabling problems.[20]
- In Utah, Medicaid HMOs are required to evaluate children with special health needs through a multidisciplinary team that develops a comprehensive service plan with the child's family. The evaluations occur promptly and result in a referral to the state's program for children with special health care needs.[21]
- Washington's Medicaid agency requires its HMO contractors to refer members with developmental problems (as identified by a screening) to a neurodevelopmental center or to another provider for developmental evaluation and treatment. The HMO then follows up to verify that the services have been received.[22]

Element 4: Individual and Group Health Education

Definition and purpose

Individual and group health education targeted at children and families with chronic conditions involves a combination of methods intended to effect improvements in self care and appropriate use of health care services. Since limited time is allotted during preventive care visits to address many of the concerns of families of children with chronic conditions, it can be important to supplement this with more intensive and interactive approaches. Using nurses and mental health professionals to talk with children and families individually or in group sessions may be cost-effective in allowing parents and children more opportunity to discuss problems and receive advice. Other health education methods include educational handouts and videotapes. In general, the success of health education is largely determined by the extent to which the agendas of parents and children are addressed.

Implementation issues

Health education programs sponsored by HMOs have tended to focus on adult enrollees, addressing such topics as smoking cessation, weight reduction/maintenance, pregnancy and childbirth, and stress reduction. Where children are concerned, plans have tended to rely almost exclusively on their primary care providers to offer individual health education during preventive care visits, which focus mostly on physical health. Consequently, attention to the developmental and behavioral issues of chronically ill children (specifically, counseling about parent-child interactions, advice about growth and development, and behavioral issues affecting adolescents) is usually insufficient, given these children's needs.

HMOs may want to consider the following implementation issues in expanding their health education efforts. How can the anticipatory guidance offered during regular preventive care visits be strengthened? How can more intensive individual and group health education strategies be designed? Who should provide these services? In what settings should they be offered? Which children with chronic conditions and their families should be targeted?

Examples

- Kaiser Permanente, Northwest Region, offers an asthma management educational program called Open Airways for children ages 4 to 14 and their families. Topics addressed include what is asthma, compliance with medications, keeping healthy, how to manage an attack, when to go to the doctor, making doctor visits easier and better, recognizing and controlling asthma triggers, and solving problems about school and asthma.[23]

- In Massachusetts, Medicaid HMOs must provide health education programs for special populations, including adolescents. Mental health, substance abuse, violence prevention, and wellness programs are offered that are responsive to specific community issues or enrollee needs.[24]

Element 5: Flexible Gatekeeping Arrangements

Definition and purpose

Flexible gatekeeping arrangements include policies that allow children and their families to access certain services on a limited basis without prior authorization from their primary care providers. For example, a plan could allow self-referral for a set number of outpatient mental health services or for certain covered out-of-plan services, such as family planning or school-based health services. Flexible gatekeeping arrangements also can include simplifying regular service authorization rules, allowing standing orders to be given for a specific amount and duration of services, so that families of children with chronic conditions would not have to obtain repeated authorizations for each individual service. The use of a specialty provider to gatekeep might also be considered for at least some services likely to be required by children with chronic conditions.

Children with chronic conditions and their families often experience barriers to appropriate care within the present HMO gatekeeper system. It may be that the family has limited understanding about how to access specialized services within an HMO or that the gatekeeper is inaccessible because of location or scheduling problems. Moreover, the more specialty services for which a primary care provider is at financial risk, the less likely he or she will be to authorize multiple specialty services for a given child, particularly if many such children are in the practice or the capitation amount is not enhanced.

Implementation issues

HMOs' cost-saving achievements are due in part to their success in managing service utilization through gatekeeping mechanisms that operate at the plan level and at the level of the individual primary care provider. Because these mechanisms have successfully reduced the utilization of unnecessary services, HMOs have been reluctant to revise them to allow for more flexibility and responsiveness to individual enrollee needs. Yet, without some modifications, children with chronic conditions may miss critical opportunities for accessing necessary services.

Implementing flexible gatekeeping arrangements will require HMOs to examine a number of issues. For example, which services are underused by children with chronic conditions and to what extent would allowing self-referrals and certain out-of-plan services improve utilization patterns and access to care? Which families with children who have chronic conditions are unnecessarily burdened by having to secure authorization for specialty services that they require on a routine basis, and to what extent would standing orders for certain services reduce barriers to necessary services? What restrictions should be imposed on these flexible gatekeeping policies? What specialists are trained and interested in assuming responsibility for gatekeeping some or all services for children with chronic conditions? How can flexible gatekeeping approaches be monitored to control unnecessary use of health care services?

Examples

- Medica, in Minnesota, serving mostly Medicaid recipients, allows affiliated pulmonologists to perform the gatekeeping role for children under their care due to a chronic health problem.[25]
- Wisconsin Independent Physicians Group allows gatekeeping for children with special health needs to be done by specialists at the family's request.[26]
- The Massachusetts Medicaid agency requires that its HMOs permit direct access to mental health and substance abuse providers by self-referral, as well as state agency, school health personnel, and primary care provider referral.[27]

Element 6: Comprehensive Case Management Services

Definition and purpose

Comprehensive case management is the assignment of a nurse, social worker, or other professional to certain families of children with chronic conditions in order to provide them substantial support and guidance in managing health problems and improving their overall health and functional status. This type of active case management usually involves an assessment and ongoing monitoring of the child's needs, the development of recommendations for referral to plan and nonplan services, frequent contact with the child and family, emotional support, and advocacy assistance. Case managers must have excellent interpersonal skills, working knowledge of related community-based programs, effective problem-solving abilities, and relevant experience with different cultural groups.

Implementation issues

Many HMOs have implemented high-cost case management programs for children with complex or chronic physical or emotional problems typically following a lengthy hospitalization. Yet, few have expanded their case management models to include a less severe population of children and to incorporate a preventive focus. Rather, the job of comprehensive case management has been assumed in many localities by public health, schools, and social service agencies, with health care providers playing a limited role.

Plans considering offering comprehensive case management services for children with chronic conditions, focusing more on primary and secondary prevention and less on immediate cost issues, may want to examine the following issues. How can the highest-risk children be identified? What case management approaches, standards, and protocols should be used for children at highest risk? Who should provide the service and what is an optimal caseload? What kinds of training might be provided? What internal administrative systems need to be created or modified to identify certain children with chronic conditions in need of comprehensive case management services?

Examples

- Harvard Community Health Plan (HCHP), in Massachusetts, has created the Special Needs Program for children who have chronic or complex medical conditions. To operate this care coordination program, HCHP draws on the expertise of developmental pediatricians, social workers, a community resource specialist, pediatric physical therapists, a pediatric speech-language pathologist, and their Down Syndrome Program coordinator.[28]
- Maricopa County Health Plan, in Arizona, subcontracted with Southwest Human Development to provide case management for children at risk of abuse or neglect. A Southwest social worker with expertise in child abuse intervened with families, ensuring medical compliance, and submitted reports of abuse or neglect back to the plan.[29]

Element 7: Coordination with Public Health, Education, and Social Services

Definition and purpose

Coordination by HMOs with public health, education, and social services can include a variety of collaborative arrangements, ranging from simple referral agreements, to the exchange of medical information, to the joint development of public education and information campaigns. Numerous public programs exist at the state and community level to serve children with chronic conditions. Prominent among them are the program for children with special health care needs, the early intervention program for children from birth to three, the special education program for school-aged children, various social service programs, the foster care and adoption assistance program, and the Ryan White program for children with AIDS.

Implementation issues

Although HMO providers have sometimes coordinated a specific child's care with the public agencies also serving the child and family, HMOs generally have not established any coordination protocols or mechanisms for routine use with children with chronic conditions. As a result, interventions for these children may be more fragmented or duplicated than they need be. Moreover, plans may be losing opportunities to draw upon community resources that could improve health and functional status outcomes for these children. Given the nature and extent of the risk factors that today's child enrollees, the commercially insured as well as those covered by Medicaid, are likely to have, HMOs may want to work more collaboratively with community-based public providers in the future.

An HMO that wants to establish more formal coordination arrangements with public health, education, and social service programs will want to examine the following issues: What public programs are its child enrollees likely to be eligible for? How are the programs organized locally and what are their strengths and weaknesses? Are there any existing local interagency organizations in which a plan representative could participate? What kinds of policy guidelines or referral protocols might the plan need to develop to promote a more coordinated approach to care by primary care providers? Would any financial or other incentives need to be established?

Examples

- HealthPartners, in Minnesota, employs a pediatric social worker as part of its care management services for special-needs children and their families. The social worker makes referrals to community agencies, provides information on potential community resources, and coordinates with school and community resources.[30]
- In Illinois, its HMO contractors for Medicaid children must have formal coordination agreements with public programs, such as local public aid offices, schools, Head Start programs, mental health and developmental disability programs and providers, early intervention providers, substance abuse treatment programs and providers, and the federal Healthy Start Program. Linkage agreements specify referral procedures and detail the points of cooperation, sharing of client information, and timely response to requests from other programs and services.[31]
- The Massachusetts Medicaid agency requires its HMO contractors to coordinate with school-based services. At a minimum, HMOs have a referral mechanism and internal triage systems to ensure timely ac-

cess for children referred by school health providers. In addition, the HMOs have a systematic process for coordinating care and creating linkages with state agencies (such as the Departments of Mental Health, Social Services, Youth Services, and Mental Retardation), community services, and consumer groups.[32]

In designing future policies for serving children with chronic or disabling conditions, HMOs may want to consider a number of other issues as well. For example:

- the appropriate capitation and risk-sharing arrangements with public and private payers;
- the best new quality improvement measures for children with various chronic physical and mental conditions, including conditions that are rare; and
- the introduction of research and demonstration projects to continuously enhance service delivery for such children and to bring about improvements in their health and functional status.

As a growing number of children with chronic conditions are enrolled in managed care plans, HMOs must find new and effective ways to serve them. Seven such approaches which can be used alone or in combination have been presented here. By enhancing preventive and primary care services in these ways, HMOs can achieve a more efficient utilization of plan resources, effect improved health and functional status outcomes for children with chronic conditions, increase family satisfaction and quality of care, and realize cost savings.

REFERENCES

1. McManus, M.A., Fox, H.B., and Newacheck, P.W. "People with Disabilities: How Far Can the Managed Care Model Be Extended to Address Groups with Special Needs?" In *Strategic Choices for a Changing Health Care System*, ed. L. Humphrey. Washington, D.C.: Association for Health Services Research, 1996.
2. Fox Health Policy Consultants. Personal communication with the Health Care Financing Administration and the General Accounting Office, June 20, 1995.
3. Fama, T., Fox, P.D., and White, L.A. "Do HMOs Care for the Chronically Ill?" *Health Affairs* 14(1) (1995):234–243.
4. Fox, H.B., and Nadash, P. *State Medicaid HMO Contracting Policies Affecting Children.* Washington, D.C.: Fox Health Policy Consultants, 1995.
5. Newacheck, P.W., and Taylor, W.R. "Childhood Chronic Illness: Prevalence, Severity, and Impact." *American Journal of Public Health* 82 (1992):364–371.
6. Zill, N., and Schoenborn, C.A. "Developmental, Learning, and Emotional Problems: Health of Our National's Children, United States, 1988." *Advance Data* 190 (1990):1–18.
7. Newacheck, P.W., and McManus, M.A. *A Current Profile of Children with Disabilities.* San Francisco: Maternal and Child Health Policy Research Center, 1994.

8. Newacheck, P.W., Budetti, P., and Halfon, N. "Trends in Activity Limiting Chronic Conditions Among Children." *American Journal of Public Health* 76(2) (1986):178–184.
9. Newacheck, P.W., McManus, M.A., and Fox, H.B. *Epidemiology of Childhood Chronic Illness and Disability.* San Francisco: Maternal and Child Health Policy Research Center, 1994.
10. Newacheck and Taylor, "Childhood Chronic Illness."
11. Newacheck, P.W. Tabulations of unpublished data from the 1992 National Health Interview Survey, 1995.
12. DiVerde, M. "Effective Strategies for Working with Managed Care Programs: An Arizona Practice Shares Its Experiences." *CATCH Quarterly.* Elk Grove Village, IL: American Academy of Pediatrics, 1995.
13. Florida Agency for Health Care Administration. *Florida Medicaid Prepaid Health Plan,* 1994.
14. Green, M., ed. *Bright Futures: Guidelines for Health Supervision of Infants, Children, and Adolescents.* Arlington, VA: National Center for Education in Maternal and Child Health, 1994.
15. Meisels, S.J., and Provence, S. *Screening and Assessment: Guidelines for Identifying Young Disabled and Developmentally Vulnerable Children and Their Families.* Arlington, VA: National Center for Clinical Infant Programs, 1992.
16. Kiernan, J.G., Watters, P.J., and Yates, A. "HEADS-SET: A Tool for Testing Adolescent Risk." *HMO Practice* 7 (1993):166–167.
17. National Center for Clinical Infant Programs. *Summary of Kaiser Temperament Program.* Arlington, VA: National Center for Clinical Infant Programs, 1995.
18. Florida Agency for Health Care Administration. *Florida Medicaid Prepaid Health Plan,* 1994.
19. Fox Health Policy Consultants. Personal communication with Harvard Community Health Plan, 1994.
20. Fox Health Policy Consultants. Personal communication with Medica, 1994.
21. Utah Division of Health Care Financing. *Model HMO Open Panel Contract,* Attachment C, 1994.
22. Washington Department of Social and Health Services. *Model Contract,* 1994.
23. Moe, E.L., et al. "Implementation of Open Airways an Educational Intervention for Children with Asthma in an HMO." *Journal of Pediatric Health Care* 6(5) (1992):251–255.
24. Commonwealth of Massachusetts Department of Public Welfare. *Contract between Mental Health Management of America and Commonwealth of Massachusetts,* 1992.
25. Fox Health Policy Consultants: Personal communications with Medica, 1994.
26. Fox Health Policy Consultants: Personal communications with Wisconsin Independent Physicians Group, 1994.
27. Commonwealth of Massachusetts, Department of Public Welfare. *1995 Purchasing Specifications,* 1995.
28. Harvard Community Health Plan. Special Needs Program Brochure.
29. McManus Health Policy, Inc. Personal communication with Maricopa County Health Plan, 1995.
30. McManus Health Policy, Inc. Personal communication with HealthPartners, 1995.
31. Illinois Department of Public Aid. *Healthy Kids Provider Manual.* 1994.
32. Commonwealth of Massachusetts Department of Public Welfare. *Contract between Mental Health Management of America and Commonwealth of Massachusetts,* 1992.

14

Caring for Children with Special Needs in HMOs: The Consumer's Perspective

Betsy Anderson

Can HMOs provide appropriate care for children with special health needs? While families and professionals have probably not agreed upon the questions to be asked and while the data are not in to show that HMOs can provide the necessary care for special needs children, there are many positive benefits and features of care in most HMOs. Addressing areas of importance to families—information needs, case management support, access to pediatric specialty care, quality practice, and member partnerships—will certainly strengthen the quality of care for children with special health needs and their families.

HMOs may come to see themselves as partners with families in developing programs and policies specifically targeted to the needs of children with special health needs. In fact, HMOs have the potential to serve this population for several reasons: they can offer coordinated systems of care, with a focus on case management, and a continuum of care emphasizing community-based models of care; their premiums are affordable to many families; and they usually emphasize patients as active partners in their own care.

However, no data are available to aid families in choosing HMOs that have services and case management systems especially designed to meet the distinct needs of children with special health needs. Moreover, many HMOs place special needs children in the same medical management

Source: Reprinted from B. Anderson, Caring for Children with Special Needs in HMOs: The Consumer's Perspective, *Managed Care Quarterly*, Vol. 4, No. 3, pp. 36–40, © 1996, Aspen Publishers, Inc.

model as adults or children without special needs. As a result, families who base their decisions about which HMO plan to join on word-of-mouth rather than on public "report cards" that can help them compare across health plans services and coverage may be disappointed and inadequately served.

MEETING INFORMATION NEEDS

In a survey conducted in 1986 of 910 families with disabled children, families said their most important need was information on services available; their second greatest need was for assistance in accessing services.[1] Because families of children with special health needs require significantly more information than other families prior to joining a health plan, an HMO should provide clearly described, written information to individuals prior to their enrollment.

The typical HMO brochure often does not include specific information on the type of special child health care services offered and the way to access them. Families often find it difficult to get this type of information, which they need if they are to understand what care and services are offered, the process by which they can access such services, and what services are not covered. This type of information would help families compare coverage and services across plans.

As a supplement to this written information, HMOs should have available an experienced individual who is knowledgeable about pediatric chronic illness and disability and can respond to families' questions and help them sort through the HMO's terminology and procedures. In some cases, families are referred to the HMO's member services staff person, who is usually not equipped to respond to such questions. Rather, someone who is familiar with the health plan's clinical issues, such as the HMO's case manager, might be better able to serve this function. The case manager, for example, will be better able to initiate a planning process, help families make telephone calls, investigate resources, and help expedite paperwork. Some HMOs might make such a person available initially for all children with special health needs and regularly for those with complicated or high-cost care.

The case manager may be able to clarify the HMO's written materials. In some instances, for example, when written material says that home nursing is provided, that might mean daily, shift nursing provided for months or years for a child who uses a ventilator, or only limited nursing hours provided after an acute care in-hospital episode.

After a family joins an HMO, the health plan must be aware of the variety of needs and issues that families face. For instance, an HMO will need to be able to respond to families' questions and initiate discussion about specifics such as the availability of a certain form of medication that minimizes side effects, a type of wheelchair especially designed for rugged activities, or a new genetic test that has implications for all family members. Families also need information about services beyond health care, but which are inextricably linked to and have an impact on them and the child's health (e.g., educational, social, and recreational needs).

There are numerous resources that HMOs can turn to for more information in meeting these needs: State Title V programs, which have been involved in assessing families' special health needs, and the federal Bureau of Maternal and Child Health, which publishes a document outlining assessments.[2] Children with special health needs are also often, though not always, children who are entitled to special education and related health services either through the Individuals with Disabilities Education Act (IDEA) or Section 504 of the Rehabilitation Act and the Americans with Disabilities Act. These laws and regulations offer many resources.

The case manager's role could also be part of a process of empowering the family and creating a patient partnership with the family. Together with the case manager, families can then help create a planning process that fits their needs and their child's. This plan should delineate what the HMO will provide and what resources will need to be collected from other sources. However, families themselves are often able to describe the kinds of training or components of care they anticipate they or their children will need. For instance, a family with a ventilator-dependent child at home might need formal training for maintaining ventilator support and care.

In some cases, families of children with special health needs may be already well acquainted with specialty care and services. Families may also be very familiar with health care research, new treatments, drugs, and equipment because of their special diagnoses or circumstances. Families may learn about specific care and treatment options or philosophies through contact with other families, in clinical, educational, or other settings, as well as through parent organizations.

In some instances, HMOs with extensive in-house resources are offering specialty services such as clinics for children with Down syndrome or multidisciplinary clinics for those with various chronic illnesses. These specialty clinics can easily offer a variety of specialists and ancillary care providers who coordinate and carry out individual care plans. This kind of approach supports the communication required and is respectful of families' and providers' time.

No matter what approach is used, however, an HMO should guide specialists and primary care providers to communicate and collaborate with other providers for services available outside of the plan's provider network. HMOs sometimes offer other supportive resources such as parent group meetings, specially designed educational sessions, family resource centers, or libraries.

ENSURING ACCESS TO SPECIALTY PEDIATRIC CARE

Access to specialty care and services is the area of greatest anxiety for families. For families new to HMOs, the role of primary care providers is likely to be viewed cautiously. Parents are particularly concerned about the practice in some HMOs of providing specialty care by staff caregivers whose expertise is with adults, not children. Families assume that since adult patients are more numerous, HMOs may be saving dollars by hiring solely practitioners whose area is adult health. Because many children with special health needs have received most or even all of their care in specialty settings, their families are well aware that certain kinds of care and services will always be needed which may only be available from specialists, usually in tertiary settings.

Care for children should be safeguarded by HMO policies that specify pediatric caregivers and define the circumstances under which adult, nonpediatric practitioners may provide care to children. HMOs should be prepared to give families information on the experience its primary caregivers have with their children's conditions and disability and also provide its clinical staff with opportunities to access specialized information or consultation, especially if these services involve out-of-plan resources. Chronic conditions in children are rare and consequently few practitioners will have extensive knowledge or experience.[3] HMOs should be prepared to give families information on which pediatricians specialize in caring for children with disabilities.

Another access issue is provider support. HMOs should support the primary care providers and case managers in their roles as patient advocates by ensuring that providers' paperwork or procedures do not become administratively burdensome. This assumes a system that routinely offers providers ongoing education, support, reinforcement, flexibility, decision making ability, and financial control over many aspects of children's care.

DESCRIBING PROTOCOLS AND QUALITY PRACTICE

Trust is at the heart of health care and families need to know that the HMO they have joined supports and provides "best practices" for their children. One proposal suggests a rationale for establishing a standard for pediatric care.[4] Families should be provided with the HMO's own policies and practices with regard to quality in pediatric care and some families will also want to have access to information from consumer groups or other organizations that look at practices within or across HMOs. For example, families may want to know if the HMOs' standards for childhood immunizations or other measures differ from standards recommended by organizations such as the American Academy of Pediatrics.

Currently, HMOs group families of children with special health needs in together with its general membership. HMOs, however, should define their members by their specific health needs in terms of the plan's specified medical decision making processes and parameters for determining what specialty care will be paid for and when. In fact, HMOs should inform families about how its policies, procedures, and standards apply to children with special health needs. They may, for instance, provide families with scientific validation of HMO practitioners' recommendations, especially because families often receive advice from others. They also should know how and when outcomes will be measured and should have the opportunity to express their satisfaction with the HMO caregivers and the process of obtaining care.

Families may want to approach consumer organizations regarding standards that HMOs must meet in this area. For example, the National Committee for Quality Assurance, the national accrediting commission for managed care organizations, includes consumer representation on its board, and may provide some guidance in this area.

Such standards should also include guidance on conflict resolution, including the HMO's formal dispute resolution and grievance processes. Families of children with special health needs might find it important to know from the outset if an HMO they are thinking of joining has frequent grievances in areas that are important to their child's care. They also may need to know the process for obtaining second opinions, which may become especially important when differences occur.

Some families are concerned that although they may have been successful in obtaining specific care or service for their child, the decision may have been made as an "exception to policy" and therefore would not be applicable to other families in the same or similar circumstances. This is the kind of issue that an advisory board might investigate and follow up on.

Many HMOs emphasize consumer satisfaction in their public relations materials and may even make such information available to the general public.[5] While it may be helpful to know about others' satisfaction, HMOs should be able to describe to families how it defines and measures quality, and even more specifically, how the plan addresses quality for those with special health needs, whose lives or quality of daily life depend upon the care provided. Moreover, a plan should be able to explain whether children with special health needs are separately clinically tracked to better address their concerns, and how categories of these children are defined. The National Association of Children's Hospitals and Related Institutions are beginning to develop a definition.

Families' perspectives should be sought in discussion of the kinds of issues to be tracked and in the development of tools used. Families should be part of focus groups or other mechanisms which analyze or discuss care for special needs children.

One way for HMOs to ensure that family perspectives are being considered is to create a consumer advisory board focused on children with special health needs. The opportunity for HMO members to advise and shape the policies and programs of a given HMO is generally far ahead of practices in other settings. Some children's hospitals and state Medicaid programs include family input into advisory boards, but seldom do conventional insurance plans include provision for direct consumer participation. Many HMOs view themselves as partners with consumers and have instituted a variety of programs and approaches to reinforce this effort.

CREATING PATIENT PARTNERSHIPS

While advisory boards in some plans may be more active than others, there is a history and a mindset behind many HMOs that emphasizes members as active partners with HMOs in their care.

Beyond the role that families take in the care of their own children there are a number of ways HMOs can work with family members as partners in program and policy development to address the care children need. A recent report of family participation with state Title V programs identifies several key areas, some of which are also likely to be relevant to HMOs: parents as participants on advisory committees to discuss and design services and policies; parents as participants in staff in-service training; parent or parent organizations as resources of information for other families; and parents hired as staff or consultants, something some HMOs are already doing.[6] A list of resources for contacting existing parent groups and families is available from the Federation for Children with Special Needs.

In any one of these efforts, families may be able to work with the health plan to determine an HMO's priorities with regard to what services families need at a program and policy level, and opportunities for families to contribute knowledge about resources they have found useful. Some families, for example, can provide an HMO with information about home adaptations that encourage children to become more independent, summer camps that all family members might enjoy, or after-school job opportunities for young adults with disabilities.

THE PLANNING PROCESS

Families of children with special health needs are likely to benefit from a planning process, whether available only initially, episodically, or ongoing. This kind of assistance should address, in a comprehensive way, both the child's and family's needs. Families' own needs are important not only because they are immediately affected by a child's special needs, but also because family members, especially parents, are likely to be the primary caregivers. In many cases, these families need information, training, and support.

HMOs can also develop partnerships with other organizations active on behalf of children with special health needs and with other health care providers in their states and communities: specialty children's hospitals, the state Title V program, and the state Academy of Pediatrics chapter (including the subcommittee on children with special needs). Other important, though perhaps less familiar partners might be parent and family organizations and advocacy groups for children with special needs.

These groups are usually very knowledgeable about existing resources, may know what gaps or inadequacies in services presently exist, and can offer good information to the plan to help it understand new and emerging issues in the community. These organizations may, in essence, become a two-way street with HMOs for referral and information.

Finally, as HMOs assume a greater role in the care of children with special needs they may want to—and may be expected to—be visibly and actively part of special initiatives for children with special needs in their states and communities. HMOs have generally espoused a philosophy of comprehensive coordinated care for their members. For children with special needs, this philosophy may involve some new issues and some new partners.

LOOKING AHEAD

As more Americans receive their health care as members of HMOs, these individuals will increasingly include children—and adults—with chronic illnesses and disabilities. Family Voices, a national grassroots organization for families of children with special health needs and their advocates, has identified the following issues as important: that care is specially tailored to children; that care is timely, appropriate, of high quality, affordable, and cost-effective; that coverage is comprehensive; that services are broad and flexible, and include preventive, acute, specialty, and rehabilitative services; that choice, access to specialists, and the opportunity to work in partnership with health professionals remain critical parts of the plan; that standards, outcome measures, uniform billing, and data collection are continuous functions of plan operations; and that community-based, family-centered care becomes the cornerstone for caring for children with special needs.[7]

HMOs may use these issues as the basis for discussion with families to determine how a particular HMO meets these areas, and to chart future directions for children with special health needs.

REFERENCES

1. *New Directions: Serving Children with Special Health Care Needs in Massachusetts.* Boston, MA: Project Serve, 1985.
2. Work Group on Systems Development. *Needs Assessment for Improved Systems of Care: Focus on Children with Special Health Care Needs.* Washington, D.C.: National Center for Education in Maternal and Child Health, 1994.
3. Hobbs, N., et al. *Chronically Ill Children and Their Families.* San Francisco, CA: Jossey-Bass Publishers, 1985.
4. Wehr, E., and Jameson, E. "Beyond Benefits: The Importance of a Pediatric Standard in Private Insurance Contracts to Ensuring Health Care Access for Children." *The Future of Children* 4 (3) (1994):115–133. Los Altos, CA: Packard Foundation, 1994.
5. Atlantic Marketing Research Co. *Attitudes toward Health Plans: A Statewide Survey of Consumer Opinion and Published Research on Health Care Quality.* Boston, MA: Atlantic Marketing Research Co. for the Massachusetts Association of HMOs, 1995.
6. Wells, E., et al. *Families in Program and Policy: Report of a 1992 Survey of Family Participation in State Title V Programs for Children with Special Health Care Needs.* Boston, MA: Federation for Children with Special Needs, 1993.
7. *Ten Key Issues of Health Care Reform for Children with Special Health Needs.* Algodones, NM: Family Voices, 1994.

VI

Mental Health

15

Evolution of Services for the Chronically Mentally Ill in a Managed Care Setting: A Case Study

Steve Stelovich

Key factors have shaped the rapid evolution of mental health and substance abuse care in HMOs and managed care settings in the last 25 years. The development of a broad spectrum of services, treatment allocation algorithms, and outcomes measurement has been directly linked to patient care. Other factors are indirectly related to patient care: negotiated dollar amounts allocated to mental health and substance abuse services, the exploration of alternative service delivery models, and the use of diverse reimbursement models.

At Harvard Pilgrim Health Care (HPHC), an HMO in Boston, with staff, group, and independent physicians association (IPA) components, practitioners have witnessed significant changes in mental health and substance abuse service delivery as it relates to these factors. The HPHC experience is worth studying given its growth and history. Founded in 1969 as a staff model HMO called Harvard Community Health Plan (HCHP), the health plan became HPHC following a 1995 merger with Pilgrim Health Care. Harvard Pilgrim Health Care now serves approximately one million members throughout Massachusetts, Rhode Island, New Hampshire, and Maine. HPHC consists of four divisions: a salaried staff model component, the Health Centers Division, with 300,000 members; a capitated group model component, the Medical Groups Division, with 185,000 members; a blended staff and group model component, the New England Division,

Source: Reprinted from S. Stelovich, Evolution of Services for the Chronically Mentally Ill in a Managed Care Setting: A Case Study, *Managed Care Quarterly*, Vol. 4, No. 3, pp. 78–84, © 1996, Aspen Publishers, Inc.

with 94,000 members; and a predominantly IPA component, the Pilgrim Health Care Division, with 385,000 members.

The changes HPHC experienced in Massachusetts illustrate many of the problems and opportunities a managed care organization faces when expanding services to a more broadly based patient population. In this paper, the HCHP and HPHC experience will be used to illustrate the challenges related most directly to clinical practice and the implications for service delivery planning.

SPECTRUM OF CARE DIVERSITY

Many aspects of managed health care's recent mental health service development can be seen as transfer of the community mental health center movement into the private domain. Thirty years ago, a federal law, The Community Mental Health Centers Act of 1963, and its amendment of 1975, called for a spectrum of services to be provided to patients in the public sector, many of whom were chronically or severely disabled. Frequently ignored in the private sector, that legislation called for a number of service provisions: emergency care; screening services; consultation/ education services; inpatient services; follow-up and outpatient care; partial hospital, and transitional housing. Further, the acts stipulated that services be provided to child, adult, and geriatric populations as well as to those suffering from alcoholism or drug abuse.

Among the essential services called for in these federal acts was "transitional housing." The provision of these services, however, has never been fully implemented and remains controversial even today.[1] Nonetheless, in face of the fact that housing can have a major impact upon the course of illness and resource utilization, various ad hoc approaches to the problem in managed care settings have been attempted:

- Payment for housing through benefit exception following formal case review when the cost of housing can be anticipated to offset mental health resource utilization.
- Cost sharing with families, particularly useful for halfway houses where the managed care organization pays for a "treatment" component with the family assuming responsibility for a "lodging" expense.
- Payment for housing during the time it meets criteria for providing an alternative to acute inpatient hospitalization.
- Refusal of payment for housing while advocating for the patient with municipal or state agencies "charged" to provide such services.

With the growing number of patients from Medicaid and Medicare transferring into managed care settings, the issue of housing responsibility can be expected to assume increasing importance in the next three to five years.

At its inception, HCHP did not envision a full spectrum of mental health services. Psychiatric consultation was provided to primary care clinicians as appropriate. For the most part, as with many early HMOs, treatment of serious and chronic mental illness was simply not undertaken or even seen as part of the benefit. In 1976, however, the Commonwealth of Massachusetts mandated a benefit of at least $500 annually or up to 20 visits for outpatient mental health services and removed exclusions for "chronic conditions" that were not further defined by either legislation or regulation.

In the face of legislative and regulatory confusion regarding "chronic conditions," "medical necessity," and a poorly defined inpatient benefit, an uneasy peace existed for a number of years between managed care systems and the Massachusetts Department of Mental Health, which covered the cost of care when people had "exhausted benefits" and had no further personal resources. From 1976 until the late 1980s, persons with serious and chronic mental health problems enrolled in managed care programs could not expect to receive consistent services. Frequently, administrative bickering regarding where responsibility for care rested led to fragmented or insufficient support.

During the late 1980s, Massachusetts experienced a period of significant economic downturn. Public financial support for mental health services, both hospital and community-based programs, was increasingly constrained. At that time, the Massachusetts Division of Insurance issued an interpretation of the 1976 benefits legislation that favored a wider exposure for managed care programs, effectively requiring unlimited inpatient care for acute psychiatric conditions. At the same time, the Massachusetts Department of Mental Health began to clarify the nature of chronic custodial services for which it would bear responsibility.

HCHP began to establish its own comprehensive mental health service delivery program in 1976. Psychiatrists, psychologists, psychiatric nurses, and licensed independent social workers were hired to work together in each of its centers. In addition, care was provided using modes that differed from traditional long-term insight oriented psychotherapy, which was the treatment of choice in Massachusetts. Group psychotherapy as opposed to individual work was encouraged when appropriate. Time-limited psychotherapy, cognitive therapies, health education, and behavioral interventions were promoted. For persons not responding to short-term interventions, "continuing care" support groups were established employing group psychotherapies, medication management, counseling regarding activities of daily living, and education regarding symptom management. In practice, benefit limits were informally extended through a process of clinical case reviews when it was thought that additional outpatient support would offset costly hospitalization. Because short-term inpatient hospitalizations and day treatment programs providing true alternatives to inpatient stays were not available in the private sector, HCHP elected to develop its own programs. Such endeavors were generally successful: Hospital stays were reduced, alternatives to hospitalization were utilized, and patients with increased psychiatric morbidity could be cared for.

By the late 1970s, almost a decade after HCHP began enrolling Medicaid beneficiaries, the majority of Medicaid individuals' care could be provided within the HCHP system. However, managed care was still relatively new, and the concepts of criteria-driven resource allocation, provider profiling, gatekeeping, and outpatient and inpatient utilization review criteria were not included in creating a quality mental health system.

Initially, program development at HCHP was done in the context of staff model operations only. Serious shortcomings with this approach, however, quickly became evident. In 1986 HCHP merged with the MultiGroup Health Plan and began to provide services through capitated groups in its new Medical Groups Division. Many of the services that had to be built by HCHP only five years previously had by then begun to become available for purchase in the community at large. With one division relying upon a salaried staff based in clinics and another providing services through a distributed network of contracted providers and programs, advantages and disadvantages associated with each model became evident.

Staff model programs initially proved highly successful: They established a common philosophy of care and uniformity of practice across programs; referrals between programs were efficient in such a single "system"; clinical information could be transferred relatively easily among staff; and close integration with primary care providers could be assured. Yet problems remained in the staff models that were easily addressed in a network: Patient appointment availability was constrained; a lack of geographic access and cultural diversity existed as a result of limits imposed in staffing the centralized clinics; and salaried staff often presented an "I was not hired to do that" attitude when asked to participate in service delivery modification.

TREATMENT ALLOCATION ALGORITHMS

Between 1987 and 1990, HCHP developed a Mental Health Redesign Project to reassess its mental health program, specifically to examine how a mental health benefit could be expanded to include the most appropriate treatment for psychiatric and substance abuse problems, and at the same time limit fiscal risk and avoid blanket entitlements. Particularly at issue was the definition of the term "appropriate treatment."

Health plan practitioners felt that both clinical conditions and treatment options should be clearly delineated in order to develop algorithms best linking patients to services. They knew that relying upon diagnosis or clinical judgment alone to formulate treatment plans and allocate treatment resources usually results in extreme variability. The limits of diagnostic classification alone was documented 10 years ago in studies on the feasibility of using diagnosis-related groups (DRGs) in psychiatry to determine prospective hospital payment. In one study, researchers reported that grouping patients in 15 psychiatric DRGs reduced variance in length of stay by only 3.9 percent. "We conclude that DRGs do not adequately predict length of stay or costs in psychiatric hospitals," according to the study.[2] Moreover, in 1980 the DSM-III, the American Psychiatric Association's Diagnostic and Statistical Manual, recognized the limitations in using traditional diagnosis for treatment planning. This third edition proposed a multiaxial system, which coded diagnoses according to five axes: clinical syndromes, developmental and character disorders, physical disorders and conditions, severity of psychosocial stressors, and global assessment of functioning.[3]

HCHP found these axes to be of use, but insufficient to guide careful and consistent treatment planning. To address this problem, the health plan developed a Patient Assessment Tool (PAT), which established scales for eight variables: substance abuse; duration of abstinence; severity of diagnosis; lethality; scaled limitation of function; change in limitation of function; stressors; and impairment of support system. In this system, all scales rank order results from zero through nine with regard to the degree of impairment (Figure 15–1). And in practice, the PAT can be scored in less than two minutes following a well-structured standard psychiatric interview. No formal test administration is required.

Treatment options had to be defined likewise. The HCHP Mental Health Redesign Project ultimately shaped its recommendations around specifications for access, intensity of services needed, duration of services, and the modality of service.

The PAT and a codification of components of care enabled algorithms to be developed guiding patient treatment decisions. Under this system, for example, a person with schizophrenia automatically qualifies for a score on the severity of diagnosis scale associated with the unlimited provision of medical management for the illness as well as specific individual and group supports for the patient with no increasing copay. An individual with an adjustment disorder receives a lower severity of illness score and does not automatically have unlimited access to the full spectrum of medical management/support that the schizophrenic would have. However, elevated scores on lethality, social support difficulties, or other scales could qualify the patient for such services.

Allocation algorithms and an expanded spectrum of services at HCHP offered the possibility of both more comprehensive and appropriate treat-

Lethality Scale (LTH)

In using this scale, the clinician should assign the patient **the highest or most severe rating** appropriate to the patient's clinical presentation.

Note: Scale evaluates patient presentation **at the time of evaluation** with the exception of factors concerning history of attempt of gesture.

0. No suicidal ideation or evidence of self-destructive or aggressive thoughts or behaviors

1. Occasional self-defeating or aggressive thoughts or feelings

2. Persistent self-defeating or aggressive thoughts or feelings

3. Occasional passive wishes to be dead or questioning of the value of living or occasional feelings of resentment toward specific individuals or groups

4. One or more of the following:
    a. Fleeting active suicidal/homicidal ideation. No intent or plan.
    b. Frequent exposure to significant risk through life-style (drives car fast, rides motorcycle, etc.)
    c. Chronic exposure to physically abusive situation (as victim or abuser)
    d. Past history of suicide attempt or gesture
    e. Persistent passive wishes to be dead or questioning of the value of living, persistent feelings of resentment toward individuals or groups

5. One or more of the following:
    a. Intermittent suicidal/homicidal ideation. No intent or plan. Able to contract for safety
    b. Persistent self-destructive or aggressive behavior without conscious suicidal or homicidal intent (getting into fights, placing oneself at risk for assault)
    c. Occasional superficial cutting or scratching

6. One or more of the following:
    a. Suicidal/homicidal ideation present on a daily basis. No plan or intent. Able to contract for safety
    b. Persistent superficial cutting and scratching

7. One or more of the following:
    a. Continual preoccupation with suicidal/homicidal ideation. No specific plan or intent. Can contract for safety
    b. Serious, nonlethal, self-mutilation

8. One or more of the following:
    a. Suicidal/homicidal preoccupation and plan. No immediate intent. Cannot contract for safety

9. One or more of the following:
    a. Suicidal/homicidal preoccupation and plan with intent. Cannot contract for safety
    b. Uncontrollable assaultive behavior secondary to mental disorder
    c. Command hallucination instructing either self-harm or harm to others

Figure 15–1. Order results ranked from zero through nine. *Source:* Copyright © 1994 Harvard Community Health Plan. Used with permission.

ment to those needing it, at least in the traditional medical sense of the term. In particular, enrollees with severe and chronic disorders could access unlimited amounts of medical care if conditions warranted. During the first two years of implementation, contingency funds were set aside to cover budget overruns should they occur, which did not. Longer hospitalizations and individual psychodynamic psychotherapies decreased while alternatives to hospitalization, groups, cognitive, and other special modality therapies increased.

Still, a number of unresolved problems remained. For example, while the Mental Health Redesign Project had sought to create a mechanism by which to make appropriate treatment allocations, it may have achieved a far more limited goal of creating a system that made orderly and replicable allocations alone. To determine whether such allocations were truly appropriate, the outcomes associated with such allocations would need to be evaluated.

OUTCOMES IN MENTAL HEALTH

Early forays into the realm of outcome evaluation in managed care settings were, in fact, almost exclusively measurements of costs expended. Over time, however, as managed care organizations grew to serve more and more patients, medical outcomes and associated population health status evaluations have emerged as a focus of concern. In addition, large purchasers of care became interested in issues beyond direct cost savings, and the scientific community at large began to focus upon outcomes as a key factor in evaluating health care service delivery.

In its own attempt to deal with the increasing interest in outcomes measurement, Harvard Pilgrim Health Care has taken several steps. Within the past year, a mental health steering committee has been created and charged with developing corporate recommendations regarding mental health outcome activities and associated measures, which have incorporated the most common currently employed in the field, including patient and provider satisfaction, symptom reduction, general health status, direct service costs, and indirect costs.

Conditions that entail significant morbidity, afflict patients in all settings, generate significant expenditures in time and money, and which have a chronic course have been assigned highest priority. Major initiatives are now under way in the area of depression and alcohol abuse, including projects for early screening, diagnosis, and primary care treatment for major depression and alcohol abuse as well as a collaborative study of depression in high users of medical services. As opposed to an approach that only five years ago was limited to count units of service as a measure of quality or outcome, such as admission rates and hospital days per thousand, current approaches consider comprehensive treatment of specific disease states within the population at large, and evaluating results upon multiple axes.

In the near future, one can anticipate that totally new questions will be posed to managed care programs in the face of such measurements. For example: Is clinician or patient satisfaction the more important factor? How much of direct and indirect costs should be allocated to the improvement of general health status in the absence of patient dissatisfaction? If symptoms can be relieved by a demonstrably superior and low-cost intervention, which is associated with poor satisfaction, how is the problem to be handled?

PERIPHERAL ISSUES

Other factors less directly associated with clinical practice also play substantial roles in shaping the development of broadly based clinical delivery systems: resources, models of delivery, and payment incentives.

Resources

During the national debate on health care reform in 1993 and 1994, there was widespread agreement that current spending patterns in managed care organizations could not be expected to cover care for substantial numbers of severely and chronically ill individuals were they to be moved into managed care settings. Moreover, few managed care organizations are willing or able to devote such resources to mental health care.[4,5]

Delivery Models

Different managed care models can also have significant impact upon the provision of care. Early managed care programs, mostly HMOs, frequently relied upon salaried staff specifically hired to deliver mental health services. Shortly thereafter, totally independent and comprehensive service delivery networks emerged. As managed care became less dominated by staff model HMO operations, it increasingly turned to such independent specialty networks to manage the mental health and substance abuse benefit. Such arrangements, known as *carve-outs*, generally relied heavily upon prior authorization and utilization review to control costs.

Most recently, blended service delivery models have evolved. In such models, low-intensity or short-term care is referred to an extended network with less intense utilization review. High-intensity work or longer-term care is referred into smaller provider groups with more intense utilization review or into staff model operations. HPHC has experience with both staff and network operations and is currently exploring a blended service model to help provide quality care to seriously disturbed patients.

Mental health carve-outs have been hotly disputed within the managed care community. Those arguing against carve-outs point to the advantages enjoyed through a close integration between mental health and primary/specialty care. Supporters, however, say mental health carve-outs can deliver care at lower costs. Moreover, carve-out programs have generally developed greater specialization within service delivery networks and utilization review activities and have paid particularly close attention to member/purchaser preferences when delivering services. In the final analysis, however, the lack of comparative outcome studies precludes a definitive recommendation of one model over another at this time.

HPHC has consistently felt that the arguments for integration outweigh those for carve-out and manages its own programs. As increased focus has been placed upon screening, early identification, and support to primary care settings, it has been felt that a close working relationship between primary care and mental health and substance abuse services needs to be maintained.

Diverse Payment Models

Reimbursement models also have profound effects upon services delivered. Salaries, discounted fees for service, capitations with risk bands, and performance bonuses have all been used to shape practice. They also have the potential to exert important influence upon the provision of services to seriously and chronically ill patients.

LESSONS LEARNED

In 25 years, HPHC has undergone significant expansion in services delivered to patients experiencing serious and chronic mental illness and substance abuse. Three clinically-based factors have repeatedly influenced and informed those developments, and lessons have been learned from each.

First, an expanded spectrum of services modeled upon the Community Mental Health Centers Acts of 1963 and 1975 is needed to provide such services and must include: emergency care; screening services; consultation/ education services; inpatient services; follow-up and outpatient care; partial hospitalization; and possibly transitional housing. Such services must be planned for children, adults, geriatric patients, and those suffering from substance abuse problems.

Second, the use of diagnoses alone does not adequately support treatment planning and resource allocation. At HCHP, algorithms have been developed to consider: substance abuse; duration of abstinence; severity of diagnosis; lethality; scaled limitation of function; change in limitation of function; stressors; and impairment of support systems in defining patient characteristics necessary for appropriate treatment planning.

Third, a broad spectrum of services provided within the context of treatment allocation algorithms still requires outcomes measurement examining a host of factors, including patient and provider satisfaction, symptom reduction, general health status, and direct and indirect costs.

Three less fully understood and clinically based influences have exerted major influence on service planning and delivery and invite cautious exploration:

- a concern that the total dollars allocated to mental health services in managed care programs are probably insufficient to underwrite large-scale integration of seriously and chronically disturbed patients into such settings given current reimbursement arrangements
- the optimal blend of staff and network operations
- the role of reimbursement mechanisms being used to influence both quantity and quality of services provided.

Of all these factors, only the first—an expanded spectrum of services—is reasonably well understood at this time. Despite this, important decisions in program planning for seriously and chronically mentally ill patients in managed care settings are made daily and must continue to be pursued.

REFERENCES

1. Carling, P. "Housing and Supports for Persons with Mental Illness: Emerging Approaches to Research and Practice." *Hospital & Community Psychiatry* 44(5) (1993):439–449.
2. Schumacher, D.N., et al. "Prospective Payment for Psychiatry—Feasibility and Impact." *New England Journal of Medicine* 315(21) (1986):1331–1336.
3. American Psychiatric Association. *Diagnostic and Statistical Manual of Mental Disorders,* (DSM-IIIR). 3rd ed., rev. Washington, D.C.: American Psychiatric Press, 1987.
4. McGuire, T. "Predicting the Cost of Mental Health Benefits." *The Milbank Quarterly* 72(1) (1994):3.
5. Arons, B., et al. "Mental Health and Substance Abuse Coverage under Health Reform." *Health Affairs* 13(1) (1994):196.

16

A Medicaid Mental Health Carve-Out Program: The Massachusetts Experience

Christopher W. Counihan, Deborah Nelson, and Elizabeth Pattullo

In the late 1980s and early 1990s the Medicaid program in Massachusetts had become derisively referred to as a "budget buster" expense item that state government officials of both Democratic and Republican administrations found difficult to control. These rising costs were fueled by the rate of inflation in health care and the unlimited and unmanaged benefit of the Medicaid program.

Several factors contributed to rising costs. First, payments for Medicaid reimbursable services were negotiated on a fee-for-service basis. These rates, established by an independent state agency, reflected that organization's policies of cost accounting principles that governed most of the hospitals and clinics that delivered mental health care to Medicaid recipients. "Class rates" were eventually established for the outpatient services provided by community mental health centers, and only minimal utilization review was conducted for inpatient and outpatient care. Moreover, the rate-setting process for hospital-based services was conducted separately for each provider, and hospital administrators identified inpatient mental health care as one of the primary means of increasing hospital revenue. Sophisticated lawyers and accountants who were hired by hospitals to negotiate these rates easily dominated the state regulators, who did not have the resources to match these experts.

Source: Reprinted from C.W. Counihan, D. Nelson, and E. Pattullo, A Medicaid Mental Health Carve-Out Program: The Massachusetts Experience, *Managed Care Quarterly*, Vol. 4, No. 3, pp. 85–92, © 1996, Aspen Publishers, Inc.

A second, and perhaps most disturbing, factor was the lack of available data. Government public policy managers had few answers when asked what services the state was buying with its Medicaid dollars and what quality indicators, if any, were being measured. In short, little accountability existed for a growing public sector program for some of the state's neediest residents.

Third, Medicaid recipients' access to inpatient mental health care was uneven. Hospitals had sole discretion over admissions; difficult clients could be denied admission at one after another private hospital and ultimately sent to state-funded community mental health centers and hospitals. A few hospitals marketed their programs to attract a high volume of Medicaid recipients. While access was high for most recipients, attention to quality was often lacking. These hospitals were criticized for overmedicating unruly recipients, discharging the homeless to shelters, and letting others leave despite active symptoms. These hospitals became known as "Medicaid mills."

A fourth factor for rising Medicaid costs was the reduction in federal funding under the Community Mental Health Center Act. These funds, administered by the Massachusetts Department of Mental Health (DMH), covered acute inpatient and outpatient mental health services for uninsured residents, intermediate and long-term hospital care, and rehabilitation services for residents of the state with a major mental illness. DMH sought to make up for federal reductions by directing its case managers to enroll uninsured individuals into Medicaid and requiring its emergency screening teams to refer any clients in need of acute care who had insurance to be treated at private hospitals so that use of state-funded facilities could be reduced.

Finally, many private insurance companies had begun to experiment with firms that specialized in capitated risk-based mental health "carveouts." These firms were paid a flat fee on a per-member per-month basis and in turn agreed to manage the mental health benefit with an incentive to earn a profit if they spent less than their flat fee. The management involved a review of level of care decisions made by providers. However, "managed care" was not universally accepted by providers, researchers, or advocates. In fact, it was labeled as "managing cost, not care," and several respected authors raised very fundamental questions about the ability of managed care organizations to accomplish cost savings without reducing quality and access.[1,2]

CHOOSING MANAGED MENTAL HEALTH

In 1990 the Medicaid director at that time, Bruce Bullen, proposed applying private sector managed care to the Medicaid program to resolve these issues. With support from the governor and human services policy makers, Bullen applied for and eventually obtained a Section 1915 demonstration waiver from the Health Care Financing Administration (HCFA) to implement a Medicaid mental health managed care program.

After the review process, Mental Health Management of America (MHMA), a small Nashville, Tennessee–based company, was selected as the contracting managed care organization. The firm had experience in utilization review for state Medicaid departments. The company's founder, the late Richard Sivley, had been the commissioner of mental health in Tennessee.

Under the terms of the mental health carve-out contract between MHMA and Medicaid, a "cap" was established for the benefit that was paid out to MHMA on a per-member per-month basis. If the cost of services exceeded the cap, the contractor was obligated to pay eight cents on each dollar spent above the cap up to a maximum risk of $2 million. Savings generated below the cap accrued to the contractor along the same formula.

This capitated managed care program was the first example of a statewide capitation for mental health and substance abuse services applied to a Medicaid population. Still, MHMA faced numerous challenges during the program's development:

- Establishing clinical protocols that met the needs of a population more chronically ill than populations previously served by managed care.
- Managing the cost without limiting the benefit or shifting it to a delivery system run by the state.
- Improving access and quality for the individual without increasing cost.
- Developing a network of services that could provide quality and access at a reasonable price.
- Implementing managed care in partnership with other state agencies that provided vital services for many of the Medicaid recipients.
- Building support among individuals and potential partners who were skeptical about the viability of the project serving such a vulnerable population.
- Measuring and improving the processes and outcomes of service delivery so that the Division of Medical Assistance and the public could be satisfied with quality, access, and outcomes of the program.

From the beginning, MHMA and Medicaid made clear that managing costs by reducing or limiting benefits would not be acceptable. As a result, a utilization review (UR) process was created and communicated to all MHMA staff and network providers; all UR decisions would be based solely on clinical appropriateness. Inpatient providers would be required to initiate active and timely discharge plans from the time of admission, while at the same time payment would only be denied for clinical reasons. This combination of a drive for aggressive discharge planning and a strict adherence to clinical levels of care was designed to ensure that patients received necessary, but not excessive, inpatient care.

MHMA clinical managers and mental health experts convened and developed an extensive provider manual clearly spelling out these principles as well as the level of care criteria that would guide the managed care contractor and their providers in making clinical decisions. Two strongly emphasized themes were that chronic mental illness required ongoing treatment and that recipient benefits would not be arbitrarily capped.

Provider contracts also required that access to health care services be direct, open, timely, and universal for Medicaid recipients. This provision assured that individuals would have the same type of access to any private hospital as recipients of private insurance policies, a situation that many managed care critics often noted was lacking.

To prevent cost shifting to the public sector, which historically occurred when private benefits ran out, MHMA developed a working agreement with the Massachusetts DMH that addressed two principles: (1) clinical criteria govern the responsibilities of each entity and (2) lines of direct communication among MHMA, Medicaid, and DMH were to be created at all levels. An interagency agreement addressed continuity of care: MHMA agreed to provide the acute mental health services, including inpatient, outpatient, and other alternative services; DMH agreed to provide intermediate and long-term inpatient care and rehabilitative services for DMH clients whose mental health benefits were managed by MHMA.

Clinical protocols were then developed to ensure that acute care patients could be easily transferred from the MHMA network hospitals into intermediate care facilities run by DMH. These protocols established clinical care criteria, pathways to evaluation, review and decision making, and avenues for higher level appeal, all steps created to further the goal of continuity of care between MHMA and DMH.

CREATING THE NETWORK

MHMA adopted three strategies for a timely and cost-effective development of a service network. The first strategy was to make provider contracting an open and competitive bidding process for inpatient care. The provider network would be limited to hospitals that could meet service needs in terms of quality and cost, reflecting the view that not all of the 76 hospitals licensed to provide inpatient mental health care were equally capable of providing high-quality care, nor were all necessary to meet the network's capacity needs. Moreover, this competitive process would allow MHMA to be an aggressive purchaser that could bargain with providers based on quality and price.

Network management staff sought input from inpatient providers in designing the network application and selection criteria. Staff also visited applicant hospitals, reviewed sample records, and checked the hospital's track record with the chronically mentally ill.

The second contracting decision was to develop alternative and diversionary levels of care that had not been previously available to Medicaid recipients:

- mental health acute residential treatment programs for children and adolescents
- acute residential programs for substance abusers, including people with chronic mental illness and substance abuse
- crisis stabilization programs
- extended assessment observation and holding beds
- partial hospitalization
- intensive clinical management and community support programs.

The third contracting decision was to allow all existing outpatient providers to become part of the network without a competitive bid process, in contrast with the inpatient process. This decision was made due to the recognition that the community mental health centers had a long and credible history of serving many of the uninsured and poor chronically mentally ill. Community providers had become skilled in the important art of linking these individuals to rehabilitative and support services, working with them in a variety of crises, and being accessible to violent, noncompliant, and high-risk cases. Including all of the community health centers in the early years of the program would help promote access to the least restrictive level of care and maintain continuity of care by keeping patients with their same providers, avoiding confusion and chaos.

Network management staff with experience in mental health services in Massachusetts were recruited. These individuals brought a great degree of credibility to MHMA, as an out-of-state managed care organization. Key managers with experience serving Medicaid recipients with chronic mental illness were also recruited. They included community mental health center providers; administrators from state departments of mental health, social services, and youth services; and community advocates, who were somewhat skeptical of applying managed care principles to the Medicaid population.

ADDRESSING BARRIERS

Several factors posed potential barriers to successful implementation of the managed mental health and substance abuse program in Massachusetts. First, private managed care organizations had a negative reputation. They were seen as single-mindedly focusing on reduced rates of admission and shorter lengths of stay that would reduce costs but also neglect quality. Second, difficult-to-treat clients were often discharged quickly into the community with no discharge planning and readmitted within days, often to another hospital, and thus "bounced around" the mental health system. Third, managed care clients who were ready to leave the hospital generally languished as inpatients because community or long-term inpatient resources were not readily available. Finally, lack of service and cost data left administrators with no means of tracking quality, cost, and outcomes.

According to critics, applying managed care UR to these already existing problems would only exacerbate these conditions. Hospitals, they noted, would admit only cooperative individuals and avoid disruptive clients who might require more staff resources during the course of treatment and extend beyond the average length of stay, thus limiting access. Moreover, UR, they said, did not take into consideration the complex mental and social conditions of these patients.

MHMA sought to address the barriers to smooth and successful implementation by including an assessment of the inpatient recipients' level of functioning during routine utilization review. Additional care was approved if it was shown that a patient was not yet stabilized and if further specific inpatient interventions and treatment were necessary.

As clinicians conducting UR for MHMA gained more experience, they realized that stabilization of psychiatric symptoms was not the only goal of inpatient hospitalization for the chronically mentally ill recipient. Addressing homelessness, transiency, and diverse chronic conditions influenced how inpatient social workers developed a sound discharge plan. Resolving these issues would increase or maximize the benefits of inpatient treatment, increase continuity into the community, and potentially prevent or reduce subsequent hospitalizations.

UR staff turned to the network department and the regionally based treatment services specialists for assistance in addressing these psychosocial stressors. This collaboration resulted in a more thorough discharge plan for the patient's return to the community. Moreover, managed care gained more credibility among its initial skeptics, especially those who experienced first-hand the attention to enhanced linkages that MHMA facilitated.

In time, an "alert" system was created among network providers via computer, whereby client-specific crisis plans were developed. These alerts enabled any user of the system to coordinate services for an individual and to collect individual case data into an aggregated form to highlight broader systems issues around access to other types of care within the MHMA network or the DMH service system.

Staff were also encouraged to forward to MHMA and DMH relevant patterns and trends that affected lengths of stay in the organization. The nature of the risk-based contract and the freedom from bureaucratic constraints contained in state agency procedures enhanced this organizational decision making process within MHMA.

MEASURES OF SUCCESS

Some of the Medicaid program results to date show positive results with respect to the goals of the Medicaid waiver: improved access and quality and reduced costs. Others address the process of care: the development and use of a broader continuum of care for chronically mentally ill adults resulting in more effective interventions; utilization review decision making; the relationship among the managed care partners (i.e., MHMA, DMH, providers, Medicaid recipients, and advocates); and collection and use of the data gathered to improve care.

A final issue addresses the actual management of the mental health and substance abuse care that was received by recipients: identifying, measuring, and improving quality with data generated from the managed care reporting mechanisms.

The findings are drawn mostly from an external evaluation of the first and second years of the program that was conducted by Brandeis University.[3] Other sources include another independent study of the third program year by Suffolk University and data generated by MHMA, principally a client satisfaction survey and level of functioning data.[4]

According to the Brandeis study, in terms of access, the number of Medicaid recipients being served in outpatient services per 1,000 recipients increased from 118.5 to 131.2, or 10.6 percent. Clinic medication use, which is one measure of illness severity, increased from 24.7 recipients per 1,000 to 31.9, or 29.1 percent. Penetration, defined as the number of recipients using any of the mental health or substance abuse services per 1,000 recipients, increased from 212.7 in 1992 to 222.6 in 1993. The number of Medicaid recipients using inpatient services per 1,000 recipients declined from 16.5 to 16.1, less than 3 percent.

Contrary to the fear that the managed care company would use denials and diversions as a primary means to save money, the Brandeis researchers found that diversions and denials "generally declined." The MHMA service network also expanded the range of programs to include partial hospitalization, community support, and structured outpatient addictions, none of which were available to individuals under the traditional Medicaid benefit. The Brandeis team concluded that access had increased slightly.

Another measure of access is the severity of the population served. The Brandeis study found that the clients served by the program had more severe problems than the clients served before the project started. The expected cost shift of difficult clients to DMH programs was not documented, and the trend toward treatment of a more severely disabled population continued in the third year.[5,6]

In terms of quality, in the areas of treatment recommendations, aftercare plans, length of stay, and "settings decisions" (i.e., level of care), providers reported slight increases in quality along some dimensions and equal outcomes along others. The Brandeis researchers concluded that quality was "about the same" as before managed care. The Brandeis report also examined the readmission rate as a measure of quality and found a slight drop despite a shorter length of stay. The Brandeis study reports that the readmission rate for the population of Medicaid recipients who were disabled was reduced from 25.8 percent to 22.5 percent.

In September 1995 MHMA completed a pilot project with six hospitals to reduce the readmission rate. A team at MHMA had determined that 72 percent of all adult readmissions were made up of recipients in the disabled aid categories who had a diagnosis of psychotic or affective disorder. The goal of the pilot intervention was to provide enhanced services to link these patients with their respective hospital's outpatient programs. These enhanced services included holding an outpatient meeting on the unit before discharge and making available a community support worker to assist the client in obtaining clinical, self-help, and rehabilitation services in the community after discharge. The statistical analysis identified the individual hospital to which the recipient was admitted as the best predictor of reducing readmission in the pilot project. Three hospitals had dramatically reduced readmission rates. When hospitals were interviewed about their implementation of the pilot, the following factors were associated with the hospitals that had reduced readmission rates during the pilot: lower patient to social work staff ratios, broader integration of the pilot from line staff to management, and greater experience of staff in continuous quality improvement projects.

The second best predictor of readmission was a shorter length of stay. There was a significant difference between the lengths of stay of readmitted recipients and non-readmitted recipients. The overall readmission rate during the pilot was 16.7 percent, down from 19.6 percent for the same population in the previous year, a reduction in the rate of 25 percent.

Another measure of quality and of outcome is client satisfaction. MHMA completed a client satisfaction survey of recipients in outpatient care and found the following:

- 3,000 surveys were mailed, out of which 29 percent were completed. If those surveys returned as undeliverable were omitted (a common problem with this population) the resulting response rate rose to 38 percent.
- The majority of persons (85 percent) reported satisfaction with their outpatient treatment, and noted that their day-to-day functioning improved.
- The most important predictors of satisfaction were the respect shown for patients by the therapist and agency and the self-confidence gained from participation in therapy. Staff communication with the client about the treatment options and not being disappointed with the clinic were important, but less so.
- The strongest predictors of quality were client respect and staff communication.
- Being friendly and courteous is the single most important way a clinic can improve satisfaction, followed by staff working together in partnership with a client, and the clinic being clean, answering the phone on time, and having appointments begin and end on time.
- No differences existed along gender lines or by race group on overall satisfaction.
- The six sampled clinics varied in their satisfaction ratings. The clinic with best overall satisfaction and best access rating also operated within the outpatient utilization parameters that were established by MHMA.

In terms of cost savings, the Brandeis team found the following results:

- The projected 1993 cost without managed care was estimated to be $209 million. Under managed care the total costs were $162.7 million, with $10 million in administrative cost and the balance in direct care services.
- The net cost of direct care services in the program was $184.5 million in 1992 and $151.7 million in 1993, resulting in a savings of $33.8 million, or 18.3 percent.

- Because enrollment increased from 1992 to 1993, the cost per enrollee was reduced from $488 to $402, or 17.6 percent.
- Inpatient care costs fell from $76.8 million in 1992 to $60.0 million in 1993, or 24.5 percent, and outpatient mental health was reduced from $79.1 million to $76.9 million, or 2.7 percent.

Inpatient cost savings were generated by a combination of shorter lengths of stay in 24-hour care, reductions in the per diem costs negotiated between MHMA and its inpatient provider network, and shifts from inpatient substance abuse to detoxification programs. The reduction in outpatient cost occurred because MHMA eliminated the practice of physicians billing for services to inpatients as an outpatient expense. The doctors' fees were instead included in the per diem rates.

PROGRAM PROGRESS

The Massachusetts Medicaid managed care program for mental health and substance abuse had other success factors. First, only a private organization could have prompted such far-reaching changes in so short a period of time. Unsaddled by politics, MHMA was accountable for and was able to: contract at favorable rates for services in a competitive environment; respond to financial incentives for meeting deadlines for creating a provider network; publish a provider manual; and establish a computerized clinical case management system. The financial targets in the capitated contract also provided the momentum to make decisions on programming and policy quickly.

Second, an emphasis on collaborations among program participants, and hiring key staff with experience in the Massachusetts mental health system were critical strategies that allowed an out-of-state company to be accepted in a skeptical and resistant environment. Third, making providers the primary clinical decision makers for developing UR clinical protocols enhanced the ability of clinicians to treat and place individuals with especially complex cases into the most appropriate treatment settings.

Fourth, because of the federal waiver, existing services were added to better meet program participants' needs, including partial hospitalization, crisis stabilization, 24-hour observation beds, acute residential treatment for substance abuse, and mental health acute residential treatment programs for children and adolescents.

Fifth, claims data were used to give providers information on basic measures such as length of stay and on more sophisticated measures, such as length of time to outpatient care after inpatient discharge and 30-day readmission rate. Sharing these measures with providers has helped expand MHMA's quality improvement plan to include such measures.

Still, challenges remain in a program targeting a chronically mentally ill Medicaid population. For example, while providers were included in the design of the inpatient selection document, they were not included in all of the changes made in billing formats, reporting forms, and program specifications. Moreover, initial telephone system problems made it difficult for providers to call in to the clinical department for approvals for urgent care and review of ongoing cases.

MHMA's system of payment to providers went smoothly in the initial stages of the program. However, as the volume and complexity of the program grew, significant delays arose, confusing providers and payers. In addition, entering and retrieving data in the MHMA computerized case management system was sometimes cumbersome and time-consuming.

Numerous Medicaid policies and procedural issues beyond the control of MHMA also had an impact on the care patients received. For example, all providers were required to determine a person's MHMA Medicaid eligibility in order to get authorization and payment for services. Yet, because of the complex nature of the methods in which individuals qualified for disability and AFDC benefits, the eligibility status for the benefit managed by MHMA sometimes changed without any prior notification to MHMA, the provider, or Medicaid recipient.

APPLYING THE MODEL

The MHMA program indicates the potential of managed care applied to a Medicaid population with chronic mental illness, particularly where UR standards for hospital care are designed to promote thorough discharge planning to move clients to the most appropriate level of care on a timely basis. In addition, it has demonstrated that specialized interventions for individual recipients using a provider network and assistance by network staff to hold hospitals accountable to certain care standards enhance the continuity of care.

Over time, for example, providers and staff made more use of the collected data. Individual providers received data on cost per case and length of stay. Quality issues such as the rate of readmission within 30 days were calculated for each provider and across levels of care. The availability of objective information allowed providers to be held accountable for their performance and to compete among themselves.

By requiring its contractor to report this information, the Division of Medical Assistance identified areas of improvement in both the process and outcomes of care. The division worked with MHMA to develop the principles of continuous quality improvement (CQI) in its management and problem-solving functions. Eight quality improvement teams within MHMA are using the information to improve care. Introducing the concept of managing with such data represented a major cultural shift in the delivery of mental health care to the chronically mentally ill for all parties.

Can the Massachusetts model be applied in other states? The model may be adapted, but several key conditions for success must be present. States and private managed mental health care companies must be as committed to the needs of Medicaid recipients as they are to managing costs. They must also ensure that individuals retain some choice of provider and geographic access, while closely managing a provider network for quality care. In addition, states and their partners must be able to handle crises and stresses within the public policy arena, with the managed care organization including community providers and policy makers in problem-solving. They must also collect and use claims data to help identify and solve problems such as how to treat the clients who are high users of service, and to improve overall administrative and clinical processes.

Industry observers will be watching the outcome of similar programs in Iowa, Colorado, and Ohio. If Medicaid directors can implement programs despite numerous legal, procedural, political, and bureaucratic pitfalls and are able to measure the quality and outcomes of mental health projects, a mental health carve-out for Medicaid has a potential future for any number of states.

REFERENCES

1. Dorwart, R. "Managed Mental Health Care: Myths and Realities in the 1990s." *Hospital and Community Psychiatry* 10 (October 1990):1087–1091.
2. Edinburg, G., and Cottler, J. "Implications of Managed Care for Social Work in Psychiatric Hospitals." *Hospital and Community Psychiatry* 10 (October 1990):1063–1064.
3. Callahan, J., et al. *Evaluation of the Massachusetts Medicaid Mental Health/Substance Abuse Program.* Heller School for Advanced Studies in Social Welfare, Brandeis University. January 1994.
4. Beinecke, R.H., et al. *An Assessment of the Massachusetts Managed Mental Health/Substance Abuse Program: Year Three.* New York, NY: Suffolk University, May 1995.
5. Ibid.
6. Callahan et al., *Evaluation.*

17

Commentary: Managing Care for Mental Illness: Paradox and Pitfalls

Leslie J. Scallet

The potential for applying "managed care" techniques in caring for people with mental illnesses and disorders seems at once the most natural development possible and the most dangerous. Managed care fits beautifully with the direction of the field toward comprehensive systems of care (community mental health centers, community support systems, case management). However, its threat to the existing service structures and programs creates a very real possibility that in making the shift, vital elements will be lost and the most vulnerable populations once again will be ill-served.

This seeming paradox is deeply rooted in some basic realities of the mental health care system, how it has differed from the rest of health care, and why those differences present somewhat distinct challenges and opportunities. Today's choices—public versus private responsibilities, scope and design of benefits, integrated or carve-out models—grow directly from the particular history and structure of mental health care. In turn, that history gave mental health care an early introduction and long experience with many of the key elements of managed care now sweeping the entire health care field.

Massachusetts has played a pioneering role in the ongoing drama of mental health care, so it is no accident that the two articles presented here focus on how managed care programs are evolving in that state. These two examples in fact represent the two current leading choices in managed

Source: Reprinted from L.J. Scallet, Managing Care for Mental Illness: Paradox and Pitfalls, *Managed Care Quarterly,* Vol. 4, No. 3, pp. 93–99, © 1996, Aspen Publishers, Inc.

care systems for people experiencing mental disorders: the integrated model (Stelovich) and the carve-out model (Counihan et al.). Their history is extensive enough to provide a basis for some observations.

TWO DUAL SYSTEMS

Historically, mental health care has been regarded as separate from physical health care. Following World War II, this traditional pattern began to break down. However, the history of segregation remains a powerful current in health care and health policy today.

While the medical model dominated in mental health, the disorders and their treatment as well as their funding and reimbursement mechanisms remained largely separate from medical care in the minds of practitioners, patients, and the public. For example, mental health care had strong public sector support for well over a century before the advent of significant public responsibility for physical health conditions. Separate treatment facilities were the rule. In addition to psychiatry, a whole coterie of separate specialty professionals developed.

Within the mental health sector a second duality historically obtained: between a public system, largely hospital-based and often involuntary, and a private-practice system, largely office-based and voluntary. However, both remained over many years essentially distinct from the physical health care domain.[1-3]

After World War II the growing popularity of psychoanalysis and psychotherapy, the appearance of the first effective medications for the symptomatic relief of severe mental disorders, and, somewhat later, a growing recognition of the civil rights and dignity of individuals suffering from mental disorders combined to begin bringing mental health care into the mainstream. However, this development was shaped in significant ways by two underlying dualities: mental/physical and public/private.

In the private sphere, acknowledgment grew that mental disorders affected large numbers of people, that there was a wide spectrum of disorder ranging from transient and minor problems to very severe and dysfunctional conditions, and that effective treatments could help people to recover. The spread of private health insurance, along with employer recognition that mental problems affected productivity and absenteeism fueled an expansion of mental health coverage as an element of health insurance. However, these benefits typically were circumscribed through differential limitations.

Throughout the private health insurance market, an assumption prevailed that policies could be limited safely for mental health, because anyone needing additional care could (and should) turn to the public sector safety net. Early models of managed care, such as health maintenance organizations (HMOs), incorporated this view.[4,5]

The public mental health system, however, had a life of its own, and increasingly diverged from that assumption. From the 1950s on, the projected costs of state mental hospitals spurred an exploration of less expensive alternatives and an imperative to define priorities for limited public dollars. These changes retained the separate public role but significantly reduced its capacity to provide the safety net assumed by the health system in general and private insurance in particular.

Two developments of the 1960s—the creation of Medicaid and the Community Mental Health Center (CMHC) movement—illustrate the converging mental health and health systems tempered by the ongoing influence of historical dualities. Today's managed care models, including the two in Massachusetts, grow directly from these forces.

COMMUNITY MENTAL HEALTH CENTERS, MEDICAID, AND MANAGED CARE

The Community Mental Health Center movement was in many respects a forerunner of managed care.[6] Its avowed purpose was to contain or reduce costs while providing more appropriate and less intensive care. It postulated a defined population, limited dollars, flexible coverage of care for a spectrum of disorders, a focus on prevention and early intervention, and a team of multidisciplinary providers implementing an organized plan of care for an individual.

The CMHC also was designed as a bridge between public and private mental health care. It created an alternative system to serve people with severe and chronic illness who might otherwise spend years in the state institutional system, as well as a broad range of people in the community who might have limited or no access to insurance or who might need something other than the traditional model of private office-based therapy. The network of local centers was to be established with federal seed funds, declining over time, and eventually replaced by a mix of state and private insurance dollars.

CMHCs (along with civil rights lawyers) have sustained often bitter criticism for the "failure of deinstitutionalization" and the suffering of many people with severe and chronic mental illnesses who never received the care and services in the community that were supposed to replace the comforts of the state hospital. That subject deserves more attention than this brief treatment can offer. Suffice it to say here that the failure to establish even half the planned number of centers, and the gross underfunding of an ever-increasing array of required services, represented a failure of political will that doomed the centers' attempt to fulfill their mandate.[7]

States discharged many patients to communities but also resisted funding upstart "independent" centers at the expense of state-run institutions with politically powerful constituencies. Survival instincts drove many centers to focus on insured or paying populations, and later toward provision of contract services such as employee assistance programs (and now, managed care).

In sum, while one of the most effective arguments for creating a community-based system was the goal of replacing expensive and often horrific state hospitals, the ultimate result was that the population previously served in the hospitals too often were ill-served by the new community-based system. However, by the late 1970s this problem was well understood, and steps were taken by both the federal and state governments to address it.

The resulting Community Support System (CSS) concept drew on the CMHC model: defining a target population, designing services needed by that group, and providing a flexible, individualized plan of service. Instead of bypassing the states or decreeing a one-size-fits-all approach, starting in 1977 it engaged them in a participatory process that identified essential common elements but accommodated differences among state environments. Direct federal funding to CMHCs was replaced over time by block grants to the states focused exclusively on the target population but "grandfathering" the CMHCs as service providers, drawing the community mental health centers and the states into alliance around a target population of individuals with severe and persistent mental illnesses.[8–10]

This 10-year effort (1977–1987)[11] provides one of the best examples of a true federal-state partnership. A related effort focused on children with severe emotional disturbances. The Child and Adolescent Service System Program (CASSP) conceptualized a "system of care" for children living in communities and utilizing multiple service systems, e.g., education, juvenile justice, child welfare as well as mental health and health. The Federal CSP program has continued to the present time. However, beginning in 1988, it shifted toward a research demonstration model rather than the catalyst/learning community model.

A key element of both the CSS and CASSP strategies was to maximize Medicaid as a source of payment for community-based mental health and support services. When Medicaid was created in the mid-1960s the drafters, like their contemporaries designing expanded private health insurance policies, recognized that the general run of beneficiaries might need mental health care and included a measure of general coverage as part of the mandatory package. Also like their counterparts, they had no desire to assume the safety net responsibility traditionally belonging to the states. Therefore they limited most mental health services to the optional category, and carefully excluded coverage for people over 22 or under 65 residing in "institutions for mental disease" (IMDs), that is the population thought to be resident in state mental hospitals. States continued to reflect the separate sense of public responsibility for mental health, retaining separate departments of mental health even as they established large health bureaucracies to administer the new Medicaid program.

However, by the late 1970s much of the population formerly residing in state hospitals for years actually now lived much or all of the time in the community. Also the growth of health insurance, including mental health benefits (despite limitations) had encouraged the expansion of private hospitals specializing in mental health care but not eligible (since they were IMDs) for Medicaid reimbursement for nonelderly adults. The interests of public and private sector mental health interests found common ground in advocating effectively for the expansion of Medicaid plans to cover inpatient reimbursement for eligible populations (children/adolescents and the elderly) and community-based services under the clinic option and later the rehabilitation option.[12–14]

At the same time, private insurance coverage for the employed population was also expanding in response to greater acknowledgment of the needs and benefits of such care for both employees and employers. For a brief time in the mid-1980s, it appeared that public and private roles in both health and mental health were stabilizing and converging and that mental health had established its place within both public and private health care financing systems. However, accelerating cost pressures in both public and private sectors derailed that progress and threatened to turn back the clock.

MANAGING MENTAL HEALTH CARE

The timing of mental health's advances could not have been worse. During the 1980s health costs assumed crisis proportions in the minds of private sector payers. The recent expansion of mental health benefits had produced disproportionately large percentage increases in costs, since they started from such a small base, creating a perception that those costs were out of control and perhaps one of the chief causes of the overall problem. Well-publicized abuses of insurance, particularly for long-term hospitalization for adolescents covered under their parents' policies and for substance abuse treatment, added fuel to the fire.

Mental health benefits became one of the first targets of "managed care" in the private sector, with the avowed goal of containing and reducing costs. Strategies included higher deductibles and copayments, lower limits on annual and lifetime benefits, and more limits on inpatient and outpatient visits for mental health than for physical health care.

Soon specialty firms began to appear, offering to "manage" mental health benefits to save even more. Some focused on utilization review, primarily for hospital admissions and length of stay and for long-term psychotherapy. Others developed a more flexible approach, willing to waive specific benefit limits and cover additional or newer forms of service that offered the promise of containing total costs. However, the primary focus was clearly on cost management rather than care management.[15]

In the public sector, state and local mental health services had come to rely increasingly on Medicaid dollars in order to obtain shared federal financing.[16] As costs rose, and political pressures protected hospital budgets, state mental health agencies managed costs by increasingly limiting their priorities (and most access to public services) to individuals who could qualify for Medicaid and those few others who could gain a claim on the state through the justice system or as a "state [hospital] patient."

As hospitalization was discouraged and lengths of stay decreased, fewer and fewer patients could meet admission criteria, which usually now required an extreme form of illness or demonstration of dangerousness even for voluntary admission. Public hospital emergency rooms began to face barriers in sending people to state hospitals. Individuals who exhausted their private insurance benefits simply could not access public services unless they became indigent and enrolled in Medicaid or demonstrated extreme or dangerous behavior. By the mid-1980s the old, comfortable assumption that a state mental health system was available to back up private health insurance, HMOs, and public hospitals had become obsolete. Instead, both the public and the private systems were managing the costs of mental health care by limiting services and access.

However, both sectors also provided models of "care management." It is no accident that many of the early developers of "managed behavioral health care" came out of the community mental health center movement, or that private sector–managed behavioral health care companies today are competing vigorously for talented staff from state mental health agencies and national nonprofit organizations. Aside from representing the one area of growth in the field today, managed care offers what many see as a new and in some ways better way to pursue their professional goal of rationalizing and improving care.

The Community Support System (CSS) and Child and Adolescent Service System Program (CASSP)—public sector models for adults and children, respectively, with severe mental disorders—demonstrated effective strategies to both assemble resources and provide a flexible array of services geared to the changing needs of a long-term and often very expensive population. Some progressive private employers pioneered a flexible, managed mental health benefit that allowed reimbursement for essentially any mental health service that was cost-effective in the long run.[17] Some progressive HMOs (as illustrated in the Stelovich article) began to experiment with including a broader range of mental health services than the original, intentionally limited design, including services for people with severe mental illnesses.

In the late 1980s and 1990s, managed care advanced rapidly in all areas of health, receiving a boost from the national health care reform debate of 1993–1994. Private insurance increasingly incorporated managed care for all benefits, and HMOs and insurers competed on ways to handle the mental health benefit. Some HMOs and newer forms of managed care chose an integrated strategy; others a specialized "carve-out" for all mental health care or for long-term mental health care. Managed behavioral health care firms grew rapidly in response to these opportunities, shaping their approaches to meet the needs of their customers—primarily large corporations. In 1993 these firms were responsible for over 86 million covered lives. By 1995 the total was almost 111 million covered lives.[18,19]

States began to believe that managed care could be the answer to their escalating Medicaid budgets, and developed such lucrative contracts that managed behavioral health care firms jumped into this new market, immediately challenging the expertise and livelihood of long-standing public "care management" providers, such as CMHCs and psychosocial rehabilitation centers.

DILEMMAS AND DOUBTS

Read in this context, the two articles here present acute dilemmas for the future development of managed care for individuals with mental illnesses. Managed care, as traditionally understood, would seem to offer the potential to further goals long promoted by reformers in the mental health system: reducing service fragmentation, increasing access to individualized care, establishing accountability, reducing costs, and shifting from unnecessary institutional care to more appropriate and less restrictive community services. However, experience to date in both the mental health and health arenas underscores significant risks.[20]

Underfunding

Mental health traditionally has been underfunded in relation to its impact on the population, in public systems, insurance, and HMOs.[21-23] Cost estimates today are suspect, since they are highly skewed by the current dualities and their opportunities for cost shifting (e.g., "dumping" of expensive patients onto the public mental health system, or out of all mental health care and into the criminal justice system or the street). The usual assumption of cost savings engendered by a move to managed care simply may be unrealistic, and attempts to wring savings from the system may produce dangerous cuts in services.

No Net

A casualty of the move toward increased reliance on private, for-profit managed care may be the public sector safety net. In the early years of managed mental health care, big profits nurtured the development of the managed behavioral health care industry. They now are rapidly taking over many of the functions formerly provided by public agencies and a large network of not-for-profit providers. In some cases they are in fact "buying up" key staff and incorporating service providers into the for-profit networks. But as both private sector and then public sector learn better how to estimate costs, and the profit margin falls, companies may simply withdraw from a market and move on to greener pastures. What service structures will be left to serve the people who need care the most?

Going Backwards

The field has made significant advances in the past 15 or 20 years.[24] A lot is known about the constellation of services and supports needed to serve individuals with severe mental illnesses and children with severe emotional disturbances outside hospitals and institutions. However, the applications of this knowledge have occurred within publicly dominated service and financing structures. Now the rush is on to replace these structures with contracts to managed care companies whose experience was shaped by serving a private sector, employed population base—an experience largely devoid of focus on the populations with the most complex needs. The rapidity of change risks failure to translate the substantive learning about how best to serve seriously disabled populations into this new environment.

For example, it took long years of effort in the public sector to gain understanding and acceptance of the vital role of "ancillary" support services for the success of medical services provided by Medicaid. In an era of Medicaid cutbacks, and loss of visibility for mental health constituencies within an integrated public financing system, how long will it be before

Medicaid managed care contracts include adequate community support requirements in their definitions of "medical necessity?"

Loss of Focus and Memory

The prospect of integration of mental health with health care strikes chords of ambivalence in the field. On the one hand, mental health has struggled mightily for recognition as a serious, medical concern. The long and ultimately successful battle to return the National Institute of Mental Health to the National Institutes of Health vividly illustrates the determination to be a part of the larger health structure. On the other hand, many fear that integration would mean a loss of visibility and focus on mental health problems. They note the low priority and prestige of mental health in many academic, clinical, and policy settings concerned with health broadly. They believe in integration, but not yet.

Part of this struggle involves habit and established ways of thinking and relating with each other and with the relevant environment. Part is also a pragmatic fear of losing resources that they have now.[25] The risk involved in integration is that mental health must put its hard-won categorical funding (state, federal, local, as well as private insurance) on the table, with no assurance and often little confidence that they will break even in the political and popularity contest. If national and state mental heath agencies disappear or become low-level bureaus within giant health financing and contracting structures, what kind of priority will go to the needs of people with severe and persistent mental illnesses? Will we have to learn the lessons of deinstitutionalization again?

Institutional memory is a fragile commodity, now at great risk. Faced with the assault of managed care, the federal agencies and organized constituency groups are so busy trying to cope and protect their current program budgets that precious little attention is devoted to thoughtful consideration of long-term trends or opportunities. Few private foundations focus on mental health, or recognize the interrelationship of mental health over time with their priority concerns in physical health or social problems.

MANAGED CARE IS NOT A PANACEA BUT AN OPPORTUNITY

As daunting as these dilemmas may seem, they yet do not obviate the potential benefits of the managed care revolution. First, a primary institutional memory about mental health services is that the old system has never been very good for individuals with the most serious and chronic conditions. Yes, over the past couple of decades we have done better, and now have a good deal of confidence that we know what both adults and children need. But in practice, model systems have been few. We simply have never found a way to bring the benefits of our knowledge to most people in need.

Managed care, at least, offers an opportunity to rethink and restructure, to test a different approach. This experimentation entails real risks. The unfamiliar hazards of managed care seem even greater than those posed by the current system; many in the field would prefer "the devil they know."

One prime example of the new equation of risk and opportunity will be the role of consumer responsibility and choice. For the past 20 years, mental health consumers and families have demanded, and finally attained, a significant measure of participation in decisions affecting their care and their lives: the development of patients' rights charters in states and facilities; the spread of protection and advocacy programs to assist consumers; the establishment of consumer affairs offices in state mental health departments; and the vocal representation of consumer and family groups on planning, advisory, and governing councils.

Managed care posits an active and responsible consumer role for patients, entailing active participation in their own treatment as well as monitoring the system's performance through complaints and grievances. How will the consumer activism of the mental health field translate into the context of managed care? On the one hand, the acceptance and reliance on consumers to participate will strengthen and extend a role that was won only with great effort and political pressure in the old system. On the other hand, what will private sector managed care do to assure that people receiving mental health care have access to the decision processes, information, and advocacy assistance they may need to play their designated role as responsible consumers? This challenge will help to define the success of managed care for mental health.

REFERENCES

1. Grob, G. N. *Mad Among Us: A History of the Care of America's Mentally Ill.* New York, NY: Free Press, 1994.
2. Rochefort, D. A., ed. *Handbook on Mental Health Policy in the United States.* Westport, CT: Greenwood Press, 1989.
3. Goldman, H.H., and Morrissey, J.P. "Alchemy of Mental Health Policy: Homelessness and the Fourth Cycle of Reform." *American Journal of Public Health* 75(7) (1978):727–731.
4. P.L. 93-322, Health Maintenance Organization Act of 1973.
5. Stelovich, S. "Evolution of Services for the Chronically Mentally Ill in a Managed Care Setting: A Case Study." *Managed Care Quarterly* 4(3) (1996):78–84.

6. Feldman, S. "Managed Mental Health—Community Mental Health Revisited?" *Managed Care Quarterly* 2(2) (1994):13–18.
7. Scallet, L.J. "Mental Health and Homelessness: Evidence of Failed Policy?" *Health Affairs* 8(4) (1989):185–188. Review of Torrey, E.F. *Nowhere to Go: The Tragic Odyssey of the Homeless Mentally Ill.* New York, NY: Harper and Row, 1988.
8. Mulkern, V. *Community Support Program: A Model for Federal-State Partnership.* Washington, D.C.: Mental Health Policy Resource Center, 1995.
9. Carling, P.J. *The National Institute of Mental Health Community Support Program: History and Evaluation.* Burlington, VT: University of Vermont, 1984.
10. Turner, J.C., and TenHoor, W.J. "The NIMH Community Support Program: Pilot Approach to a Needed Social Reform." *Schizophrenia Bulletin* 4(3) (1978):319–348.
11. Mulkern, *Community Support Program.*
12. Toff-Bergman, G. *Medicaid Plans and Mental Health: 1992 Profiles of State Options and Limitations.* Washington, D.C.: Mental Health Policy Resource Center, 1993.
13. Folcarelli, C., and Law, C. *Medicaid Plans and Mental Health: 1994 Updated Profiles of State Options and Limitations.* Fairfax, VA: Lewin/VHI, 1994.
14. Koyanagi, C., and Goldman, H.H. "Quiet Success of the National Plan for the Chronically Mentally Ill." *Hospital and Community Psychiatry* 42(9) (1991):899–905.
15. Trabin, T., and Freeman, M. A. *Managed Behavioral Healthcare: History, Models, Strategic Challenges and Future Course.* Tiburon, CA: CentraLink Publishers, 1995.
16. Counihan, C.W., et al. "A Medicaid Mental Health Carve-Out Program: The Massachusetts Experience." *Managed Care Quarterly* 4(3) (1996):85–92.
17. England, M.J., and Vaccaro, V.A. "New Systems to Manage Mental Health Care." *Health Affairs* 10(4) (1991):129–137.
18. Oss, M.E., ed. *Managed Behavioral Health Market Share in the United States, 1993.* Gettysburg, PA: Behavioral Health Industry News, Inc., 1993.
19. Oss, M.E., et al. *Managed Behavioral Health Market Share in the United States, 1995/1996.* Gettysburg, PA: Behavioral Health Industry News, Inc., 1995.
20. Iglehart, J.K. "Health Policy Report: Managed Care and Mental Health." *New England Journal of Medicine* 334(2) (1996):131–135.
21. Frank, R.G., and McGuire, T.G. "Estimating Costs of Mental Health and Substance Abuse Coverage." *Health Affairs* 14(3) (1995):102–115.
22. Stelovich, "Evolution of Services."
23. Counihan, "Mental Health Carve-Out."
24. Mechanic, D., Schlesinger, M., and McAlpine, D.D. "Management of Mental Health and Substance Abuse Services: State of the Art and Early Results." *Milbank Quarterly* 73(1) (1995):19–55.
25. Stelovich, "Evolution of Services."

VII

Using Data to
Design Programs

18

USQA Health Profile Database as a Tool for Health Plan Quality Improvement

*Nicholas A. Hanchak, James F. Murray, Alex Hirsch,
Patricia D. McDermott, and Neil Schlackman*

Managed care organizations (MCOs) assume responsibility for both the financing and delivery of health care. In addition to maintaining financial solvency, MCOs have accepted an explicit commitment to monitor and actively improve the care delivered to their members. Because MCOs have been active in controlling resource utilization, they have come under increased scrutiny from patients, employers, and accrediting organizations for the quality of care delivered to their members.[1] The assessment of care is challenging because the organizational arrangements between providers and MCOs vary. MCOs must be innovative in measuring physician performance and quality of care, and in implementing quality improvement programs. A key requirement of managing the financing and delivery of health care services and assuring the quality of care is a sophisticated information system.[2]

This article explores the relationship between cost and quality for patients with chronic diseases, and the role information systems play in measuring and reporting performance. We describe the development of a patient-centered approach for chronic diseases, and its integration with the analysis of providers to assess the quality of medical care delivered in a managed care setting.[3] The methodology was developed by U.S. Quality Algorithms (USQA), a subsidiary of U.S. Healthcare (USHC). USQA directs the performance measurement of and provides information used in

Source: Reprinted from N.A. Hanchak, J.F. Murray, A. Hirsch, et al., USQA Health Profile Database as a Tool for Health Plan Quality Improvement, *Managed Care Quarterly*, Vol. 4, No. 2, pp. 58–69, © 1996, Aspen Publishers, Inc.

the quality improvement programs for USHC, a two million-member HMO operating in 13 states in the Northeast and Mid-Atlantic regions as well as the District of Columbia. We relate the development and implementation of a patient database, the USQA Health Profile Database (HPD), for the purposes of quality improvement and patient management. We also provide an in-depth example of the identification criteria for diabetes mellitus and use examples of a patient-centered approach to measure the quality of care for diabetes, using the MCD Database. In addition to quality issues, we demonstrate results that compare the financial liabilities of and among different chronic diseases within the health plan.

QUALITY, COSTS, AND INFORMATION SYSTEMS

Traditional quality assurance (QA) relies on identifying cases and particular practice patterns of physicians that may represent problem areas. Traditional QA uses retrospective review and the abstraction of medical charts as its mainstay methodology. Although these approaches still have benefit, the approach to quality management in the era of managed care is rapidly changing.[4] Quality of care activities can be enhanced by data collected by the MCO, which can be quite extensive, with different data obtained from multiple sources. For example, financial and administrative data systems, such as billing and membership information, contain important clinical data that can help contribute to measuring the quality of care delivered to patients. The challenge for MCOs is to link the multiple sources of data to obtain relevant clinical information and apply it to the MCO's quality assessment and improvement efforts.[5-8] Efficiently managing patients with certain chronic conditions has considerable impact on both quality and cost. A key aspect of improving quality and controlling costs is to be able to identify and manage patients with specific needs due to certain clinical conditions. The starting point for accomplishing this is the MCO's information systems.

Several database sources can potentially provide important clinical information, each with their own strengths:

- An encounters database provides information about the diagnoses and procedures of patients who seek care from their capitated providers, both primary care physicians and capitated specialty providers.
- Claims databases gather diagnostic information about patients who utilize noncapitated resources, and provide insight into the number and types of procedures that providers use to treat certain conditions. Both outpatient claims, generally submitted on a HCFA 1500 standard claim form, and inpatient claims, which utilize the standard

UB82/UB92 formats, have diagnostic and procedural information. They also furnish information about the episodes of care, including the dates of service and the responsible providers.[9]

- A membership database allows clinicians to target certain demographic and benefits variables that may influence access to care, identify the utilization patterns of specific health care resources, and help identify increased risk for certain conditions or adverse outcomes.
- Pharmacy data in some cases allow providers to identify specific disease states, as well as important information about the prescribing patterns in the treatment of specific diseases.
- Laboratory data allow the plan to identify patients with specific diseases and to understand the outcomes of certain processes of care.

Most approaches to using administrative databases to evaluate the quality of medical care have taken a provider-focused approach to profiling the quality of care, with administrators relying solely on claims data. Services received by a patient are aggregated to the provider level and utilization patterns for individual providers are compared with other providers. The availability of data on multiple providers yields a reference for determining expected or normative behavior. Deviations from the norm are flagged as potential problems. Using providers as the unit of analysis is a necessary part of a quality assessment program, but it is not sufficient. A comprehensive approach requires integration with other analyses that focus on the patient as the unit of analysis and incorporates all available data. Without this integration of provider and patient-centered analyses, and without the inclusion of information from multiple data sources, there are limitations to the conclusions that can be drawn about the delivery of quality medical care.

SELECTING CHRONIC DISEASES FOR INCLUSION IN THE DATABASE

The intent of the HPD is to profile members within the health plan who have certain diseases that are chronic in nature and for whom their conditions will likely need ongoing medical care management. The quality of care that providers within a health plan are able to deliver is best demonstrated by their ability to take care of members with chronic diseases. The costs of caring for members who suffer from these illnesses represent significant costs to a health plan. This is not to negate the importance of acute conditions. Acute illnesses represent a significant burden to the members within a health plan, yet because they are of limited duration and are therefore difficult to identify from retrospective claims data with sufficient timeliness, they do not allow for assessing and improving the quality of care of specific patients. Acute illnesses are critical for analyzing such activities as provider practices.

We are currently developing methods to incorporate multiple sources of data for identifying episodes of acute illnesses, and ultimately a comprehensive view of the burden of illness in a primary care provider's patient panel.

There were no prior assumptions made about the inclusion or exclusion of certain conditions into the HPD. The selection of illnesses is an ongoing process. The selection process first began with an analysis of individual claims and illnesses that were identified as either prevalent in terms of number of members with or health care encounters for the disease. The prevalence criterion was secondary to the cost requirement, so that the need for high prevalence was relaxed for diseases in which there were high costs per patient.

A second consideration was that selected diseases be candidates for improvement in the processes of care that would ultimately lead to better outcomes.[10] In other words, preference was given to diseases in which practice guidelines have been developed and proven to be both efficacious and effective in improving the health of a population with a given disease. By having providers follow these performance standards, the health of a specific at-risk patient population can potentially be improved. High-cost chronic conditions were then identified and their potential for improved processes and outcomes was evaluated. The results of a literature search were incorporated with clinical judgment to identify and quantify those diseases with potential for improved outcomes. In addition to medical conditions that are chronic in nature, certain other conditions have been incorporated because of the interest in the care obtained by patients with those conditions (e.g., lung cancer, breast cancer). A total of 36 different chronic diseases were identified to be of sufficient import within the USHC membership to track. The list of chronic conditions currently included is presented in Exhibit 18–1. We will continue to extend this list with other conditions that present opportunities for improvement in quality, cost, or both.

METHODS FOR DISEASE IDENTIFICATION

This stage involved developing clinical selection criteria for each disease using all clinically relevant databases. The HPD was developed using disease-specific specifications developed by USQA. The current specifications used the following information to identify members with certain chronic disease:

Exhibit 18–1 List of Diseases Included in the U.S. Healthcare Health Profile Database

1. AIDS	19. Hemophilia
2. Alcoholism	20. Hypercholesterolemia
3. Asthma	21. Hypertension
4. Atrial Fibrillation	22. Hyperthyroidism
5. Back Pain	23. Hypothyroidism
6. Benign Prostatic Hypertrophy	24. Iron Deficiency Anemia
7. Breast Cancer	25. Ischemic Heart Disease
8. Cerebrovascular Disease	26. Kidney Stones
9. Cholelithiasis	27. Lung Cancer
10. Chronic Obstructive Pulmonary Disease	28. Migraine and Other Headaches
11. Chronic Renal Failure	29. Multiple Sclerosis
12. Colon Cancer	30. Nonspecific Gastritis/ Dyspepsia
13. Congestive Heart Failure	31. Osteoarthritis
14. Crohn's Disease	32. Otitis Media
15. Depression	33. Peptic Ulcer Disease
16. Diabetes Mellitus	34. Rheumatoid Arthritis
17. Diverticular Disease	35. Sickle Cell Anemia
18. Epilepsy	36. Systemic Lupus Erythematosus

- ICD-9 diagnosis codes from claims and encounter files
- CPT-4 procedure codes from claims and encounter files
- Medispan GPI pharmacy codes (Medispan is a mapping of all NDC codes into similar drug classes based on a proprietary grouping system)
- utilization patterns of certain laboratory tests
- patient demographic data

The selection criteria may draw from any or all of these sources. The patient demographic data help to protect the algorithm from unreliable data by ensuring that the identification of a disease is appropriate (e.g., females are not identified with benign prostatic hypertrophy). An example of the selection criteria for diabetes mellitus is presented in Exhibit 18–2.

The methodology currently in place can easily expand to include any additional diseases or other clinical variables, such as procedures or screening tests that are identified as being important to track. Currently, USHC is developing a process whereby clinicians will be able to determine whether a lab test has occurred and its result by checking the laboratory results database.

Exhibit 18–2 Diabetes Mellitus Selection Criteria

Diagnosis Criteria (ICD-9 Codes)
250–250.93 (diabetes mellitus with various manifestations)
357.2 (polyneuropathy in diabetes)
362.0–362.02 (diabetic retinopathy)
366.41 (diabetic cataract)
Procedure Criteria (CPT-4 Codes)
82985 (glycated protein) and/or 83036 (glycated hemoglobin) occurring
    twice in any 12 consecutive months, at least 90 days apart
J1820 (diabetic injectable medications)
W0070 (oral hypoglycemic medications)*
W0071 (antidiabetic products—miscellaneous)
5190D (registered nurse diabetic visit)*
5205D (certified diabetes educator)*
9890A (diabetes education program)*
E0607 (home blood glucose monitor)*
Pharmacy Criteria (NDC Codes)
Insulin
Sulfonylurea
Not Included (ICD-9 Codes)
648.8 (abnormal glucose tolerance test in pregnancy)
790.2 (abnormal glucose tolerance test)
962.3 (poisoning by insulin or antidiabetic agent)

*U.S. Healthcare internal billing codes.

THE USQA HEALTH PROFILE DATABASE

Using the disease selection specifications, the identification program used to populate the HPD queried the encounters, claims, pharmacy, and laboratory databases. A record was generated for any member who met the necessary specifications for one or more diseases. This data file is matched against the U.S. Healthcare Enrollment File to add selected demographic data while additionally generating a record for U.S. Healthcare members without any of the currently specified chronic diseases.

Each database record consists of two basic components—the demographic(s) section and the disease section. The demographic(s) section includes the following fields: U.S. Healthcare member number; number of diseases from 0–36; age; sex; date of birth; Social Security number; membership enrollment dates; and primary care physician. The disease section lists one segment per disease. Included within each disease segment are the following: date first identified; date last identified; how the disease was first identified; when this disease was added to the member's chronic disease record; diagnosis code identifier; procedure code identifier; prescription identifier; lab test utilization identifier; lab test result identifier; claims database identifier; encounter database identifier; and disease-specific tags (e.g., diabetics on insulin). Various override codes exist in certain instances, such as when the member or member's physician specifies that member has or does not have the disease in question.

Updates occur on a monthly basis with all the demographic data being fully replaced each month to keep the database consistent with the enrollment data. Information on disenrolled members is maintained in the database with an indication of the inactive status of the member.

In the future databases will be updated and used by the Patient Management case workers in real time.[11] This will enhance the capture of disease identification information primarily collected by case managers from their interactions with patients and physicians. The access to disease information will enable case managers to more appropriately direct additional medical care through proactive disease management programs.

VALIDATING THE SELECTION CRITERIA FOR THE USQA HEALTH PROFILE

As with any system of quality measurement that relies solely on administrative data, there is the need to determine the accuracy of the data and the methodologies employed in analyzing the data as it is converted into meaningful information.[12,13] The process of validating the HPD will be illustrated using diabetes mellitus. As of October 1994, USQA identified 39,331 U.S. Healthcare members believed to have diabetes, who were profiled in the HPD. To begin to validate the selection criteria used in the identification of diabetic patients, all U.S. Healthcare primary care physicians were sent a list of the members in their practices who were identified as having diabetes by the administrative selection criteria. Offices that found errors on their lists of diabetics were asked to identify false positives (i.e., those on the list who do not have diabetes), and false negatives (i.e., those who were not on the list, but who have diabetes).

A total of 292 physician offices responded to the questionnaire for a response rate of 8 percent. This low response rate is probably because only offices with significant error rates were asked to respond. The number of diabetic patients identified by the initial selection criteria in the panels of these responding physicians was 4,172, and the total number of capitated patients taken care of by these physicians was 220,298. The positive predictive (e.g., percentage of positive tests that accurately reflected the disease state) value for the selection criteria was 84.2 percent, and the sensitivity (e.g., the percentage of the time that the presence of a disease state was accurately reflected by a positive result) was 97.3 percent based on a total of 115 diabetic patients that were added based on the physician reports. Although the sensitivity and specificity of the individual criteria can be calculated, the results must be interpreted with caution because of certain biases in physician responses. The error rates are likely magnified due to selection bias, whereby physicians with a higher error rate will tend to have greater incentive to respond to the request to have their errors corrected.

Moreover, the ratio of false positives to false negatives was likely inflated. This is due to the fact that it is easier to recognize a patient as not having a disease, when presented with the patient name, as opposed to identifying patients from a panel who were inappropriately left off the list. Figure 18–1 demonstrates the additive effect of pharmacy data, primary care physician encounters data, and laboratory test utilization data on improving the detection of members with diabetes. The ability of administrative data alone to identify disease may vary. For instance, diseases such as diabetes can be specifically identified by several database sources (i.e., claims, encounters, pharmacy, lab). Others, such as osteoarthritis or sickle cell anemia, are only diagnosed by ICD-9 diagnosis codes from claims or encounters.

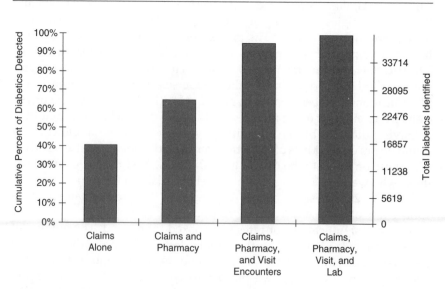

Figure 18–1. Incremental detection of various databases.

THE USQA HEALTH PROFILE DATABASE: APPLICATIONS FOR EPIDEMIOLOGICAL STUDIES AND ASSESSING QUALITY OF CARE

The applications of the MCD Database for assessing physician performance and quality will also be illustrated using diabetes mellitus. Within the group of chronic diseases, diabetes mellitus provides one of the most significant opportunities for effective patient management. The recent release of the Diabetes Control and Complication Trial provides firm evidence that good glycemic control leads to better outcomes. Diabetic patients are at risk not only for complications resulting from hyperglycemia and hypoglycemia, but also for cardiac and peripheral vascular disease, end-stage renal disease, retinopathy, and peripheral neuropathy. The USQA HPD was used to conduct a study to assess the prevalence and costs of diabetes in the U.S. Healthcare member population. The quality of care provided to diabetic patients by U.S. Healthcare's contracted providers was an important consideration. The results of the study have many important implications for management decisions aimed at providing improved care to diabetic members.

The calculation of the prevalence of diabetes is complicated by the time lag between when a member joins the health plan and when the data that identify the disease reach the administrative databases. This time lag in acquiring the necessary data from administrative databases can lead to an underestimate of the true prevalence. The prevalence estimate of 3.1 percent has been calculated by limiting the denominator and numerator to those members belonging to USHC for at least 12 months. This calculation is further limited to those members on the pharmacy plan to improve the sensitivity of selection criteria using this database. This estimate is consistent with other reports of the estimated prevalence of diabetes appearing in the medical literature.[14,15] Figure 18–2 shows a graph of the calculated prevalence for members who are currently enrolled and who have been enrolled for each of the specified minimum time periods. Limiting the prevalence calculation to those members who were health plan members for at least one year begins to address the decreased sensitivity of administrative data associated with a shorter period of active time in the health plan. Note that the prevalence curve continually increases and never appears to flatten. This occurrence may be influenced by the incidence rate for the USHC population. Further investigation is being done to evaluate this hypothesis.

In addition to the prevalence and utilization statistics outlined above, we analyzed measures that evaluate the degree to which care delivered to diabetic patients follows the accepted standards as promoted by the

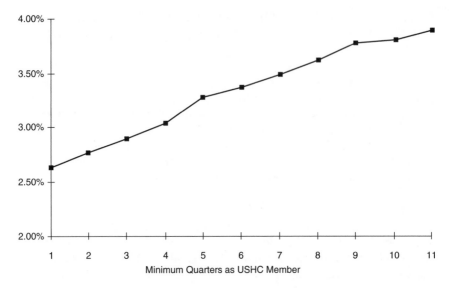

Figure 18–2. Prevalence based on varying membership time periods.

American Diabetes Association. Exhibit 18–3 shows an example of a diabetes report that evaluates important process and outcome measures.[16] These measures can serve as indicators of the quality of care provided by participating physicians to their capitated members. This version of the report provides results for U.S. Healthcare overall. The measures include physician use of various preventive tests as supported by practice guidelines advocated by the American Diabetes Association. Measures include issues related to the percentage of diabetics who visit their primary care physician, the average number of visits per diabetic member, and the use of glycated hemoglobin testing. Regional and U.S. Healthcare overall rates of performance can be used to set practice-based benchmark levels of performance, of hemoglobin A_{IC}, retinal eye exams, microalbuminuria, and cholesterol tests. Outcome measures include the number of diabetes-specific emergency room visits and hospitalizations, admission for DKA/HHNK/diabetic coma, hypoglycemia, and cellulitis. Other measures, which are easily calculated using the HPD, are the prevalence of ischemic heart disease and end-stage renal disease in diabetic patients. The annual occurrence of lower extremity amputation, diabetic nephropathy, and blindness/impaired vision has also been calculated.

Along with evaluating the above measures for U.S. Healthcare as a whole, USQA has calculated the same measures for each U.S. Healthcare

Exhibit 18–3 U.S. Healthcare Diabetes Performance Report

Prevalence Measures

1	Actual number of current members identified with diabetes	39,331
2	Estimated overall prevalence of diabetes*	3.1%
3	Diabetics with pharmacy plan on insulin*	25.1%

Clinical Measures*

4	Average number of annual primary care visits per diabetic	4.0
5	Diabetics who visited their physician at least once in reporting period	84.4%
6	Average number of annual glycated hemoglobin tests per diabetic	0.8
7	Diabetics with at least 2 glycated hemoglobin tests during reporting period	21.4%
8	Diabetics receiving retinal exams during previous year	30.4%
9	Diabetics receiving cholesterol screening test during previous year	33.8%
10	Diabetics who had a microalbuminuria screening test during previous year	2.6%

Outcome Measures*

11	ER visits specifically for diabetes/1,000 diabetics/year	8.2
12	Total admissions (acute) specifically for diabetes/ 1,000 diabetics/year	24.8
13	Admissions for DKA, HHNK, or diabetic coma/ 1,000 diabetics/year[†]	6.5
14	Admissions for hypoglycemia/1,000 diabetics/year	3.0
15	Admissions for cellulitis/1,000 diabetics/year	6.0
16	Prevalence of ischemic heart disease in diabetics	17.2%
17	Prevalence of end-stage renal disease in diabetics[†]	1.5%
18	Annual incident detection of lower extremity amputations[†]	0.2%
19	Prevalence of neuropathy in diabetics[†]	0.6%
20	Prevalence of retinopathy in diabetics	13.7%

*Based on members who were in the study for the full 12 months
[†]Results should be interpreted with caution because of small numbers

regional health plan to identify opportunities for improvement. USQA has calculated the measures at individual primary care physicians' offices to provide educational feedback to help physicians better understand their own performance and how it compares with their peers. The ability to evaluate the epidemiology of chronic diseases and measure the performance of network physicians on important process and outcome measures is crucial to the success of managed care plans. Such analyses can help improve decisions on whether and how to apply resources to physician education and patient management programs. These analyses can also help determine the potential impact from proposed interventions and justify anticipated costs of these interventions. Studies of the epidemiology of the other disease in the databases are planned together with performance reports to evaluate the care provided by physicians.

APPLYING THE USQA HEALTH PROFILE DATABASE TO FINANCIAL MANAGEMENT

Costs related to diabetes in the health plan constitute an important proxy for the burden of illness experienced by diabetic patients. These costs can also help to estimate the proportion of health care resources used by diabetic patients. The total noncapitated costs for these patients can be calculated using the HPD. The direct facility and professional costs for inpatient care, emergency room care, short procedure unit care, and outpatient care are shown in Figure 18–3, for diabetic patients versus the average U.S. Healthcare member. For the purpose of this preliminary analysis, we have combined indirect and unrelated costs. Indirect costs are for conditions related to diabetes, such as kidney disease and heart disease. Unrelated costs are all costs other than direct (for diabetes) and indirect costs. In addition, we have excluded the following costs (both medical and societal): capitation paid to primary care physicians, radiologists, laboratories,

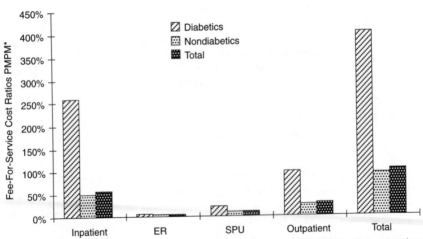

*Adjusted scale equates total fee-for-service costs for average U.S. Healthcare member at 100 percent.

Figure 18–3. Comparison of total fee-for-service costs.

podiatrists, and mental health providers; pharmacy costs; nursing home costs; costs for undiagnosed diabetics; and foregone income due to illness, disability, and premature death. These cost estimates represent one advantage of using a patient-centered approach rather than a claims-centered approach to evaluate the quality of care. By using a claims-centered approach, only direct disease-related costs can be calculated since members with a disease were not first identified.

Figure 18–4 presents the cumulative diabetes-specific costs associated with the 2,000 most expensive and presumably sickest diabetics during the 12-month reporting period. Although these 2,000 diabetics represent only 4.9 percent of the U.S. Healthcare diabetic population, they account for 91.9 percent of the yearly direct diabetes-specific expenditures. The top 400 sickest diabetic patients (1 percent of diabetics) account for 58.7 percent of the yearly noncapitated diabetes-specific expenditures. This highly disproportionate utilization of medical resources suggests the potential return to be gained by concentrating aggressive case management efforts on the sickest diabetic patients.

Table 18–1 shows estimated prevalence statistics for USHC members with the diseases currently in the USQA HPD along with a cost factor. This cost factor is the ratio of noncapitated costs for members identified with

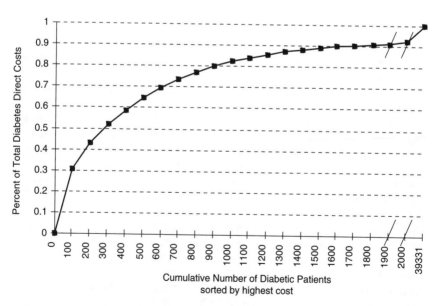

Figure 18–4. Incremental costs of diabetic patients.

Table 18–1 Unadjusted Cost Ratios for Pharmacy, Inpatient Days, and Total Noncapitated Cost (as a Percent of the Average for All USHC Members)

Disease classification	Prevalence (%)	Rx PMPM (%)	I/P Days (%)	Total PMPM (%)
Chronic renal failure	0.2	722.9	2181.3	1772.9
Hemophilia	0.0	103.1	449.1	1617.4
Lung cancer	0.1	411.1	2224.6	1241.6
Congestive heart failure	0.7	547.2	1584.4	1044.8
AIDS	0.1	1018.5	1101.0	944.3
Atrial fibrillation	0.5	503.7	1394.7	811.7
Cerebrovascular disease	0.7	451.3	1134.3	787.3
Colon cancer	0.1	295.0	1490.5	774.8
Iron deficiency anemia	0.2	378.8	1045.4	749.2
Chronic obstructive pulmonary disease	0.7	495.3	1067.2	672.8
Systemic lupus erythematosus	0.1	412.7	793.6	620.8
Sickle cell anemia	0.0	68.6	920.1	611.7
Crohn's disease	0.1	410.7	991.2	572.3
Ischemic heart disease	3.0	442.8	718.0	525.1
Breast cancer	0.4	350.0	568.7	514.0
Peptic ulcer disease	0.5	402.4	762.1	476.6
Alcoholism	0.4	225.9	472.1	462.2
Multiple sclerosis	0.1	310.0	634.4	450.9
Epilepsy	1.7	297.0	511.2	449.2
Cholelithiasis	0.9	252.4	635.7	413.7
Kidney stones	0.9	218.7	448.3	368.4
Diverticular disease	0.7	330.8	568.8	363.2
Osteoarthritis	1.3	354.0	367.8	353.5
Diabetes mellitus	3.2	395.0	446.2	353.4
Benign prostatic hypertrophy	0.9	348.8	430.0	344.9
Depression	4.7	367.1	291.7	300.4
Nonspecific gastritis/dyspepsia	10.2	325.8	343.7	298.4
Hyperthyroidism	0.3	220.5	313.4	264.9
Hypertension	10.0	325.0	271.5	247.5
Hypercholesterolemia	4.9	380.8	242.6	246.1
Hypothyroidism	2.2	299.2	220.3	237.3
Low back pain	8.3	209.1	207.8	205.3
Migraine and other headaches	5.0	220.6	196.8	202.2
Asthma	7.6	191.0	164.5	161.8
Rheumatoid arthritis	1.5	127.5	128.8	140.8
All USHC members	**N/A**	**100.0**	**100.0**	**100.0**
Otitis media	17.4	83.2	69.1	85.2
USHC members w/o disease	N/A	30.2	37.0	41.2

the disease compared with the noncapitated costs of the average U.S. Healthcare member. Although limitations exist among the variable sensitivities of administrative data for different diseases, depending on relative seriousness of the disease and the coding biases by physicians for different disease processes, these results are a snapshot of the percentage of USHC members who can be identified with certain diseases despite the limitations. Consequently, the use of administrative data has great cost advantages over the need for primary data collection. Moreover, the cost ratios are an attempt to quantify diseases that tend to be relatively more expensive, to help clinicians prioritize diseases to address in their patient management programs.

There are many strengths in a patient-centered approach to profiling clinical administrative data, and the HPD serves as a tool in following this approach. It tends to be more all-inclusive, with a more complete capture of members with important conditions than a claims-centric approach. The ability to use data from five or more years and provide the common linkage (i.e., the member identification number) improves the sensitivity of identifying members with certain diseases. Because this approach does not rely on just one type of database, the limitations of some databases may be overcome by the strengths of others. The development of the USQA HPD can be used as a starting point to define the burden of illness in the member population of the health plan.[17,18] Because the HPD is developed and maintained in an ongoing fashion, its data regarding the prevalence and distribution of members with specific diseases across physician offices are current. It can be queried as needed, and members who are capitated to specific physician offices can be identified.

As with any methodology that relies heavily on administrative data, there will be error rates from miscoding (e.g., overcoding and undercoding). For example, the present ICD-9 coding system is limited in cases of medical visits that occur for the diagnostic work-up of yet undiagnosed symptoms. Therefore, further development and validation of the HPD through chart review and feedback from physicians and their patients is desirable.

Another factor is that the algorithms used for different diseases will vary in their sensitivity and specificity. In diseases that have a broad range of selection criteria (i.e., diabetes where there is a series of ICD-9 diagnosis, specific pharmacy criteria, and laboratory criteria), the sensitivity can be considered to be quite good and likely better than a disease where the only specific selection criteria are ICD-9 diagnosis codes (e.g., sickle cell anemia and osteoarthritis, which only have ICD-9 diagnosis criteria).

USQA and U.S. Healthcare are developing further several specific areas. The first set of projects, to be driven by the USQA HPD, is a series of performance measures for all significant conditions that are currently profiled. Using the Diabetes Performance Report as an example (see Exhibit 18–3), performance reports will be developed for a variety of other specific disease states.

The work that USQA has just begun in the understanding the epidemiology and costs of members with specific diseases will continue, and will help to define those conditions for which the provision of additional health care resources appears justified. The information will be enhanced through physician and patient disease surveys in which the sensitivity and specificity of the various selection criteria can be further refined. The USQA HPD will also provide the data necessary to identify factors that are important to member satisfaction and reenrollment, as well as termination studies to understand the impact having a chronic disease has on these measures. Finally, correlations will be investigated regarding the impact that certain diseases have on members' overall health status outcomes.

The USQA HPD can be used to profile problem lists of medical conditions for patients. On-line electronic medical records will greatly improve the accuracy in the capture and further the development of more clinically relevant databases. The HPD, however, is an important start, and the lessons learned will move the field of health plan quality improvement further ahead by the time electronic medical records are commonplace. Even with the widespread use of electronic medical records, there will be limitations to drawing clinical conclusions. Rather than being paralyzed by the limitations and inaccuracies of the present state of administrative data, however, the HPD is being used in a constructive and meaningful way to provide the type of medical management information that helps providers improve the care they provide to their patients.

REFERENCES

1. Siu, A., et al. "A Fair Approach to Comparing Quality of Care." *Health Affairs* 10 (1990): 62–75.
2. Ginsburg, P., and Hammons, G. "Competition and the Quality of Care: The Importance of Information." *Inquiry* 25 (1988): 108–115.
3. Donabedian, A. "The Quality of Care: How Can it Be Assessed?" *Journal of the American Medical Association* 26 (1988): 1743–1747.
4. Roos, L., and Brazauskas, R. "Outcomes and Quality Assurance: Facilitating the Use of Administrative Data." *Quality Assurance in Health Care* 2 (1990): 77–88.
5. Hidalgo, J. "Development of a Model Longitudinal Data Base to Measure Outcomes and Quality of Care Among Persons with AIDS." *Quarterly Review Bulletin (Chicago)* 16 (1990): 355–364.
6. Weiner, J.P., et al. "Applying Insurance Claims Data to Assess Quality of Care: A Compilation of Potential Indicators." *Quarterly Review Bulletin (Chicago)* 16 (1990): 424–438.

7. Leatherman, S., et al. "Quality Screening and Management Using Claims Data in a Managed Care Setting." *Quarterly Review Bulletin (Chicago)* 17 (1991): 349–359.
8. Goldfield, N. "Measurement and Management of Quality in Managed Care Organizations: Alive and Improving." *Quarterly Review Bulletin (Chicago)* 17 (1991): 343–348.
9. Gottlieb, L., Margolis, C., and Schoenbaum, S. "Clinical Practice Guidelines at an HMO: Development and Implementation in a Quality Improvement Model." *Quarterly Review Bulletin (Chicago)* 16 (1990): 80–86.
10. Siu, A.L., et al. "Choosing Quality-of-Care Measures Based on the Expected Impact of Improved Quality of Care for the Major Causes of Mortality and Morbidity." *RAND HMO Quality of Care Consortium* JR-03 (1992): 1–73.
11. Pryor, D., and Lee, K. "Methods for the Analysis and Assessment of Clinical Databases: The Clinician's Perspective." *Statistics in Medicine* 10 (1991): 617–628.
12. Green, J. and Wintfeld, N. "How Accurate Are Hospital Discharge Data for Evaluating Effectiveness of Care?" *Medical Care* 31 (1993):719–731.
13. Nordstrom, D.L., Remington, P.L., and Layde, P.M. "The Utility of HMO Data for the Surveillance of Chronic Diseases." *American Journal of Public Health* 84 (1994): 995–997.
14. Rubin, R.J., Altman, W.M., and Mendelson, D.N. "Special Article: Health Care Expenditures for People With Diabetes Mellitus." *Journal of Clinical Endocrinology and Metabolism* 199(78) (1992): 809A–809F.
15. Rendell, M., et al. "The Health Care Status of the Diabetic Population as Reflected by Physician Claims to a Major Insurer." *Archives of Internal Medicine* 153 (1993): 1360–1366.
16. Hanchak, N.A., and Schlackman, N. "The Measurement of Physician Performance." *Quality Management in Health Care* 4 (1995): 1–10.
17. Iezzoni, L.I., et al. "Chronic Conditions and Risk of In-Hospital Death." *HSR: Health Services Research* 29 (1994): 435–446.
18. Von Korff, M., Wagner, E., and Saunders, K. "A Chronic Disease Score From Automated Pharmacy Data." *Journal of Clinical Epidemiology* 45 (1992): 197–203.

19

Using Clinical Data in Program Design: A Family Support Program for Families with Preterm Infants

Maryjoan Ladden

IMMEDIATE AND LIFETIME COSTS OF PREMATURITY

Prematurity is the number one perinatal and neonatal problem in the United States today. While significant advances have been made in the survival rate of preterm and other medically complex infants, these "survivors" are at increased risk for medical complications, chronic illness, and developmental delay compared with normal birthweight infants.[1-3]

The newborn costs of caring for these infants is significant, too. Average costs for a neonatal intensive care unit (NICU) stay for a very low birthweight infant (less than 1,250 grams at birth) may reach more than $200,000.[4] Continuing medical care costs for these infants are also high since many of them develop chronic conditions. Fifty-nine percent of the total health expenditures for children are accounted for by only five percent of the children, those with chronic health conditions.[5]

The physical, emotional, and financial costs to the families of these infants can also be extensive. Families with preterm infants have difficulty in several areas, such as meeting the infant's daily care and monitoring needs, maintaining marital and family relationships, integrating the infant into the family, and coping with the disruption of the parents' careers and depletion of their financial resources.[6-8]

Source: Reprinted from M. Ladden, Using Clinical Data in Program Design: A Family Support Program for Families with Preterm Infants, *Managed Care Quarterly*, Vol. 4, No. 3, pp. 30–35, © 1996, Aspen Publishers, Inc.

Preterm infants have a variable prognosis after discharge from the neo-natal intensive care unit. Depending on factors such as gestational age, birthweight, and other clinical issues, preterm infants may have health outcomes ranging from normal growth and development to developmental delay to cerebral palsy and other neurological disorders.

As a national health problem, premature births present a challenge to the health care system: The physical and emotional consequences place both the infant and family at increased risk not only for later health problems but also for increased and potentially inappropriate use of the health care system. HMOs are in a prime position to lessen the impact of premature births by creating supportive interventions for these families, efforts that have generally been proven to be effective in improving clinical and functional outcomes in the infant and family members.[9,10]

Clinical intervention programs, however, must be based on valid and reliable data. These data will help HMOs define the clinical areas of concern, identify the target population, and provide clinical indicators on how to provide the most high-quality, cost-effective care. Two types of data—primary and secondary clinical data—offer this capability. Primary clinical data include information used from interviews with patients and clinicians; secondary clinical data are collected from medical records, claims forms, or other administrative records. Data collected specifically for the purposes of the research are primary data, while secondary data are those data sets that were originally collected for another reason.

GROUNDWORK: CREATING THE DATA RESEARCH QUESTIONS

At Harvard Pilgrim Health Care in Boston, Massachusetts, clinicians and administrators used both primary and secondary data to design an intervention program to support, educate, and conduct follow-up on families with preterm infants.

The first and perhaps most important stage in collecting data to develop a clinical intervention program is identifying the problem, the characteristics of the target population, and the areas toward which the interventions can be aimed.[11] This stage began at Harvard Pilgrim Health Care in 1988 with clinical observations and research questions generated by a perinatal-neonatal team consisting of a maternal child nurse case manager, a neonatologist, and a neonatal clinical nurse specialist.

The research team noted that, at NICU discharge, parents of preterm infants are often very stressed by the high-risk pregnancy, the preterm birth experience, and the long infant stay in the NICU. Moreover, families have described these infants as intense and difficult to feed and console. Also, many of the infants are discharged home with equipment needs, such as apnea monitors and oxygen, as well as multiple follow-up appointments with their primary health care providers and medical specialists. Thus in the first months at home, the parents, already stressed at NICU discharge, may be overwhelmed with the daily care needs of the preterm infant.

The team then sought to answer several questions based on their observations, including: What are the characteristics of families who deliver preterm infants at the HMO; what are the health outcomes of these preterm infants in the first few years of life; and what in-house resources are used most often by these infants and their families? Answering these and other questions early on helps the clinician/researcher to project more accurately the issues involved at each stage of the research process, ultimately saving everyone time, energy, and money.

To help answer these questions, the Harvard research team adopted what is known as the Double ABCX Model of Family Adaptation.[12-14] This model, derived from family stress research, suggests that a family's vulnerability to crisis depends upon the interaction of the stressor (in this case the preterm infant) with both a family's existing resources (physical, emotional, and financial resources) and a family's perceptions (of the preterm infant). For example, when the preterm infant is discharged from the NICU, a family crisis may occur if the family's resources and perceptions interfere with their ability to cope and adapt to the care of the infant and family.

To answer the questions regarding family characteristics, health outcomes, and resources, the who, what, where, when, and why issues needed to be addressed.

The first question is, *what* is the purpose of the research? What types of data are necessary and available? The data should be distinguished between primary data (collected primarily for research purposes, such as patient interviews) and secondary data (data collected for other purposes such as from medical records or claims files). Secondary clinical data can be helpful because they contain health information on patients and their families but they may not contain all the variables needed to answer the questions.

Why are the clinical data necessary? Given the limitations of secondary clinical data, such as issues of reliability and lack of flexibility, can the clinical research questions be answered sufficiently using other data sources? *Where* are the data currently available? Are the data for specific patient encounters only available in the traditional handwritten format? If they are available in a less labor-intensive format, such as on computer disk, does the reporting format allow the research team to examine all the important variables? In addition, does the data need to be changed from its original format, such as from individual to family level data?

The *who* relates to the sample. Is the sample for the research easily identifiable in the data set or is manipulation of a larger clinical data set necessary? For data collection and analysis, questions also relate to who will collect the data and provide methodologic and statistical consultation, and what are these associated costs. In addition, is approval needed for access to the clinical data for research?

Finally, *when* are the data needed? Is there a timeline for the research process, and where do the primary and secondary data sources, including the use of clinical data, realistically fit into this timeline? For example, if the research findings from the analysis of the clinical data are needed to support a grant application for funding, the timeline should accurately reflect the issues in using a clinical data set for research.

USING RESEARCH TO DEFINE THE PROBLEM

In the first Harvard Pilgrim Health Care study examining infant health outcomes in the first year of life, the team found that the families who delivered preterm infants between 1987 and 1989 were different from those described previously by other investigators in the literature. The majority of the mothers were white, had an average age of 29 years at the preterm birth, and were married, reflecting families who are employed and have health insurance. In contrast, other previous research has described a high incidence of preterm births among African American adolescents.[15,16]

This first study illustrated several points. First, since the literature mostly described clinical interventions for families who were different from those delivering preterm infants at Harvard, those interventions may not be applicable to the health plan members. Second, the health plan preterm infants were consuming a high level of plan resources in their first year of life. Third, further research on this population was needed to confirm the sample characteristics, to examine health care use in the preterm family members (mother, father, siblings), to determine which health plan resources were used most frequently, and to quantify the impact of the preterm family on the plan by comparing them with families who delivered infants at term.

The team was then able to make several conclusions about the health outcomes and service use of the preterm and term families and their impact on the health plan over the first four years of life. First, the demographics of the preterm families remained consistent from the first study. Second, compared with term babies, preterm infants are seen more frequently for well visits and chronic visits in the first two years of life. In particular, the very low birthweight infants, less than 1,500 grams at birth, used the health plan's resources most frequently.

Third, although preterm infants need to be monitored more closely for growth and development, these infants also had many additional well visits to the health plan for guidance and parental reassurance related to feeding difficulties and temperament issues. Fourth, preterm infants and their families experienced a higher rate of acute illness and mental health problems than term infants and their families, especially in the first two years of life. Also, the areas of greatest use (well and chronic visits) can be the most amenable to clinical interventions. Fifth, the families of the preterm infants appeared to be stressed and experiencing a pile-up of demands, as measured by family health care service use.

The health plan research team determined that a supportive clinical intervention program in the first two years of the infant's life could benefit the families and the health plan. For the families, a family support program would provide support, education, and follow-up to improve family functioning and decrease adverse health outcomes in family members over the first two years after the birth. For the health plan, this intervention would potentially increase the family's satisfaction with their care and quality of life, while achieving economies by replacing many of the health center visits with close follow-up through home visits and telephone calls.

ISSUES IN USING CLINICAL DATA

Using a clinical data set for research, even one that is computerized, has advantages and limitations. Secondary data such as medical records can be helpful at the start of a research program to test ideas prior to undertaking a larger study.[17] Reliance on secondary data is less expensive than primary data and allows clinicians to track data over time and to use a larger sample size.

The clinical data set, however, has limitations. Measurement errors can occur during several phases: during the original data collection and documentation process, during the extraction of the data from the written encounter form into the computer and onto the data research forms, and during the last research phase as data are being interpreted.[18]

Inconsistencies were found in the health plan's clinical and demographic data, such as figures on infant birth parameters, race, parental occupation, and socioeconomic status. For example, specific infant birth parameters, such as apgar scores and length of stay in the nursery, were not consistently entered into the HMO computerized record of the infants born at term. The race of the infant was not always consistent with that reported for both parents.

Likewise, parental occupation was not consistently documented or updated even though there is a specific field for this variable on the encounter form. In addition, the socioeconomic status of families was difficult to determine from the medical record, since standard variables such as maternal and paternal education are not collected or recorded. As a result, socioeconomic status was not chosen as a variable. However, infant birth parameters, race, and parental occupation were used when they were found to be reliable for all members of the family.

Another consideration is whether secondary clinical data contain all the variables needed to answer the research questions. In fact, new variables may need to be created to portray important concepts, such as the pile-up of demands on the family as described by the Double ABCX Model of Family Adaptation. According to the model, *pile-up of demands* is an accumulation of demands on the family that occurs after they adjust to a crisis and involves the family's resources, perceptions, and behavioral responses.

To create a yearly family pile-up score, a health plan can calculate the number of visits each family member made to the HMO each year from the medical records of the infant, mother, father, and sibling(s). The Harvard Pilgrim Health Care team sought to determine not only the health care use of each family member but also the service use of the family as a whole.

The team also examined the intensity of the family pile-up demands. A new family variable was created by assigning weights to each type of visit according to its intensity (i.e., well visit = 1, least intense, to hospitalization = 5, most intense). For each family member for each year the number of visits were multiplied by their weights and divided by the number of people in the family that year. The final score reflected both the intensity and the frequency of health services used by the family each year.

Using clinical data for research and program planning also raises patient confidentiality issues. The federal government and most organizations have strict guidelines around the use of clinical data for research. However, when clinical data are collected to answer specific clinical questions related to practice, there may be confusion about whether this is practice improvement or research. As these clinical questions and projects arise they should be discussed with the health plan's institutional review board, which reviews research protocols involving human subjects.

ADDITIONAL DATA SOURCES

As the Harvard experience illustrates, secondary clinical data from medical records have limited ability in describing the full parameters of a problem and in targeting an area for intervention; primary data collection may be necessary. Perhaps the most important data source in designing a clinical intervention program such as a family support program is the target group: the family of the preterm infant. Especially important are family members' perspectives on the issues facing them individually and as a family and their suggestions on areas the intervention could target.

Parents noted that support from their family and friends was less than they would have liked during the infant's NICU experience and even up through the first year of life.[19] They sensed that people were afraid to congratulate them on the birth and ask them about the infant's progress for fear of not being able to provide adequate support. The parents also commented that professional support was readily available and appreciated while the infant was in the NICU; however, after discharge they felt alone, as if they had "dropped off into the vast nothingness." Early intervention services were helpful but sporadic and did not always meet the parent's needs.

When asked how the infant's pediatric primary care provider could be more helpful, family members expressed a need for more age-adjusted developmental counseling and a more realistic discussion about potential health and developmental issues. For example, they noted that the primary care providers were often so eager to avoid a potential vulnerable child syndrome that they extensively reassured the parents that the preterm infant was "normal." However, the parents noted that reassurance was not enough; they also wanted acknowledgement that their infant's developmental progress may be different than for those born at term and guidance in assessing the infant's progress over time.

Another source of primary data are the clinicians who care for these preterm infants and their families. Clinicians in pediatrics, obstetrics, mental health, case management, and specialty pediatric programs can provide an important perspective on the most difficult times for families and the interventions that seemed to be most effective. Ultimately, they help determine whether a family support program is needed and what it will look like.

In individual and group interviews, the clinicians described areas of improvement. For example, the pediatric clinicians said that in caring for medically complex infants they often "feel as overwhelmed as the family." Because these infants are seen in many different pediatric practices, individual clinicians do not have a large enough caseload to allow them to feel completely comfortable in managing complex clinical issues in this special population, such as reading pneumograms and manipulating multiple medications. They also noted that, because their focus was often on the medical issues of the preterm infant, they were perhaps not as sensitive to family issues as they should be. Therefore, any family support program for preterm infants should include both clinician-centered and family-centered interventions.

ADDITIONAL DATA USES

The Harvard data collection process demonstrates that primary data from preterm families and their clinicians and the quantitative analysis of the secondary clinical data regarding family health outcomes and service use were crucial in defining the scope of the problem and determining an effective intervention. Clinical data are also useful in other steps in designing a clinical intervention program. For example, one might expect that if parent support groups were to be used given the demographics of the plan's preterm families (thirties, working couples), the groups would have to be creative and flexible in their structure. They would have to be held in the evening; provide child care arrangements; and, because the HMO coverage area is geographically diverse, be held in different regions.

Clinical data can also serve to build internal support for the intervention. The findings from research can serve not only to convince clinical managers that an intervention is needed but also to describe better the clinical issues. At Harvard Pilgrim, clinicians in obstetrics, pediatrics, neonatology, and case management have been supportive of this research because it provides answers to some of their own clinical questions. For example, although prenatal care was not the focus of the study, the HMO's team was able to examine the differences in prenatal care for mothers who deliver prematurely. Preliminary data showed that even when adjusted for the shortened gestation, mothers of the low birthweight infants received less prenatal care than mothers of term infants. These findings will be shared with obstetric clinicians and managers.

Also important is identifying internal HMO and external community resources already available to meet the needs of families in this area. Internally, the Developmental Consultation Service provides consultation and case management services to families with medically complex infants and children. In the community, the early intervention program provides follow-up for infants at risk, and parent support groups in the hospitals provide support during the intense NICU period.[20,21]

TOWARD THE FUTURE

The Harvard Pilgrim Health Care experience demonstrates how clinical data can contribute to the design of a clinical intervention program. The effort also indicates how health plan researchers and other staff using clinical data have an important role in advising their organizations on issues such as how the data set could be improved and which new variables should be added. Moreover, the HMO's experience provides a guide to other health plans on determining the clinical indicators within their organizations for improving care for chronically ill populations.

REFERENCES

1. McCormick, M. "Longterm Follow-up of Infants Discharged from Neonatal Intensive Care Units." *Journal of the American Medical Association* 261 (1989):1767–1771.
2. Hack, M., et al. "Rehospitalization of the Very Low Birthweight Infant: A Continuum of Perinatal and Environmental Morbidity."*American Journal of Diseases in Children*, 135 (1981):263–266.
3. Office of Technology Assessment. United States Congress. *Neonatal Intensive Care for Low Birthweight Infants: Costs and Effectiveness.* DHHS Publ.No. OTA-HCS-38. Washington, D.C.: Government Printing Office, 1987.
4. Shankaran, S., et al. "Medical Care Costs of High Risk Infants after Discharge from the Newborn Intensive Care Unit." *Pediatrics* 81 (1988):372–378.
5. Lewitt, E., and Monheit, A. "Expenditures on Health Care for Children and Pregnant Women." *The Future of Children* 2 (1992):95–114.
6. Hunt, J., Cooper, B., and Tooley, W. "Very Low Birthweight Infants at 8 and 11 Years of Age: Role of Neonatal Illness and Family Status." *Pediatrics* 82 (1989):596–603.
7. Affleck, G., Tennen, H., and Power, J. "Mothers, Fathers and the Crisis of Newborn Intensive Care." *Infant Mental Health Journal* 11 (1990):12–25.
8. Gennaro, S. "Maternal Anxiety and Problem Solving Ability in Mothers of Premature Infants." *Journal of Obstetric, Gynecologic and Neonatal Nursing* 15 (1986):160–164.
9. Brooten, D., et al. "A Randomized Clinical Trial of Early Hospital Discharge and Home Follow-up of Very Low Birth Weight Infants." *New England Journal of Medicine* 3(15) (1986):934–939.
10. Elmer, E., and Maloni, J. "Parent Support through Telephone Consultation." *Journal of Maternal Child Nursing* 17 (1988):13–23.
11. Dumka, L., et al. "Using Research and Theory to Develop Prevention Programs for High Risk Families." *Family Relations* 44 (1995):78–86.
12. Feetham, S. "Conceptual and Methodological Issues in the Research of Families." In *Family Theory Development in Nursing: State of the Science and Art*, ed. A. Whall and J. Fawcett. Philadelphia, PA: F. A. Davis, 1991.
13. Gilliss, C. "Family Research in Nursing." In *Toward a Science of Family Nursing*, ed. C. Gilliss, B. Highley, and I. Martinson. Menlo Park, CA: Addison-Wesley, 1989.
14. McCubbin, H., and Patterson, J. "Family Transitions: Adaptation to Stress." In *Stress and the Family, Volume I: Coping with Normative Transitions*, ed. H. McCubbin and C. Figley. New York, NY: Bruner/Mazel, 1983.
15. Brown, L., et al. "A Sociodemographic Profile of Families of Low Birthweight Infants." *Western Journal of Nursing Research* 11 (1989):520–532.
16. Combs-Orme, T., et al. "Rehospitalization of Very Low Birthweight Infants." *American Journal of Diseases in Children* 142 (1988):1109–1113.
17. Woods, N., and Cantanzaro, M. *Nursing Research: Theory and Practice.* St. Louis, MO: C.V. Mosby, 1988.

18. Aaronson, L., and Burman, M. "The Use of Health Records in Research: Reliability and Validity Issues." *Research in Nursing and Health* 17 (1994):67–73.

19. Smith, K., et al. "Parental Opinions about Attending Parent Support Groups." *Children's Health Care* 23 (1994):127–136.

20. Zelle, R. "Follow-up of At-Risk Infants in the Home Setting: Consultation Model." *Journal of Gynecologic and Neonatal Nursing* 24 (1995):51–55.

21. Pless, I., et al. "A Randomized Trial of a Nursing Intervention to Promote the Adjustment of Children with Chronic Physical Disorders." *Pediatrics* 94 (1994):70–75.

20

Using Data to Design Systems of Care for Adults with Chronic Illness

Gerri S. Lamb, Vicky Mahn, and Rebecca Dahl

ATTEMPTS TO ORGANIZE CARE

Most health care systems are seeking effective strategies to organize care for their chronically ill members. Major efforts attempt to bridge acute care and long-term care for older adults with chronic illness. For example, the National Chronic Care Consortium, a group of 22 health care organizations known for their innovations in integrating care for older adults, has focused on developing tools and systems to improve care for the chronically ill.[1]

Like many other groups, the consortium has identified several goals of an effective delivery system:

- early identification of individuals likely to use extensive high-cost services
- timely coordination and initiation of alternative and less expensive services, including primary care and community-based programs
- improvements or slowed decline in functional independence and quality of life
- reductions in avoidable complications
- reductions in avoidable hospitalizations and emergency visits.

Source: Reprinted from G.S. Lamb, V. Mahn, and R. Dahl, Using Data to Design Systems of Care for Adults with Chronic Illness, *Managed Care Quarterly*, Vol. 4, No. 3, pp. 46–53, © 1996, Aspen Publishers, Inc.

Selecting appropriate programs to achieve these goals can be a difficult task. The current literature is filled with recommendations on how to improve the quality and costs of care for older adults with chronic conditions. In fact, popular strategies, such as risk screening, case management, critical pathways, and discharge planning teams, have vocal and persuasive advocates.

Yet while many practitioners have an appreciation of the systems and approaches needed to improve care for this population, tested guidelines and tools are not readily available, and no information is available on how one strategy complements or overlaps with another. A review of the literature on risk screening, for example, indicates that previous efforts to predict high-risk populations have had limited success.[2,3] Readily available data elements, such as age or medical diagnosis, only provide a partial picture as predictors, and the costs of automating risk screening instruments are usually significant.

Moreover, the current marketplace competition to introduce new services and products places extreme pressure on health care organizations to implement underdeveloped and untested strategies. Even the definition and practice of case management causes confusion among its users, and data supporting the efficacy of various case management models are inconsistent.[4,5] As a result, many health care organizations have implemented case management based on anecdotal data, rather than concrete evidence supporting consistent quality and cost outcomes.

DESIGNING A SYSTEM

Most health care organizations recognize that there are few quick fixes to improve systems of care and that most strategies that aim to improve care for the chronically ill adult have both significant merits and drawbacks.

Faced with the escalating costs of caring for a growing number of older adults with chronic illness, providers and payers must define their goals and implement strategies best suited to achieving quality and cost outcomes. Yet many organizations may overlook readily accessible data that will help them redesign chronic care services to define and achieve these goals and strategies.

Carondelet Health Care Network (CHN) a health care system based in Tucson, Arizona, faced this same dilemma. In its managed care contracts, CHN provides hospital, emergency room, and ambulatory services, and shares financial risk with HMOs and their affiliated physicians. Over the last five years, the organization has experienced a significant increase in the number of capitated contracts it holds with Medicare risk plans. More recently, CHN has sought to include the full set of acute and chronic care services within its capitated service package.

Although CHN historically has been attentive to quality of care issues and cost effectiveness, the shift to capitated financing led to increased awareness of outcomes such as hospital readmissions that are associated with significant financial loss. Shortly after operating with capitated financing, CHN administrators and staff noted that readmission rates for the Medicare population were higher than desired and appeared to be increasing rather than declining. The combined direct and indirect expenses associated with an 11 percent readmission rate in one Medicare risk plan of 20,000 members, for example, were approximately $7 million—all viewed as a financial loss under capitated risk-based financing.

A readmission task force was convened consisting of the medical directors of each of the system hospitals, the directors for quality resource management, and representatives from case management, home health, and social work programs. Individuals with extensive experience in discharge planning and transitional care were sought as members. The task force's ultimate goal was to reduce the rate of unplanned hospital readmissions for older adults.

Over the course of approximately six months, the readmission task force defined the scope of the readmission problem and set the stage for implementing and evaluating potential solutions. The group proceeded through four distinctive phases: examining current practices relevant to readmission rates; capitalizing on easily accessible data; conducting focused data collection; and summarizing the results of the previous phases as a prelude to selecting intervention and evaluation strategies. Key aspects of each of these phases and illustrative examples are provided in the following sections.

PHASE 1: EXAMINING CURRENT PRACTICE

The CHN readmission task force used the continuous quality improvement (CQI) approach to guide their efforts. CQI offers a systematic process to analyze, measure, and evaluate clinical problems and the impact of subsequent changes. This approach is particularly useful when an aspect of clinical care is shown to be problem-prone, high-volume, expensive, and of particular interest to a group of clinicians and administrators.[6] The care of individuals with chronic illness involves complex coordination of providers and services across multiple settings and often results in the identification of several problematic aspects of care, including hospital readmission.

As a first step, task force members identified possible reasons for the escalating readmission rates. Through brainstorming, members offered a number of factors: gaps in coordination and discharge planning; ineffective targeting of individuals at risk for readmission; premature discharge; lag in initiation of home-based services; growing restrictions on the use of home health services within capitated contracts; confusion between the roles and responsibilities of hospital-based discharge planners and payer-based case managers; and patients unable to afford medications prescribed at discharge. Initially, the medical directors suggested that the majority of readmissions were due to exacerbations of chronic medical conditions and thus, in their view, were largely unavoidable.

Several group members offered case examples to illustrate how and why the system "broke down" for individuals who were readmitted. Their stories highlighted the complexity of coordinating care across multiple services and the considerable frustration associated with fragmentation and poor communication. During this phase, however, a number of people became impatient to "do something" and began to suggest solutions to fix the readmission problem.

Often in the problem identification phase team members can get overly enamored or overwhelmed with the complexity of the task and spend too much time recounting past "horror stories." Much more problematic from a data management and outcomes perspective, however, is when the group bypasses defining and systematically analyzing the clinical problem driving the CQI process. A premature leap into implementing solutions often has several adverse effects. At some point, members recognize that they were not clear initially on what they wanted to accomplish and have wasted considerable time collecting too little, too much, or largely irrelevant data.

Information systems specialists become thoroughly frustrated with time-consuming requests for more information and customized reports than they doubt anyone will use. Potentially resource-intensive and time-consuming interventions will have been tried with little probability of demonstrating substantial impact on the problem.

After several meetings, members of the CHCC task force recognized that their shift into interventions was premature. The group leader encouraged them to identify data that would help them move forward.

PHASE 2: CAPITALIZING ON AVAILABLE DATA

The collection of meaningful data to support CQI activities for populations with chronic conditions is best carried out through automated information systems. In order to capitalize on available data, organizations first must be clear on what questions they are attempting to answer and the data required to answer the questions.

More and more, health care organizations are moving toward information systems that capture and link clinical and fiscal data across multiple settings.[7] These systems provide an ideal support for designing, implementing, and evaluating new programs of care for chronically ill adults.

In the absence of fully integrated information systems, the basic requirements for information support include the capability to:

- access demographic, clinical, and fiscal information by individual member or patient
- link demographic, clinical, and fiscal information in the same data file
- add new data elements, such as health risk items or outcome indicators
- analyze data and report results using descriptive and predictive statistics.

In most cases, it is more efficient and cost-effective to rely on data that are readily available than to create or request the entry of new data elements. Moreover, available data elements can be used in new combinations to estimate previously unmeasured events. For example, while most hospital information systems do not attempt to capture high-risk indicators, a combination of available demographic variables and utilization variables, such as age, gender, hospital and emergency room use, and discharge disposition, can provide a reasonable base from which to measure risk.[8] Recently, CHN and a partner in its integrated network combined data on use of hospital, emergency room, case management, home health, durable medical equipment, and pharmacy with physician ratings of risk for hospitalization in order to identify high-risk members in one senior health plan.

To move into the phase of data collection and analysis, the CHN readmission task force decided to begin by examining available data related to readmission rates. Easily accessible data consisted of monthly and annual readmission rates by payer group, medical diagnoses for readmissions, and time (hours or days) between initial and subsequent readmission. All readmissions that occurred within 30 days of the previous discharge were examined.

Review of these data indicated that one payer, a large HMO in southern Arizona, had a higher than average readmission rate (Table 20–1). The readmission rate for Payer 1 was 11.8 percent compared with an overall hospital readmission rate of 9.1 percent and an overall Medicare readmission rate of 11.2 percent. For this payer, the majority of readmissions occurred soon after the previous discharge and were associated with a relatively small set of medical diagnoses.

Table 20–1 Evaluation of Accessible Data

Hospital admission-readmission profile

Total hospital admissions	11,581
Average length of stay (days)	4.0
Readmissions within 30 days	1,055
Readmission rate (whole hospital)	9.1%
Readmission rate for Payer 1	**11.8%**

Readmission rates by major diagnostic category (MDC) for Payer 1 (%)

MDC 1 Central Nervous System	10
MDC 4 Respiratory	10
MDC 5 Circulatory	**15**
MDC 6 Gastrointestinal	12
MDC 8 Skeletal	12

Readmission rates by diagnosis

DRG 127 (Congestive Heart Failure)	**18%**

Readmission rates by days since last admission (%)

0–7 Days	**41**
8–14 Days	24
15–21 Days	19
22–30 Days	16

The major diagnostic categories (MDCs) associated with the greatest percentage of readmissions for Payer 1 were, in descending order, circulatory, gastrointestinal, skeletal, respiratory, and central nervous system diseases. Diagnosis-related group (DRG) 127, congestive heart failure, had the highest percentage of readmissions. Almost two-thirds of the readmissions for this one payer occurred within two weeks of the initial discharge. Forty-one percent of the people who were readmitted within 30 days came back into the hospital within one week. Approximately one-half of the readmissions within the first week occurred in the first 72 hours.

CHN staff nurses had previously used a brief four-item risk screening instrument to identify high-risk individuals during hospitalization. The screening tool was intended to trigger closer scrutiny by members of the social work department. Questions on the risk screening tool included use of hospital or emergency room services in the past month, need for assistance with activities of daily living and instrumental activities of daily living (e.g., shopping, transportation, housekeeping), difficulty managing required self-care skills like medication management, and evidence of significant difficulty coping with the demands of illness.

Since the risk screening tools were not automated, review of these data required more labor-intensive, but still relatively brief record review. The task force's examination of the risk assessment tools identified several important shortcomings. In a random review of 104 records, 16 percent of the tools had not been completed. In several instances, individuals who were subsequently readmitted were not identified as high-risk for readmission, indicating that the screening instrument had limited predictive power and that substantial modification was needed.

PHASE 3: FOCUSED DATA COLLECTION

At this point, task force members identified a need for more detailed information about clinical practice patterns and patient perceptions about readmission. Since this next phase would require the collection of less accessible data, group members elected to focus on the risk plan (Payer 1) with the greatest enrollment and the highest readmission rate, and with whom the hospital shared the greatest financial risk for readmission rates. A representative of the risk plan became an active member of the task force. The analysis conducted with the selected risk plan was expected to become a prototype for subsequent analyses of readmission patterns for all CHN contracts.

For this phase of data collection, committee members planned to supplement available data by interviewing members of the targeted risk plan who had been readmitted to the hospitals and by concurrently reviewing their medical records. The goals of the survey were to identify factors that patients believed had contributed to their readmission and to complete an audit trail of the discharge planning process to uncover patterns of care associated with readmission. In addition, the medical directors reviewed the medical care of each participant in the survey.

A questionnaire was designed to capture the patient's perspective of the events leading up to hospital admission. Patients were asked the following questions:

- Tell me what happened when you left the hospital last time.
- What brought you back to the hospital?
- When you left the hospital the last time, did you think that you might need to come back again?
- Do you think that anything could have been done differently that would have changed the need for you to come back here?

Patients were led through a chronological review of their experience beginning with the previous admission to the present. A structured interview format and data collection tool was developed to improve the consistency of data collection. The interviews were conducted by an experienced social worker.

The concurrent chart review focused on discharge planning during the previous admission and reasons for readmission (Table 20–2). A retired home health administrator with extensive experience in discharge planning and coordination of home-based services volunteered to complete the chart reviews. At the end of the chart review, this individual was asked to comment on whether, in her experienced opinion, the current admission could be considered avoidable.

The results of 25 interviews and chart reviews were illuminating. The majority of participants had not received any home-based services, although a number of people felt that they had left the hospital feeling "weak" and not yet ready to manage their own care. In most cases, the records indicated that each of the people who had been interviewed had

---

Table 20–2 Selected Indicators from Readmission Interview and Chart Review

Retrospective review from previous admission	Concurrent review upon readmission
1. Date of discharge _____	1. Date of readmission _____
2. Discharge diagnosis _____	2. Diagnosis _____
3. Evaluated by social work? ❑ Yes ❑ No	3. Reason for Readmission (patient's words): _____
4. Services arranged on discharge:	_____
Home health ❑ Yes ❑ No	_____
Nurse case management ❑ Yes ❑ No	4. Primary readmission contributors:
Community assistance ❑ Yes ❑ No	❑ Progression of disease
	❑ Recurrence of previous symptoms
	❑ Failure to address abnormal lab values
	❑ Failure to perform adequate discharge planning
	❑ Failure to provide timely home health or community services
	❑ Failure of home health or community services to provide services adequate to need
	❑ Failure to get access to needed medical care in a timely way
	❑ Patient failure to recognize or act on early symptoms of exacerbation
	❑ Other (specify): _____

been asked prior to discharge if they thought they "needed any help at home." The majority refused any assistance.

In situations where home-based services, such as home health, were ordered, the services were not always provided within the first 24 to 48 hours of discharge. More than half the participants readmitted were advised by their physicians to return to the hospital. Physician comments to the reviewer suggested that they felt that the hospital or the emergency room, rather than community services, were their best option for timely and responsive care.

In addition, the physicians reviewing the medical records identified potentially problematic trends in medical care that might have contributed to the unplanned readmissions. In specific instances, the physician reviewers questioned the accuracy of discharge diagnoses and the adequacy of treatment during the previous admission.

PHASE 4: SUMMARIZING THE DATA

The results of the data review and interview data were summarized and key points for subsequent program design were identified:

- The majority of readmissions were for three diagnoses: congestive heart failure, pleural effusion, and pneumonia. In a number of instances, the diagnoses of these conditions appeared to overlap.
- The largest percentage of readmissions occurred within the first week of discharge, and within that week the majority of readmissions were in the first 72 hours.
- Individuals who were subsequently readmitted typically refused assistance at home although they recalled feeling "weak" and concerned about being able to manage their care at home.
- Readmissions were associated with gaps in initiation of services between hospital and home.
- Readmission patterns were influenced by physician preferences for use of acute care rather than community-based services.
- The risk screening instrument currently used to identify individuals at risk of hospital readmission did not adequately predict readmission patterns.

Based on these findings, the committee decided to focus the next phase of its work on the group of risk plan members with diagnoses of congestive heart failure and pneumonia. The committee was reconstructed to include key clinical people involved in the care of individuals with congestive heart failure and pneumonia in both the hospital and community settings. This group, supplemented with consultants in information systems, finance, and outcomes measurement, was charged with designing a systematic and comprehensive approach to care for older adults with the targeted diagnoses.

All of the data collected during the problem specification phase are integral to the selection of proposed intervention and evaluation strategies. Data on the current risk identification instrument indicated that it required significant modification to improve its predictive ability. Task force members are in the process of designing more effective instruments to identify individuals with the target conditions who are at high risk of readmission (Table 20–3). The proposed risk indicators integrate clinical parameters (e.g., ejection fraction or history of myocardial infarction) and service use patterns (e.g., past history of hospital or emergency room use) with patient perceptions of their health and functional well-being.

Analysis of available data identified the period immediately following discharge as the most vulnerable time for readmission. Therefore, the initial focus of the group is on identifying and carrying out strategies that enhance timely coordination between hospital and community settings. Of particular interest are those interventions that will: improve acceptance of community follow-up as an expected component of care for high-risk individuals; maximize the likelihood that critical self-care skills, like symptom and medication management, are assessed and reinforced across service settings; and assure timely linkages between hospital and community care. The task force identified each of these areas through the collection and analysis of accessible data sources.

At the same time that the task force deliberates on response strategies, an evaluation team is working on outcome indicators that will determine the extent to which task force goals are accomplished. Performance measures will include the counts of readmission rates for the targeted conditions and percentage of readmissions within diagnosis (Table 20–4). In addition, task force members have expressed an interest in capturing process indicators, such as self-care management of symptoms and medications, that the literature and clinical experience have indicated are integral to the achievement of reduced readmissions.[9]

FUTURE OUTLOOK

Faced with an urgent need to redesign chronic care services across the continuum, organizations often overlook readily accessible and useful data. By creatively using and supplementing available data they can provide a more cost-effective foundation for selecting and evaluating programs for chronically ill older adults than is the current norm.

Table 20–3 Sample of Readmission Risk Factor Matrix

Risk factor	Measures	Definition	Formula	Source
No. hospital admissions in previous 6 months for CHF or pneumonia		Count	Total admits	ICD-9 codes, DRGs
Functional status	Selected ADL measures	Number of dependent ADLs	Total	Nursing admission assessment
Perception of health status	SF-36 (Ware, 1993)	Score on items of SF-36	Scoring instructions SF-36	Interview
Polypharmacy	No. of prescription medications at discharge	Count	Total	Discharge orders

The experiences at Carondelet demonstrate that it is possible, within the constraints of using available staff and limited resources, to use readily accessible data to systematically analyze a major clinical problem and design relevant programs in response. In order to maximize the effectiveness and efficiency of this process, organizations undertaking similar projects are encouraged to:

- clearly specify the problem and intended goal before requesting supporting data or generating solutions
- identify all possible sources of data relevant to the problem
- review the match between problem, goal, measurement indicators, and suggested solutions at regular intervals
- not underestimate the importance of understanding the clinical process underlying the problem before attempting to choose measurement indicators or initiate changes
- analyze the cost benefit of collecting additional data before undertaking any time-consuming data collection projects.

Health care organizations cannot afford to wait to analyze expensive clinical problems until the ideal information systems are in place. As dem-

Table 20–4 Sample Outcome Matrix for CHF Pilot

Outcome	Measures	Definition	Formula	Source
Readmission for CHF	Readmission: 30 days 60 days 90 days 180 days	Count	Total readmits	Discharge Diagnosis IDC-9 codes DRGs
% individuals with CHF readmitted with CHF		Count	Total no. of readmissions with discharge dx of CHF divided by total no. with discharge dx of CHF	Discharge Diagnosis ICD-9 codes DRGs
Self-care ability	Symptom management	Count	Total score	Survey
Identification of high-risk CHF individuals	Systolic ventricular function (ejection fraction)	Select ≤ 30 31–40 41–50 ≥ 51	Distribution of readmissions from each ejection fraction range	Echocardiogram Cath Lab report Medical H&P

onstrated in the Carondelet project, a simple, yet focused analysis of available data has the potential to result in more effective use of resources and substantial cost savings.

REFERENCES

1. National Chronic Care Consortium. *An Introduction to the National Chronic Care Consortium: Transforming America's Approach to Chronic Care.* Bloomington, MN: National Chronic Care Consortium, 1994.
2. Anderson, G.F., and Steinberg, E.P. "Predicting Hospital Readmission in the Medicare Population." *Inquiry* 22 (1985):251–258.
3. Corrigan, J.M., and Martin, J.B. "Identification of Factors Associated with Hospital Admission and Development of a Predictive Model." *Health Services Research* 27(1) (1992):81–101.
4. Lyon, J.C. "Models of Nursing Care Delivery and Case Management: Clarification of Terms." *Nursing Economics* 11 (1993):163–169.
5. Lamb, G. "Case Management." *Annual Review of Nursing Research* 13 (1995):117–136.

6. Mahn, V., and Heller, C. "Clinical Paths at Carondelet St.Joseph's Hospital." In *Clinical Paths: Tools for Outcome Management*, ed. P. Spath. Chicago: American Hospital Publishing, Inc., 1994.
7. Ellsasser, K.H., Nkobi, J., and Kohler, C.O. "Distributing Databases: A Model for Global, Shared Care." *Healthcare Informatics* 12(1) (1995):62–68.
8. Burns, L.R., Lamb, G.S., and Wholey, D.R. "Impact of Integrated Community Nursing Services on Hospital Utilization and Costs in a Medicare Risk Plan." *Inquiry* 33(1) (1996):30–41.
9. Dracup, K., et al. "Management of Heart Failure: Counseling, Education and Lifestyle Modifications." *Journal of the American Medical Association* 272(18) (1994):1442–1445.

Index

A

Acute care
  compared to chronic care, 6–7, 10
  Health Plan of Nevada, 84
AIDS program
  children, 209
  Community Medical Alliance,
    140–142
Asthma care, 156–172
  asthma guides, 156–157
  asthma peak flow diary, 162–163
  daily preventive treatment, 161
  data collection/analysis, 169–170
  early diagnosis, 158–159
  first site visit schedule, 158
  home care visit care, 165
  implementation issues, 170–172
  inhalation devices, 159–161
  monitoring of patient status, 161
  oral steroids, use of, 159
  patient education, 161, 164–169, 206
  second site visit schedule, 159
  See also Childhood asthma

B

Behavioral medicine, pain
  management, 176–177

Benchmarking, 117
Boundary problem, of managed care,
  15
Breast cancer, 26–29
  areas for measurement
    development, 47
  cost effectiveness of interventions, 28
  efficacy of interventions, 27
  health plan and interventions, 28–29
  improving quality of care, 27–28
  prevalence of, 26–27
Bright Futures, 203
British Chronic Care Clinic, 110–111
Bureau of Maternal and Child Health,
  215

C

Capitation, incentives related to, 4
Cards, sent by volunteers, 76
Carondelet Health Care Network
  (CHN) data system, 286–297
  collection of available data,
    289–292
  design of system, 287–288
  examination of current practice,
    288–289
  focused data collection process,
    292–294

299

future view for, 295–297
summarizing data, 294–295
Carve-outs
    and cost control, 230–231
    mental health care, 230–231, 234, 235
Case management
    assessment of patient cases,
        67–69
    chronic childhood conditions, 208–
        209
    continuum of care, 63
    data availability, 65–66
    definition of, 62
    evaluation of outcome measures,
        69–71
    financial incentives, 66–67
    of Health Plan of Nevada. See Health
        Plan of Nevada case management
    limitations to effectiveness of, 71–72
    provider relations, 64
    staffing/training, 64–65
    teams for, 97
    compared to utilization
        management, 62–63
Case Management Society of America,
    69
Child and Adolescent Service System
    Program (CASSP),
    248–249, 250
Childhood asthma, 43–46
    areas for measurement
        development, 48
    cost effectiveness of interventions,
        46
    efficacy of interventions, 44–45
    health plan and interventions, 46
    improving quality of care, 45–46
    prevalence of, 43
Children
    childhood asthma, 43–46
    disability, causes of, 199–200
    See also Chronic childhood
        conditions
Chronic benign pain syndrome,
    173–182
    assessment of, 173–174

behavioral medicine/health
    psychology, 176–177
caregiver lack of expertise, 175
Chronic Daily Headache Program,
    180–181
and health care delivery system, 175
management complications, 174
pain education group, 179–180
primary care provider attitudes
    about, 174
Skills Not Pills program, 176,
    177–179
special issues for managed care,
    175–176
successful implementation of,
    181–182
treatment as acute pain, 174–175
Chronic care
    compared to acute care, 6–7, 10
    deficiencies in, 104–106
    effective models of, 11–12,
        106–107
    evidence-based, planned care,
        108–109
    feedback in, 114–115
    future view for care, 117–118
    generalist versus specialist in,
        113–114
    in Germany, 107, 113
    in Great Britain, 107, 110–111
    integrated systems, 115–116
    and managed care, 116–117
    patient self-management in, 111–113
    practice redesign, 109–111
    profile of current care, 11
    registries, 114–115
    in Sweden, 107
Chronic childhood conditions
    access to specialty care, 216
    care challenges, 200–201
    care planning process, 219
    comprehensive case management,
        208–209
    coordination with social services,
        209–211
    educational programs, 206–207

enhancement of care, elements of, 201
enrollment of patients in HMOs, 197–198
flexible gatekeeping arrangements, 207–208
future view for, 219–220
information needs of HMOs, 214–216
information sources for HMOs, 215
management of, 200
multidisciplinary teams, 204–205
patient partnerships with HMOs, 218
protocols and quality practice, 216–218
screening and risk assessment, 203–204
specially trained providers in, 201–202
types of, 198–199
Chronic illness
and children. *See* Chronic childhood conditions
definition of, 9
managed care, optimal situation, 12–13
and modern medical treatment, 9–10
patient needs, 104
Claims database, 260–261
Class rates, 233
Colorectal cancer, 29–33
areas for measurement development, 47
cost effectiveness of interventions, 32–33
efficacy of interventions, 29–32
health plan and interventions, 33
potential for quality improvement, 32
prevalence of, 29
screening methods, 29–32
Community-based social service programs, and HMOs, 4–5
Community Medical Alliance AIDS program, 140–142
cost/utilization, 144–146
enrollment, 142–143
enrollment criteria, 138
nurse practitioner, role of, 139–140
policy context, 135–136
quality monitoring, 147–149
rationale for, 136–137
satisfaction levels, 143–144
severe physical disability program, 137–139
strategies in development of, 149–150
types of services, 137
Community Mental Health Center movement, 247–248
Community Mental Health Centers Acts, 231, 234
Community Support System (CSS), 248, 250
Complex case management
Health Plan of Nevada, 85, 86–88
indicators for referral to, 85
Comprehensive case management, chronic childhood conditions, 208–209
Computerized practice guidelines
focus group information on, 187–188
future view, 192–193
hospital system, use of, 185–186
ideal system, elements of, 191
key markers of disease progression, 188–189
multispecialty group, use of, 186–187
oversight of system, 191
provider acceptance of, 183–184, 185, 189–191
vendor capability, 191–192
Consensus building, 99
Cooperative health care clinic, 125–132
case selection, 126–128
expansion of program, 130–131
future view for, 131–132
positive outcomes from, 128–129
Coordinated care, meaning of, 93–94

Coronary artery disease, 21–26
  areas for measurement
    development, 46–47
  cost effectiveness of interventions,
    25–26
  diagnosis/treatment methods, 24
  efficacy of interventions, 21–24
  health plans and interventions, 26
  improving quality of care, 24–25
  mortality figures, 21
  risk factors in, 22–23
Custodial care, Health Plan of Nevada,
  85

D

Database
  claims database, 260–261
  encounters database, 260
  laboratory data database, 261
  membership database, 261
  pharmacy database, 261
  U.S. Quality Algorithms (USQA)
    Health Profile Database,
    260–274
Depression. See Major depression
DIABEDS program, 113
Diabetes Care and Complications
  (DCCT), 14
Diabetes Control and Complications
  Trial, 106
Diabetes mellitus, 40–43
  areas for measurement
    development, 48
  cost effectiveness of interventions,
    43
  efficacy of interventions, 41–42
  health plan and interventions, 43
  improving quality of care, 42–43
  prevalence of, 40
  types of, 40–41
Dilution, pitfall to case management,
  71
Dual task theory, 105

E

Education, asthma care, 161, 164–169,
  206
Educational programs, chronic
  childhood conditions, 206–207
Encounters database, 260
Evidence-based, planned care, 108–109

F

Family, integration into care model, 12
Family Voices, 219
Federation for Children with Special
  Needs, 218
Friendly caller volunteers, 76
Friendly companions, 76
Friendly telephone programs, 5
Functional status, and chronic care
  systems, 12

G

Germany, chronic care in, 107, 113
Great Britain, chronic care in, 107, 110–
  111
Group Health Cooperative, 108
Group Health of Puget Sound, 113–
  114, 204

H

Harvard Community Health Plan, 114,
  205, 209
Harvard Pilgrim Health Care, mental
  health care, 223–232
HEADS-SET, 204
Health Alliance Plan, 94
Health Assessment Questionnaire
  (HAQ), 67
Health fairs, 76
Health maintenance organizations
  (HMOs)
  and chronic care, 116–117, 150–151

improvement process for, 13–15
innovations related to, 5–6
issues related to, 3–4, 15–17
HealthPartners, 210
Health Plan Employer Data and
Information System (HEDIS)
quality measures in, 18
See also Quality assessment
measures
Health Plan of Nevada
home health benefits, 77
organization of, 73–74
risk assessment methods, 75
Senior Dimensions Service Center,
74–75
subacute/rehabilitative care, 77–78
volunteer program, 75–77
Health Plan of Nevada case
management, 78–92
acute institutional in-area, 84
acute institutional out-of-area, 84
complex case management, 85,
86–88
custodial setting, 85
high/moderate/low intensity
interventions, 86
improved care coordination model,
89–91
institutional case management, 81, 84
levels of intensity, 81, 82
oversight, 86
philosophy of, 79–80
program characteristics, 81
subacute skilled nursing, 84–85
timeline of events, 79, 80–81
Health psychology, pain management,
176–177
Healthy People 2000, 22
Healthy Start Postnatal Screen, 204
Healthy Start Program, 210
Henry Ford Health System, 94
Home care
integration with medical care, 11–12
types of services, 77

Housing, mental health care, 224
Hypertension Detection and Follow-
up Program, 106

I

Incentives
and case management, 66–67
related to capitation, 4
Individuals with Disabilities Education
Act, 215
Information systems
Carondelet Health Care Network
(CHN) data system, 286–297
on preterm infants, 276–284
U.S. Quality Algorithms (USQA)
Health Profile Database,
260–274
Integrated care
for chronic illness care, 115–116
meaning of, 93–94
primary care models, 115–116

K

Kaiser Permanente Colorado,
cooperative health care clinic,
125–132

L

Laboratory data database, 261
Layering, pitfall to case management,
71
Low back pain, 33–38
areas for measurement
development, 47–48
cost effectiveness of interventions, 37
efficacy of interventions, 34–36
health plan and interventions, 37–38
improving quality of care, 36–37
medical costs related to, 33
prevalence of, 33
treatment of, 34–36

M

Major depression, 38–40
  areas for measurement
    development, 48
  cost effectiveness of interventions,
    40
  efficacy of interventions, 38–39
  health plan and interventions, 40
  improving quality of care, 39–40
  prevalence of, 38
Managed care. *See* Health maintenance
  organizations (HMOs)
Maricopa County Health Plan, 209
Medica, 205
Medicaid
  and managed care, 8
  rising costs, reasons for, 233–234
Medicaid mills, 234
Medical Outcomes Study, 110
Medical Value Plan, 94
Medicare, and managed care, 8
Membership database, 261
Mental health care, 223–232
  assessment tools, 227
  and carve-outs, 230–231, 234, 235
  Child and Adolescent Service
    System Program (CASSP),
    248–249, 250
  Community Mental Health Center
    movement, 247–248
  Community Support System (CSS),
    248, 250
  consumer role in, 254
  cost reduction strategies by
    managed care, 249–250
  delivery models, impact of,
    230–231
  diverse payment models, 231
  dual system of, 246–247
  exhausted benefits, 225
  housing problem, 224
  integration with health care, 253
  medical model in, 246

outcomes in managed care setting,
    229–230
  and private health insurance,
    246–247
  resources and mental health care, 230
  scope of services, 225–226
  staff model programs, 226
  treatment allocation algorithms,
    226–229
  underfunding for, 251–252
  See also Mental Health Management
    of America
Mental Health Management of
  America
  alert system, 239
  barriers to implementation,
    238–239
  challenges to program, 235
  cost shifting, prevention tactics, 236
  model applied to Medicaid
    population, 243–244
  network creation/management,
    236–238
  progress of program, 242–243
  success measures, 239–242
  utilization review, 235–236,
    238–239
Mental Health Redesign Project, 226
Miniclinics, 107, 110–111
Multidisciplinary care teams
  in case management, 97
  chronic childhood conditions,
    204–205
  role of, 12, 97
MultiGroup Health Plan, 226

N

Narrowing, pitfall to case
  management, 71
National Chronic Care Consortium,
  goals of delivery system, 286
National Early Childhood Technical
  Assistance System, 203

National Health Interview Survey, 27, 43

National Health and Nutrition Examination Survey (NHANES II), 24

National Health Service, 107

Nurse practitioner, role in community medical alliance, 139–140

O

Open Airways, 206

Oversight, 86

P

PacifiCare, 184, 185, 192

Pain
chronic benign pain syndrome, 173–182
low back pain, 33–38

Patient Assessment Tool (PAT), 227

Patient partnerships, 218–219

Pharmacy database, 261

Population-based management of care, 108–109, 116

Practice guidelines. *See* Computerized practice guidelines

Practice redesign, 109–111
innovation in, 110–111
process of, 110

Preterm infants
challenges to health care system, 277
cost of care, 276
data for clinical intervention program, 277–279
data sources on, 277–279, 281–283
future view for interventions, 283–284
issues related to use of data on, 280–281
research on, utility of, 279–280, 283

Primary care, 5
integrated with specialty care, 11

Primary Care Delivery System, 64

Principle Health Care, intervention, focus of, 155

Program for All-Inclusive Care for the Elderly (PACE), 12

Q

Quality assessment measures
for breast cancer, 26–29
for childhood asthma, 43–46
for colorectal cancer, 29–33
for coronary artery disease, 21–26
for diabetes mellitus, 40–43
disease selection, criteria for, 19–20
for low back pain, 33–38
for major depression, 38–40
recommendations, 46–49

Quality of care, 4

R

RAND Health Insurance Experiment, 18

Randomized clinical trials, 106

Regenstreif Institute, 114

Registries, 114–115
advantages of, 114
as feedback, 114–115

Rehabilitation Act, Section 504, 215

Report cards, 4

Risk assessment
chronic childhood conditions, 203–204
questionnaires for, 75

Ryan White program, 209

S

St. Mary Medical Center, 184, 192

Self-care, 5

Senior Dimensions Service Center, Health Plan of Nevada, 74–75

Skills Not Pills program, 176, 177–179

Social Security Income (SSI),
    enrollment of patients in managed
    care, 136–137
Social services, chronic childhood
    conditions, 209–211
Specialized health care
    change/consensus building
        strategies, 98–99
    information/validation strategies,
        95–96
    intervention/education/em-
        powerment strategies, 96–98
    patient characteristics, 93–94
Subacute care, Health Plan of Nevada,
    77–78, 84–85
Sweden, chronic care in, 107
Systolic Hypertension in the Elderly
    Program, 106

T

Temperament Program, 204
Title V programs, state, 215, 218
Transportation, 5

U

Urban Medical Group, 137–138

U.S. Quality Algorithms (USQA), 259–
    260
U.S. Quality Algorithms (USQA)
    Health Profile Database, 260–274
    applications for epidemiological
        studies, 267–270
    components of database record, 264–
        265
    disease identification methods, 262–
        264
    financial management, use for, 270–
        274
    selection of chronic diseases for,
        261–262
    validation of selection criteria, 265–
        266
Utilization management, compared to
    case management, 62–63
Utilization review, Mental Health
    Management of America, 235–236,
    238–239

V

VA Cooperative Studies Program, 117
Volunteer program
    Health Plan of Nevada, 75–77
    types of services, 75–77